Milestones in Health and Medicine

by Anne S. Harding

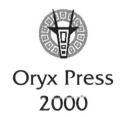

Oryx Press
2000

The rare Arabian Oryx is believed to have inspired the myth of the unicorn. This desert antelope became virtually extinct in the early 1960s. At that time, several groups of international conservationists arranged to have nine animals sent to the Phoenix Zoo to be the nucleus of a captive breeding herd. Today, the Oryx population is over 1,000, and over 500 have been returned to the Middle East.

© 2000 by Anne S. Harding
Published by Oryx Press
4041 North Central at Indian School Road
Phoenix, Arizona 85012-3397
www.oryxpress.com

Published simultaneously in Canada
Printed and bound in the United States of America

∞ The paper used in this publication meets the minimum requirements of American National Standard for Information Science—Permanence of Paper for Printed Library Materials, ANSI Z39.48, 1984.

Library of Congress Cataloging-in-Publication Data

Harding, Anne S.
    Milestones in health and medicine / by Anne S. Harding.
        p. cm.
    Includes bibliographical references and index.
    ISBN 1-57356-140-1
    1. Medicine—History. I. Title.
    R133.H36 2000
    610'.9—dc21   00-032660

Contents

8-14-00

Preface

As the twenty-first century begins, health care offers us a wealth of promise. Cures are now possible that were impossible just decades before. We have decoded the language of the genome, and, within our lifetimes, the Human Genome Project will reveal all of the text carried on our chromosomes.

But with this new knowledge and power comes risk. Many discoveries, such as the ability to grow human embryonic stem cells in culture and the possibility of predicting our future with genetic tests, bring with them difficult ethical questions. On a more mundane level, our choices in medical care have never been more complex, or expensive. This book was written to provide anyone with an interest in milestones in health and medicine—that is, just about everyone—with a historical perspective in these exciting and sometimes frightening times.

Milestones in Health and Medicine includes more than 500 entries describing advances in the treatment of disease and the understanding of human health. The world-changing discoveries, such as anesthesia, antisepsis, the X-ray, antibiotics, and the structure of DNA, have occurred in the past century, but we have been treating fractures, medicating ourselves with plants, and performing surgery since the beginning of recorded history, and possibly before. The book traces back the ancient roots of some health care practices while also describing modern advances. It is important to note that this book presents *milestones* in health and medical events. The emphasis is on significant advances in diseases, treatments, and health issues. For example, for a disease, the entry explains the first time that a disease was noted and subsequent significant advances in understanding and treating it. This book is not meant to be a comprehensive medical dictionary nor does it purport to be a full historical treatment; rather, it is a reference book that shows the significant landmarks related to each of the topics described.

Many entries are milestones in themselves, such as the discovery of circulation; the invention of the heart-lung machine; penicillin; AZT, the first drug for treating AIDS; and anesthesia. These are milestones because they radically advanced medicine and in some cases health. For example, the heart-lung machine made open-heart surgery possible, and anesthesia—as well as antisepsis—allowed surgeons to go beyond the crude, quick operations they had previously practiced, usually in emergency situations, to complex surgeries on the internal organs. The discovery of the vitamins, and the subsequent development of methods to produce them in commercial quantities, made it possible to identify and treat deficiency diseases that had plagued humanity since ancient times.

Other entries cover diseases, treatments, organizations, and issues. Entries are written to incorporate as much information as efficiently as possible. Rather than make an entry for each of the dozens of cancer chemotherapy drugs, for example, I have instead written one for each class of drugs, along with individual entries for medicines that represent a leap forward, such as nitrogen mustards, taxol, and tamoxifen. There are entries for infectious diseases, several types of cancer, psychological conditions, congenital diseases, chronic illnesses, and more. I decided whether or not to include an illness based on its historic toll and its human cost today. Entries on diagnosis and treatment include imaging techniques, drugs, diagnostic tests and tools, and surgical procedures and were chosen on a similar basis. For example, I have included the relatively simple glucose test along with more dazzling discoveries such as magnetic resonance imaging because the ability to monitor blood sugar has made a major difference in the lives of people with diabetes.

I have left out some recent milestones whose significance is not yet fully understood, such as some findings on signaling among cells and metabolism at the molecular level. I have included older discoveries in basic science, such as the role of vitamins in nutrition and the function of antibodies and T cells in immunology, because we have reached the point where we have a firm grasp of their influence on health.

These choices were often a matter of personal judgment, and other authors may have chosen differently, but I believe this book—while it is by no means exhaustive—covers a wide and informative swathe of medical history. Suggestions for topics to include for future volumes are welcome. Please direct such information to Editor, *Milestones in Health and Medicine*, 4041 N. Central Avenue at Indian School Road, Phoenix, Arizona 85012.

While the book is written from a national perspective, in that I discuss the development of public health, medical specialties, and systems for medical research in this country, I have addressed other subjects as globally as possible. Contributions to the understanding of human health and treatment of human illnesses have been made around the world. Furthermore, travel and trade across national and continental boundaries are making the planet smaller than ever—particularly in terms of infectious disease.

My main objective in choosing illustrations for this book was to find a group of interesting images representing a broad expanse of time as well as the continuum of technological development. I also chose a variety of illustrative styles, from an engraving of an early mental hospital building to electron microscope images of viruses and bacteria. My sources were generally medical libraries and archives of professional societies, both of which tend to have a rich store of engravings and photographs.

There are three finding aids for the information in this book: First, at the front of the book, there is a subject list, which presents the entry names (or headwords) by broad subject area. Second, at the back of the book, there is a timeline, which lists medical and health milestones chronologically, beginning with around 10,000 BC and ending with the year 2000. Finally, there is a general index to the contents of the entries. Within the text, **boldfaced terms** refer to other entries in this book, and there are "see" and "see also" references to other entries as well. Using these tools, the reader will be able to navigate smoothly through the book and also use it as a starting point for more in-depth research.

Each entry contains a source for additional reading, which includes the author's name, the title of the book or article, and page numbers if applicable. The bibliography provides a full citation for each of these sources and lists dozens of other books that I used in the course of my research.

I began my research for *Milestones in Health and Medicine* by reading several books on medical history, some providing overviews of medicine in general and others addressing specific areas, such as cardiology or immunology. As I read, I developed my list of entries. Once I had a reasonable number, I began more in-depth research, using primary resources whenever possible, such as the original journal article describing an important discovery. This entry list grew and shrank during the course of my work on this book, as some of my original choices turned out not to be milestones at all while other choices contained several milestones within them.

I spent a great deal of time at the Columbia University Health Sciences Library, which houses more than 500,000 books and complete sets of more than 4,400 medical journals, some of which date back to the nineteenth century. The library was extremely helpful to me for tracking down vague references in contemporary works. Web-based resources were also vital to me in helping me to fill in gaps in my research.

This book is for anyone with an interest in medical history or medicine in general, from grade-school students to professors. People are fascinated with medicine and health, as the current proliferation of consumer health news on the Internet and in newspapers and magazines suggests. My goal was to provide a book that would put all the information that's out there in context. I believe that learning about medical history is just as important as learning about health; people need to understand the ways that medicine has progressed (and in some cases, regressed). I have attempted to use simple language and to explain terms lay audiences may not be familiar with. I believe nearly everyone, from people with no medical training to physicians, will find new and interesting information here.

I received invaluable assistance from several people at libraries and historical collections in assembling the illustrations for this book, and I would like to thank them for their help: Caroline Duroselle-Melish at the New York Academy of Medicine; Lynn Parker at the Wellcome Centre Medical Photographic Library; Carol Tomer at the Cleveland Clinic Archives; Dr. Eric v.d. Luft at the Health Sciences Library Historical Collections at the State University of New York Health Science Center at Syracuse; Sue Welch and Sharon Ledbetter at the National Human Genome Research Institute; Caron Capizzano at New York University School of Medicine; Gerard Shorb at the Alan Mason Chesney Archives of the Johns Hopkins Medical Institutions; Jeff Karr at the American Society of Microbiology; Steve Novak at the Augustus C. Long Health Sciences Library at Columbia University; Chris Philips at the American Association of Neurological Surgeons; and the Armed Forces Institute of Pathology. I would also like to thank my husband, Philip Klint, for his support during the process of writing this book, as well as my editors at Oryx, Lori Kennedy, Jennifer Ashley, and Anne Thompson.

Subject List

Alternative or Non-Western medicine
Acupuncture
Alternative medicine
Chinese medicine
Chiropractic
Herbal medicine
Homeopathy
Hydrotherapy
Osteopathy

Anesthesia and analgesia
Acetaminophen
Analgesics
Anesthesia
Aspirin
Chloroform
Chloral hydrate
Cocaine
Epidural anesthesia
Heroin
Ibuprofen
Morphine
Nitrous oxide
Nonsteroidal anti-inflammatory drugs (NSAIDs)
Opium
Twilight sleep

Antibiotics
Actinomycin
Antibiotic
Cephalosporin
Penicillin
Streptomycin

Cancer
Actinomycin
Alkylating agents
Antimetabolites
Anti-tumor antibiotics
Brain tumor/spinal cord tumor
BRCA1,2

Breast cancer
Cancer
Cancer center
Cancer vaccine
Carcinogens
Cervical cancer
Chemotherapy
Colorectal cancer
Herceptin
Hodgkin's disease
Hyperthermia
Leukemia
Lung cancer
Melanoma
Nitrogen mustards
Oncogenes
Podophyllotoxin
Prostate cancer
Prostate-specific antigen (PSA)
Radiation therapy
Tamoxifen
Taxol
Tumor-suppressor gene
Vinca alkaloids

Cell biology and physiology
Apoptosis
Cell theory
Electrophoresis
Growth factors
Osmosis
Phagocytosis
Stem cell
Tissue
Tissue culture
Tumor necrosis factor (TNF)

Dentistry
Dentistry
Dentures

Subject List

Fluoridation
Orthodontia
Toothbrush

Dermatology
Melanoma
Phototherapy
Sunscreen
Tretinoin

Diagnosis
Auscultation
Percussion
Pulse watch
Sensors
Sphygmomanometer (blood pressure cuff)
Stethoscope
Thermometer

Drugs
Amphetamine
Antabuse
Anticholinesterase
Anticoagulant
Antidiabetes drugs
Antiparasitics
Antiviral drugs
Arsenic
Atropine
AZT (Azidothymidine)
Barbiturates
Chlorothiacide
Colchicine
COX-2 inhibitors
Curare
Ephedrine
Ergot
Heparin
Hirudin
Interferon
Ipecac
LSD (lysergic acid diethylamide)
Marijuana
Opiate antagonists
Physostigmine
Placebo
Prescription
Prontosil
Protease inhibitors
Purgatives
Quinine
Reserpine
Salvarsan
Six-mercaptopurine (6-mp)
Warfarin

Ears and hearing
Cochlear implants
Hearing aids

Hearing test
Otoscope

Emergency care
Air ambulance
Ambulance
Artificial respiration
Burn treatment
CPR (cardiopulmonary resuscitation)
Decompression
Endotracheal intubation
Heimlich maneuver
Hyperbaric oxygenation
Intensive care unit (ICU)
911
Poison control center
Shock
Trauma center
Triage

Endocrinology
Addison's disease
Adrenal gland
Androgens
Cortisone
Diabetes mellitus
Epinephrine
Erythropoetin
Glucose testing
Graves' disease
Hormone
Insulin
Norepinephrine
Parathyroid
Pineal gland
Pituitary gland
Progesterone
Prostaglandin
Thyroid gland

Gastroenterology
Cimetidine
Digestion
Endoscopy
H. pylori

Genetic disease
Cystic fibrosis
Down syndrome
Inborn errors of metabolism
Sickle-cell anemia
Tay-Sachs disease

Genetics
Barr body
Biochips
Chromosome
Chromosome banding
DNA
DNA fingerprinting

Subject List

Infection control
Antisepsis
Asepsis
Pasteurization
Rubber gloves
Universal precautions

Infectious disease
AIDS
Bubonic plague
Burkitt's lymphoma
Chagas' disease
Chicken pox
Cholera
Contagion theory
Cryptosporidium
Dengue
Diphtheria
Dysentery
E. coli 0157:H7
Germ theory
Gonorrhea
Hepatitis
Influenza
Leprosy
Lyme disease
Malaria
Measles
Mumps
Pertussis
Poliomyelitis (polio)
Prion
Rabies
Retroviruses
Rubella
Scarlet fever
Schistosomiasis
Serum therapy
Smallpox
Syphilis
Tetanus
Tuberculosis (TB)
Typhoid fever
Typhus
Virus
Yellow fever

Men's health
Artificial insemination
Circumcision
Condom
Impotence treatment
Prostate-specific antigen (PSA)
Sperm bank
Vasectomy

Nephrology
Bright's disease

Dialysis
Diuretics
Gout
Renin-angiotensin system

Neurology
Acetylcholine
Alzheimer's disease
Botulism toxin
Brain death
Cerebral localization
Cerebrospinal fluid
Electroencephalography (EEG)
Endorphins
Epilepsy
Head-injury treatment
Hydrocephalus
Migraine
Multiple sclerosis (MS)
Neurons
Parkinson's disease
Receptors
Reflex
REM
Serotonin
Sleep apnea
spinal cord injury treatment
Stroke
Transmissible spongiform encephalopathies (TSEs)
Trepanation

Nutrition
Beriberi
Calcium
Goiter
Kwashiorkor
Oral rehydration therapy
Pellagra
Rickets
Vitamin
Vitamin A
Vitamin B
Vitamin C
Vitamin D
Vitamin E
Vitamin K

Obstetrics and gynecology
Abortion
Amniocentesis
Apgar score
Birth control pill
Birth defects
Birthing centers
Cesarean section (c-section)
Chorionic villus sampling
Colposcopy
Contraception

Eclampsia
Egg donation
Estrogen
Fetal monitoring
Fetal surgery
Forceps
GIFT (gamete intrafallopian transfer)
Hormone replacement therapy (HRT)
In vitro fertilization (IVF)
Intrauterine device (IUD)
Lamaze method
Midwife
Pap smear (Papanicolaou test)
Pregnancy test
Pre-implantation genetic diagnosis (PGD)
Prenatal care
Puerperal fever
Tubal sterilization

Old-fashioned medicine
Cupping
Hippocratic corpus
Humoralism

Ophthalmology
Cataract surgery
Contact lenses
Corneal transplant
Eyeglasses
Glaucoma
Gonioscope
Ophthalmoscope
Refractive surgery
Rhodopsin
Tonometer
Vision test

Organizations, International
Alma Ata International Conference on Primary Health
    Care
Red Cross
UNICEF (United Nations Children Fund)
World Health Organization (WHO)

Organizations, U.S.
Centers for Disease Control and Prevention (CDC)
Environmental Protection Agency (EPA)
Food and Drug Administration (FDA)
Food Safety and Inspection Service
National Institutes of Health (NIH)
Social Security
U.S. Children's Bureau
U.S. Public Health Service (PHS)
U.S. Sanitary Commission
Visiting nurse association (VNA)
WIC

Orthopedics
Club-foot treatment

Fracture repair
Osteoporosis
Scoliosis treatment

Pediatrics
Infant feeding
Premature infant care

Plastic surgery
Cleft lip/cleft palate repair
Plastic surgery
Rhinoplasty

Psychology
Addiction
Addiction treatment
Alcoholics Anonymous (AA)
Alcoholism
Anorexia nervosa
Anti-anxiety drugs
Antidepressant drugs
Antipsychotic drugs
Anxiety disorders
Attention-deficit hyperactivity disorder (ADHD)
Behavior therapy
Behaviorism
Biofeedback
Bulimia nervosa
Convulsive therapy
Depression
Diagnostic and Statistic Manual of Mental Disorders
    (DSM)
Electroconvulsive therapy (ECT, electroshock therapy)
Hypnotherapy
Lithium
Lobotomy
Mental hospital
Mental illness
Methadone
Psychoanalysis
Psychotherapy
Rapid opiate detoxification
Relaxation response
Schizophrenia

Public health
Air bags
Industrial hygiene
Needle exchange programs
Public health
Quarantine

Surgery
Ambulatory surgery
Amputation
Anatomical theater
Anatomy
Appendectomy

Arthroscopy
Autopsy
Blalock-Taussig procedure
Cauterization
Cingulotomy
Cryosurgery
Electrocautery
Gamma knife
Gastrectomy
Laparoscopy
Laser surgery
Lithotomy
Microsurgery
Minimally invasive surgery
Ovariotomy
Robotic surgery
Stereotactic surgery
Surgical staples
Sutures
Tracheotomy

Transplants or artificial organs
Artificial heart
Artificial skin
Bone graft
Bone marrow transplant

Drinker respirator
Heart transplant
Heart-lung machine
Hip replacement
Kidney transplant
Liver transplant
Lung transplant
Prosthesis
Skin grafts
Xenografts

U.S. Government
Centers for Disease Control and Prevention (CDC)
Clean Air Act
Clean Water Act
Environmental Protection Agency (EPA)
Food and Drug Administration (FDA)
Food Safety and Inspection Service
"Healthy People"
National Institutes of Health (NIH)
Social Security
U.S. Children's Bureau
U.S. Public Health Service (PHS)
U.S. Sanitary Commission
WIC

Women's health. *See* **Obstetrics and gynecology.**

A

abortion

Abortion is the intentional termination of pregnancy. From Hippocrates' time—and probably before—through the Middle Ages, folk wisdom provided women with a number of herbs that could cause abortion. The herbs listed by Dioscorides and Soranus, two ancient Greek physicians, were roughly the same: they included soapwort, pennyroyal, and lupine. Hildegard of Bingen (1098–1117), who has been called the world's first woman doctor, mentioned the herb tansy in her book *De simplicis medicinae*. Surgical abortions, or abortions brought on by violent massage of the abdomen, were also probably performed occasionally in ancient times, but very rarely, since these methods were much more hazardous than giving herbs earlier in pregnancy. Medieval common law criminalized abortion caused by manipulation, but not abortion using herbs or other chemicals.

The controversy over whether abortion is a woman's choice or a sin against God also dates back to ancient times. The Greek and Latin church fathers distinguished between formed and unformed fetuses. Aborting an unformed fetus—which basically did not yet look human and was thought to be soulless—was condoned. Using "menses-inducing drugs" was permissible during the first 40 days of pregnancy. The Talmud's instructions regarding abortion are similar.

As the church began to toughen its stance on abortion in the Middle Ages, abortifacient drugs and the people who prescribed them came under attack. Many women were executed as witches throughout Europe, often for providing information on abortion or birth control. This resulted in the suppression of much of the ancient knowledge about herbal means of controlling fertility.

Many herbals (books collecting herbal knowledge) written during this time stated that certain herbs could produce abortion without condoning their use; an herbal of 1694 said that savin, or juniper, is "too well known and too much used by wenches."

In the nineteenth century, abortion-producing substances such as asafetida and juniper were given to women to relieve "suppression of the menses." Medicines for inducing abortion were advertised in newspapers under names like "French Renovating Pills" and "Dr. Champlin's Red Woman's Relief." The famous Lydia Pinkham's Vegetable Compound, which is still sold today, contains abortifacient herbs. Attempts were made toward the end of the 1800s to ban or regulate abortifacients.

European countries began to criminalize surgical abortion around 1800. Connecticut passed the first U.S. law against abortion in 1821. By the 1950s, all U.S. states banned abortions or allowed them only to save the mother's life, except for Alabama and Washington D.C., which allowed abortions to save the woman's health. Most abortions of this time were performed illegally, with crude surgical methods, and many women died from infection after these "back alley" abortions.

By 1970, 18 U.S. states had liberalized their laws to allow abortions by a licensed physician using the proper procedures early in pregnancy. A Texas resident named Norma McCorvey became pregnant in 1970 and could not afford to travel to a state where abortion would be legal. She sued, as "Jane Roe," arguing that her constitutional right to privacy was violated by laws that made abortion illegal. *Roe vs. Wade* was argued before the Supreme Court. The court decided in 1973 that first-term abortions were legal, and left it up to the states to regulate abortions thereafter.

Safe surgical abortions are now available in the United States to women in the first trimester of pregnancy. These early abortions generally are performed at clinics on an outpatient basis, using suction or a procedure called dilation and curettage in which the lining of the uterus is scraped away. Abortions in the second trimester require a more complex procedure.

In 1976, the Supreme Court ruled that states requiring parental consent for minors seeking abortions would have to provide an alternative by allowing them to seek consent through the courts. In 1989, the Supreme Court made a ruling called *Webster vs. Reproductive Health Services* that challenged *Roe vs. Wade* without dismantling it. The court decided that a Missouri state law banning public employees from performing abortions was constitutional.

By the late 1980s, about 95 percent of abortions were being performed using vaccuum aspiration, a method that employs suction to remove the embryo or fetus from the uterus. Although an "abortion pill," RU-486, was developed during this decade, it is not yet available for use in the United States. This artificial progestin antagonist was discovered by scientists at the French pharmaceutical company Roussel-Uclaf. It induces abortion if given in the first 47 days of pregnancy. Women can take the drug at home, and the fetus is expelled by contractions a few days later. The drug was synthesized in 1982 and became available at clinics in France in 1989. Studies in the United States have found that the drug is safe and effective, but to date no companies have been willing to distribute the drug in this country.

Today an often violent battle continues in the United States between "pro-life" advocates who oppose abortion, and "pro-choice" advocates who believe in a woman's right to choose abortion.

Although abortion remains legal in the United States, in the 1990s the procedure has become less accessible for some women, in part because fewer doctors are being trained to perform abortions and fewer still are willing to perform the procedure in the wake of attacks on clinics and doctors.

Additional reading: Riddle, *Eve's Herbs*; Riddle, *Contraception and Abortion from the Ancient World to the Renaissance.*

ACE inhibitors

Angiotensin-converting-enzyme (ACE) inhibitors are drugs that block a series of events in the body that raise blood pressure. They are used to treat hypertension and heart disease.

The kidney produces renin, an enzyme that cues the release of angiotensin, which increases blood pressure by making blood vessels constrict. ACE converts angiotensin to its active form, known as angiotensin II. ACE-inhibiting drugs stop angiotensin from becoming active.

Researchers in 1965 observed that venom from a Brazilian snake blocked the action of ACE. A drug called teprotide, the first ACE inhibitor, was based on the venom, but it was expensive and couldn't be given orally.

David W. Cushman (1939–) and Miguel A. Ondetti (1930–) at Bristol-Myers Squibb, a pharmaceutical company, began looking for a less-expensive drug that would mimic the structure of teprotide but could be taken orally. In 1975, they synthesized a substance they called captopril, which was found to be very safe and effective after two years of use in **clinical trials**.

Another drug, created in the early 1970s, mimicked angiotensin II itself and blocked its action by competitively binding to certain receptors. This drug, Saralasin, was less than perfect because it stimulated the **renin-angiotensin system** (RAS) at high doses, thus increasing blood pressure, and it also couldn't be taken orally. In 1994, Merck, a

pharmaceutical company, released the drug Losartan, which is orally administered and mimics angiotensin II without activating the RAS.

Several large clinical trials have shown that people who take ACE inhibitors after a heart attack live longer. After a heart attack, and sometimes in people who have had hypertension for a long time, the left ventricle of the heart becomes larger and weaker. ACE inhibitors can prevent this from happening, and may do so by stimulating the growth of new cells in the heart. These drugs also allow the heart to operate better with less oxygen, and when given to people in heart failure can improve heart function.

Even though these drugs are quite effective, and they have no significant side effects aside from a cough, they are not well known and are by no means used universally. Research is underway to find hypertension drugs that block the RAS in other places.

Additional reading: Acierno, *The History of Cardiology,* pp. 329–31.

acetaminophen

Acetaminophen is an aspirin-like drug, marketed as Tylenol or Datril, that kills pain and brings down fever but does not have anti-inflammatory properties.

American chemist Harmon Northrop Morse (1848–1920) synthesized acetaminophen, also called paracetamol, while he was working at Johns Hopkins University in Baltimore, publishing a description of the process in 1878.

German physicians provided the first detailed accounts of the properties and clinical use of the drug in the 1890s. But acetaminophen was neglected for decades because it was not thought to be as effective as aspirin and other related drugs.

In the late 1940s, New York University College of Medicine researchers Bernard B. Brodie (1909–) and Julius Axelrod (1912–) found that paracetamol was identical to substances metabolized in the body from the fever-reducing, pain-killing drugs acetanilide and phenaticin, but was itself much less toxic than these older drugs.

Soon after this discovery, tablets containing acetaminophen, caffeine, and aspirin went on the market as "Triogesic." Acetaminophen alone, sold as Tylenol and manufactured by McNeil Laboratories, became available without prescription in the United States in 1955.

Studies published in the 1960s showed that acetaminophen is as effective as aspirin for reducing fever, yet does not irritate the gastrointestinal tract as aspirin does. Acetaminophen is now the best-selling pain killer in the United States.

Additional reading: Prescott, *Paracetamol (Acetaminophen).*

acetylcholine

Acetylcholine helps transmit impulses through the nervous system. It was the first neurotransmitter to be discovered.

In 1898, Sir Henry Dale (1875–1968) found that a substance isolated from **ergot** (a fungus that grows on spoiled wheat), was capable of slowing an animal's heartbeat. Dale didn't believe the substance occurred naturally in humans, but he found it in the spleen 15 years later in 1913.

In 1920, Otto Loewi (1873–1961) found that some type of chemical carried nerve impulses across the gaps—known as synapses—between **neurons**. Scientists had previously thought that nerve impulses were carried through the body in a broken electrical current. Loewi published his experiment in 1921. Five years later, he showed that another naturally occurring chemical, acetylcholinesterase, broke down acetylcholine almost instantaneously so that a series of chemical impulses could be transmitted in rapid succession. Acetylcholinesterase is found in muscle and nerve cells, as well as elsewhere in the body.

Later experiments proved that acetylcholine and **epinephrine** were the neurotransmitters responsible for carrying impulses. The discovery that chemicals carried nerve impulses opened up the possibility of controlling this transmission with drugs. Loewi and Dale shared the 1936 Nobel Prize for Physiology for their work with acetylcholine.

Additional reading: O'Leary and Goldring, *Science and Epilepsy,* pp. 191–93.

acquired immune deficiency syndrome. See AIDS.

actinomycin

Actinomycins are **antibiotics** derived from the Actinomyces bacteria that are also useful for treating some types of cancer. They work by inhibiting the synthesis of RNA, the messenger that **DNA** uses to instruct cells to form proteins necessary for life.

Selman Waksman (1888–1973) and Harold Boyd Woodruff (1917–) discovered actinomycin in 1940. It was first used in patients in 1952. Actinomycins can cure Wilms' tumor, a cancer affecting children, and can also cure gestational choriocarcinoma, a cancer that strikes pregnant women. (*See also* anti-tumor antibiotics.)

Additional reading: Sneader, *Drug Discovery,* pp. 321–24.

acupuncture

Acupuncture is an ancient Chinese technique, dating back to at least 2500 B.C., for promoting health by placing needles in special points on the body. The intention of acupuncture is to restore the proper flow of *qi*, or the life force, within the body.

Acupuncture may produce its results by causing the release of neurotransmitters such as **endorphins** at acupuncture points, or by somehow strengthening the immune system.

Some historians theorize that acupuncture developed after people observed that arrow wounds produced anesthesia in certain parts of the body. Others suggest that acupuncture sprang from the use of needles to lance boils.

By about 200 A.D., moxibustion—a technique for producing heat on the surface of the body by placing burning herbs at acupuncture points—was added to acupuncture,

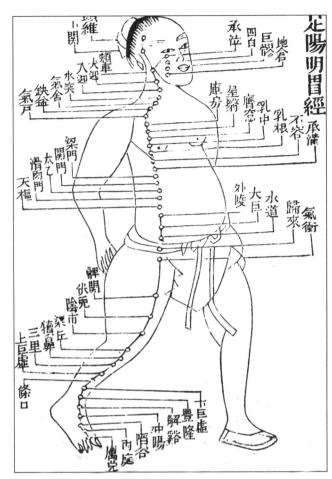

A diagram of acupuncture points from *Chin kew ta Ching,* a Chinese manuscript from 1875. (Courtesy of National Library of Medicine.)

as well as massage of acupuncture points. Chinese physicians and doctors in neighboring Asian countries used acupuncture to treat liver disease, gout, hearing loss, joint pain, and other conditions.

Today, many people in the West rely on acupuncture to help them quit smoking, cope with stress, and manage pain. In China, doctors use acupuncture as anesthesia for patients undergoing major operations, such as heart surgery.

In 1998, a panel of the **National Institutes of Health** found that acupuncture could be a useful treatment for pain, but the group did not endorse other applications.

Additional reading: Gwei-Djen and Needham, *Celestial Lancets.*

addiction

Addiction to drugs or alcohol has been understood in several different ways throughout history. In the twentieth century there was a gradual shift from seeing addiction as a character weakness to understanding it as a chronic disease that usually cannot be cured, but can be treated. At least 10 percent of the U.S. population is thought to be addicted to drugs or alcohol, and many more are addicted to tobacco.

Addiction can be both psychological and physical. A substance is considered to be physically addictive if withdrawal from it produces physical symptoms; for example, both opiate drugs and alcohol are physically addictive.

In 1925, U.S. addiction expert Lawrence Kolb (1911–1982) argued that only certain people with psychological defects would develop addictions; to put it simply, these were people for whom drugs relieved a sense of inadequacy. It is true that not everyone who uses drugs becomes addicted. Scientists increasingly believe that genetic factors may determine whether a person will develop an addiction to a drug, while environmental and behavioral factors also play a role. Addiction is generally agreed to occur when a person loses the ability to control their use of a drug. Once this happens, drug-seeking behavior and drug use becomes compulsive.

In 1957, the American Medical Association (AMA) recognized **alcoholism** as a disease. It was not until 1986 that the AMA determined that addiction to drugs is a disease as well.

In the 1990s, researchers learned a great deal about the action of drugs in the brain through advances in brain imaging. They have identified the neural circuits drugs follow as well as biochemical events that occur in neurons after exposure to a drug. They have also learned that there appear to be major differences in brain function between addicted and nonaddicted people. Leaders in this research include George F. Koob of the Scripps Research Institute and Eric J. Nestler (1954–) of Yale.

Additional reading: Austin, *Perspectives on the History of Psychoactive Substance Use.*

addiction treatment

Addiction treatment is the provision of medical and psychological assistance to help stop people from using a drug to which they have become addicted.

Success rates of addiction treatment vary depending on the substance. Roughly 50 percent of alcoholics succeed in giving up their addiction; 60 percent of opiate addicts; 55 percent of **cocaine** addicts; and only 30 percent of nicotine addicts.

Addiction treatment involves first detoxifying a person by making sure that all of the intoxicating substance has left their system. This may require hospitalization. Withdrawal from alcohol can cause hallucinations known as delirium tremens, while opiate withdrawal can be extremely physically painful. (A therapy in which the person undergoes withdrawal from opiates while anesthetized, known as **rapid opiate detoxification,** was invented for this reason.) The next step is encouraging the person to remain "clean," which usually requires a significant amount of counseling. In this intermediary stage, a person often needs residential treatment.

A popular treatment for addiction in the United States in the early twentieth century was the Towns-Lambert treatment, developed by Charles B. Towns (1862–unknown) and Alexander Lambert (1861–1939). The treatment, which the two men published in 1909, consisted of administering a mercury-based laxative to the addicted person several times. This theoretically cleared the addictive substance from the body. The rest of the treatment involved giving the person belladonna and hyoscine every half-hour to treat withdrawal symptoms.

In 1929, Congress passed laws to create a Narcotics Division within the **U.S. Public Health Service**. In 1935, federal facilities for the treatment and study of addiction were built in Lexington, Kentucky, and also in Fort Worth, Texas, in 1938. Around this time, two alcoholics, William Griffith Wilson (1895–1971) and Robert Holbrook Smith (1879–1950) founded **Alcoholics Anonymous**, a self-help program that has proved to be extremely valuable for treating addiction to alcohol as well as to other drugs.

Addiction experts agree that people with more stable lives and a higher educational and social status tend to be more successful in overcoming addiction.

A number of drugs have been developed to help people addicted to drugs or alcohol to wean themselves from their addiction. Some drugs ease the effects of withdrawal (such as clonidine for opiate addicts), others reduce the craving for a drug after a person is "clean," and others replace the addictive substance with another drug. For example, when a **heroin** addict takes the **opiate antagonist** naltrexone, they experience less desire for the drug, and if they take heroin while on naltrexone, no "high" will result. J.R. Volpicelli first reported trying naltrexone in alcoholics in 1992, with some success. Bupropion, or Zyban, was introduced in the early 1990s for people attempting to quit smoking.

One controversial drug treatment is **methadone** for opiate addicts; some argue that it replaces one addiction with another. The strategy of harm reduction, in which people addicted to drugs may not necessarily quit using a drug but instead take steps to increase their safety while using drugs, such as participating in **needle exchange programs**, are also controversial.

To cope with drug addiction treatment on the federal level, the National Institute on Drug Abuse was established within the **National Institutes of Health (NIH)** in 1980. Three years later, the California Society of Addiction Medicine developed a certification program for physicians qualifying them to diagnose and treat addicted patients, and the program was offered nationally three years later.

Currently, the leading illegal drugs of abuse in the United States, according to the National Institute on Drug Abuse (NIDA), are **marijuana**, cocaine, heroin, and methamphetamine. However, there are far more people addicted to alcohol in the United States than to any illegal or legal drug. The National Institutes of Health estimate that 14 million Americans are alcoholics. About 682,000 Americans are frequent cocaine users, according to NIDA, while the institute reports there are roughly 810,000 chronic heroin users in the United States. (*See also* alcoholism)

Additional reading: White, *Slaying the Dragon.*

Addison's disease

Addison's disease is a deficiency in secretion of hormones from the adrenal cortex, occurring when this gland is damaged by infectious disease, abnormal cell growth, or hemorrhage. The disease is named for Thomas Addison (1793–

1860), the British physician who first described the affliction.

In 1855, Addison published his observations of several patients with a mysterious disease characterized by extreme weakness and very dark brown skin. In autopsies of some of these patients, he noticed that their **adrenal glands** appeared diseased. At this point, the role of these glands was unknown.

He also noticed that the blood of the patients contained an abnormally high number of white blood cells. In his paper, Addison called the disease "bronzed skin" or "bronzed" disease. Armand Trousseau (1801–1867), a professor at the Hotel Dieu hospital in Paris, observed similar cases shortly after Addison's report was published and suggested that the condition be called "Addison's disease."

In 1893, after George Oliver (1841–1915) and Edward Schafer (1841–1915) discovered that an extract from the adrenal glands—**epinephrine**—caused **blood pressure** to rise, a few fruitless years were spent trying to cure Addison's disease with adrenaline injections. These attempts failed because Addison's disease is caused by a deficiency in other hormones produced by the adrenal glands.

In 1926, Julius Rogoff (1884–1966) and George Stewart (1860–1930) of Cleveland hit upon the real cure when they showed that dogs whose adrenal glands had been removed would survive if they ate extracts of adrenal cortex. Three years later, they reported successfully treating Addison's disease patients with these extracts.

In 1932, Robert Loeb (1895–1973) reported that people with Addison's disease had low blood sodium and chloride, and found that giving intravenous saline solutions to patients with the disease during crisis was helpful.

In 1934, Edward Kendall (1886–1972) and his colleagues at the Mayo Clinic isolated the first pure hormone from the adrenal cortex. It was not until 1945, after chemists at Merck, a pharmaceutical company, had synthesized this cortisone compound and produced enough to treat patients, that a completely successful therapy for Addison's disease became available.

Additional reading: Anderson, *What You Can Do About Adrenal Insufficiency*.

ADHD. *See* attention-deficit hyperactivity disorder.

adrenal glands

The triangular adrenal glands sit atop the kidneys and consist of two parts: an interior medulla and an external cortex. The medulla synthesizes and stores the neurotransmitters dopamine, norepinephrine, and **epinephrine**, and the cortex secretes several different hormones synthesized from cholesterol, including cortisol, cortisone, aldosterone, dehydroepiandrosterone (DHEA), **androgens**, progestins, and **estrogens**. Cortisol and corticosterone act on carbohydrate metabolism; aldosterone and DHEA handle metabolism of sodium and potassium; and the rest have various roles in reproduction.

The adrenal glands were first described in 1564 by the Italian anatomist Bartolommeo Eustachio (1520–1574); the famous Flemish anatomist Andreas Vesalius (1514–1564) missed them in his description of the kidney. Caspar Bartholin (1585–1629) described the adrenal glands as ductless glands in his *Tabulae Anatomica* in 1611. Thomas Addison (1793–1860), a British physician, proved that these glands were vital to human life in his description of a disease that came to be known as **Addison's disease** in 1855. After the publication of Addison's paper, Charles-Edouard Brown-Sequard (1817–1894) performed a series of experiments on animals showing that removing the adrenal gland was fatal in animals.

Additional reading: McCann, ed., *Endocrinology*, pp. 87–112.

aerospace medicine

This branch of medicine studies the effects of flight, both within and outside the atmosphere, on the human body. Low atmospheric pressure, temperature extremes, oxygen deprivation, and rapid deceleration and acceleration can all occur during flight, and all have physiological effects.

Paul Bert (1833–1886) of France launched the study of flight physiology with his observations of how high and low pressure affected hot-air balloon travelers and his experiments with his steel decompression chamber, outlined in his 1870 book *Barometric Pressure*. The Briton John Scott Haldane (1860–1936) made discoveries related to embolism and gas solubility in the early 1900s that helped establish safety rules for flight.

As the technology of flight developed, so did aerospace medicine. At the beginning of the 1900s, researchers began to use decompression chambers to train pilots, because pressure drops as elevation above sea level increases. From the 1920s to the 1940s, mountains became the preferred site for altitude research, but decompression chambers came back into use during World War II.

Research on aerospace medicine became particularly vital in World War II because planes were now capable of climbing quickly to great heights. Pilots could lose consciousness at these high altitudes if they weren't properly trained, and they were also in danger of developing bubbles in the blood vessels known as embolisms. Researchers developed methods for emergency breathing and examined how long consciousness lasted at various pressures (in experimental settings). At the close of the war, however, pressurized cabins that kept the pilot's environment at a constant pressure had made these techniques less important.

The first space research unit was founded in the United States in 1948. The technology developed in the 1960s for monitoring the vital signs of astronauts in space and on the Moon was put to use on Earth for monitoring patients in intensive care units. Research on the effects of lowered gravity and other aspects of space travel on health continues today. In a recent experiment, astronaut-turned-senator John Glenn (1921–) made a trip in the space shuttle in 1998, in part so that scientists could gauge the effects of weightlessness on an older person's body.

Additional reading: Franklin and Sutherland. *Guinea Pig Doctors,* pp. 287–310.

AICD (automatic implantable cardiac defibrillator)

An AICD is a device placed inside the chest of a person who suffers from ventricular tachycardia or ventricular fibrillation, two types of heart-rhythm disturbances that occur when the electrical impulses that regulate the organ malfunction. The AICD senses fibrillation and shocks the heart back into a steady beat.

Earlier versions of defibrillators were impractical because they required a person to be hooked up to a large, cumbersome device. Michel Mirowski (1924–1990) developed a smaller version, and implanted the first one in a human in 1980. A system that was easier to implant surgically became available after 1986.

Additional reading: Shorter, *The Health Century,* pp. 171–72, 177–78

AIDS

Acquired Immune Deficiency Syndrome, or AIDS, is the last stage of infection with the human immunodeficiency **virus**, or HIV. The virus infects and destroys immune-system cells, eventually leaving a person vulnerable to normally benign infections. There is currently no cure for AIDS, although new medications including **protease inhibitors** have dramatically extended the lives of many individuals with HIV infection.

In the late 1970s and early 1980s, doctors began to see an unusually high number of severe infections in apparently healthy people. Similar cases had previously only been observed in patients with very weak immune systems, such as late-stage cancer patients and premature infants. The infections included Pneumocystis carinii pneumonia (PCP), thrush, Kaposi's sarcoma, and rampant candida infection. The first report of this syndrome was written by Dr. Michael Gottlieb (1947–) at the University of California at Los Angeles Medical Center, and published in 1981 in the **Centers for Disease Control and Prevention's (CDC)** weekly bulletin, *Morbidity and Mortality Weekly Report.*

Because most of the 270 people with this syndrome described in Gottlieb's report were young homosexual men, CDC scientists named the condition gay-related immunodeficiency disease, or GRID. San Francisco and New York, cities with large homosexual populations, were the centers of early AIDS research. When it became clear that the disease did not only strike gay men, but was appearing in people with **hemophilia**, intravenous drug users, and other groups, the CDC renamed the disease AIDS in 1982.

In 1983, Max Essex (1939–) of Harvard and his colleagues reported that AIDS was most likely caused by the first **retrovirus** known to infect humans, HTLV-1, which had been discovered two years earlier by Robert Gallo (1937–) of the National Cancer Institute. Luc Montagnier (1932–) at the Pasteur Institute in Paris had discovered a similar virus, which was dubbed LAV or lymphadenopathy-associated virus, that was associated with AIDS, and reported his findings in 1983. By 1985, after the viruses and their relatives were genetically sequenced, it was clear that LAV and another virus Gallo had discovered, HTLV-III, were one and the same and did indeed cause AIDS.

An outbreak of AIDS in Central Africa, mainly among heterosexual men and women, began in the late 1970s or early 1980s and continues today. In some areas, more than half of the population is infected with HIV. The stigma associated with the disease has made efforts to prevent its spread ineffective. Because affected African nations are extremely poor, expensive new drugs for treating AIDS are basically unavailable to these men and women. The only hope for preventing the further spread of AIDS in Africa and Asia, most experts believe, is the possible development of a **vaccine** for HIV. Testing of such a vaccine began in 1998. Vaccines are also being tested in conjunction with anti-AIDS drugs in patients already infected with HIV, and studies have suggested that these vaccines may make the drugs more effective in combating the virus and restoring immune-system function.

There are two tests available to test blood for HIV antibodies: the less precise ELISA (enzyme-linked immunosorbent assay) test, and the more precise and expensive Western Blot, which is used to confirm positive ELISA tests. The first ELISA test was licensed for commercial use in the United States in 1985.

The AIDS epidemic in the United States peaked in 1985. Efforts to control AIDS, such as public health messages promoting "safer sex" and **condom** use for all, have helped to reduce the spread of HIV through sexual contact in the developed world. Efforts to make the nation's blood supply safe were not made quickly enough, however, to prevent most hemophiliacs from contracting the virus.

Treatment of HIV infection with **AZT** and protease inhibitors has helped thousands of people to live relatively healthy lives with the virus, and has also begun to prevent the spread of the disease to infants born to HIV-infected mothers. These drugs are not perfect, however; they have severe side effects and some people with HIV infection have stopped taking them for this reason.

A handful of people infected with HIV have retained completely normal immune system function for many years. Researchers are studying them in hopes that their body chemistry will yield clues to a cure or vaccine for AIDS.

In the late 1990s, several researchers gathered evidence suggesting that the HIV virus sprang from a similar virus affecting chimpanzees, which is known as SIV (simian immunodeficiency virus). Because these primates are regularly hunted and butchered for their meat, the virus could have spread to a human hunter from the ape's blood.

Additional reading: Garrett, *The Coming Plague,* pp. 283–389, 459–503; Burkett, *The Gravest Show on Earth;* Grmek, *History of AIDS.*

air ambulance

Air ambulances are helicopters used to bring injured people to hospitals.

The first known air medical transport took place in 1915, during the retreat of the Serbian army from Albania, when a French pilot flew 12 wounded soldiers to safety.

During World War II, more than 100,000 injured soldiers were transported in fixed-wing planes. In 1945, a helicopter was used as an air ambulance for the first time, evacuating an injured pilot from the Burmese jungle for medical care. Helicopters, which offered an advantage because they could be landed safely in a much smaller space than a fixed-wing aircraft, were first used regularly as air ambulances during the Korean War in the early 1950s. Patients rode in baskets strapped to the outside of the helicopters, while pilots regulated the flow of the patient's IV bottle. Eventually helicopters were designed so the wounded person could ride inside with a medic providing care, cutting the mortality rate by more than half. Helicopters were also widely used during the Vietnam War.

European countries began using helicopter ambulances for civilians in the 1960s, with West Germany leading the way. In the United States, the rural states of Alabama and Georgia began using helicopters to transport car accident victims to the hospital in the mid-1960s. Dr. Henry C. Cleveland (1924–), president of a Denver, Colorado hospital and a Vietnam veteran, launched the nation's first hospital-based helicopter ambulance program in 1972.

By 1983 there were 56 hospital-based air transport programs in the United States. Today there are about 175. Since 1972, about half a million injured Americans have been transported to a hospital by air.

Additional reading: Hart, "The Flying Rescuers."

air bags

Air bags are protective devices in automobiles that are designed to expand upon impact to protect the driver and passengers from injury.

U.S. Secretary of Transportation John Volpe (1908–1994) led early efforts to study the feasibility of equipping cars with air bags in the early 1970s. Ford was the first car maker to install them, putting front passenger-seat air bags in a fleet of Mercury sedans in 1972. The following year, General Motors equipped Chevrolets with both passenger and driver front-seat air bags. GM went on to build 300,000 full-size sedans with air bags, but the cars sold very poorly, for several reasons. The option cost about $325, and full-size cars weren't selling well because of the oil and gas shortage of the early 1970s. Also, there were concerns that the airbags might deploy by accident and be difficult to service.

The National Highway Transportation Safety Administration (NHTSA) held two series of hearings on air bags in the 1970s. It decided that for three years beginning in 1982 all new cars would have to be built with air bags.

The Reagan administration rescinded the air-bag ruling, but the Supreme Court ultimately upheld a requirement that automakers begin installing passive restraints—either automatic seat belts or air bags—by 1984. Secretary of Transportation Elizabeth Dole (1936–) set phase-in requirements for passive restraints.

By the late 1980s, a significant number of cars on the market were equipped with air bags. Volvo introduced a side-impact airbag in 1995. Air bags became mandatory for all cars sold in the United States in September 1997.

Since the mid-1980s, when manufacturers began selling cars with air bags, there have been some deaths and injuries from air bags, which deploy with such force that they can cause internal injuries. The main danger appears to be to children and small adults. Manufacturers developed an on-off switch for the airbags in the late 1990s. In 1997, NHTSA introduced regulations that allow motorists determined to be at risk of airbag injury to have on-off switches for the devices installed. The government is attempting to address this danger by developing new testing standards for air bags, set to be in place by March 2000.

Additional reading: Weiss, "Curbing Air Bags' Dangerous Excesses."

Alcoholics Anonymous (AA)

Alcoholics Anonymous is a self-help program for fighting **addiction** to alcohol. About 2 million members of AA make up 63,000 groups in 114 countries. Roughly half of all AA members live in the United States.

William Griffith Wilson (1895–1971), a New York stockbroker, and Akron, Ohio surgeon Robert Holbrook Smith (1879–1950), started AA in 1935 after they found that their conversations had helped them to avoid drinking. Their discussions and friendship formed the basis of AA, which is founded on the idea of alcoholics telling one another their stories honestly. Wilson and Smith published the first edition of *Alcoholics Anonymous,* known as the AA bible, in 1939.

AA members attend free meetings held in churches and other community spaces. Anyone who wants to stop drinking can join, and AA does not recruit people. At these meetings people acknowledge their addiction to alcohol and attempt to develop their own "program" for staying clean, and, like Bill W. and Bob S., tell their stories. People who join AA are paired with a sponsor, a recovering alcoholic who has succeeded in staying sober.

The basic rules of AA are to stop drinking, "one day at a time," and to go to meetings. Members may go to several meetings a week, and are encouraged to call other members if they feel the urge to drink. They follow a series of "12 Steps," which include admitting powerlessness over one's life and one's addiction, taking responsibility for one's actions and past mistakes, and seeking forgiveness from loved ones for these mistakes. The 12 Steps center on faith in a "higher power," which can be God or the AA group itself. Roughly half of people who join AA and continue to go to meetings for at least a year will stay sober, or "recover."

Offshoot groups use this approach to fight addictions to other substances, such as narcotics, and to activities, such as gambling or sex. (*See also* addiction treatment; alcoholism)

Additional reading: Robertson, *Getting Better.*

alcoholism

Alcoholism is an **addiction** to alcohol, and in its late stages can lead to malnutrition, brain and liver damage, and death.

Alcoholism probably has existed ever since humans began drinking alcohol. The earliest records that mention alcohol are clay tablets from Mesopotamia, dating back to about 4000 B.C. The tablets discuss the use of alcohol to dilute medicine and record how much alcohol local people consumed. The Code of Hammurabi of Babylon, of 1700 B.C., mentions restrictions on the sale and use of alcohol.

Benjamin Rush (1745–1813), an influential Philadelphia doctor, wrote in 1784 that alcohol was a drug that a person could become addicted to, that once this addiction set in a person was powerless to control it, and that total sobriety was the only cure for addiction to alcohol. The term "alcoholism" came into use during the mid-nineteenth century.

Following the influence of the temperance movement, the United States banned alcohol in 1920 with the Eighteenth Amendment. This period, known as Prohibition, did little to stop people from drinking. The amendment was repealed in 1933. It was at about this time that two alcoholic men, William Griffith Wilson (1895–1971) and Robert Holbrook Smith (1879–1950), founded **Alcoholics Anonymous (AA)**, a self-help group now considered to be the best approach to treating alcoholism. In 1956, the American Medical Association (AMA) stated that alcoholism should be considered a disease, adopting the view of AA.

Several different studies of male twins, beginning in the 1960s, have suggested that genetics strongly influence whether a person will become an alcoholic.

A number of different methods are used to determine whether or not people are alcoholics; most consist of a series of questions that people answer themselves. These include questionnaires by the National Council on Alcoholism, a volunteer group; the National Alcoholism Test (developed by researchers at Johns Hopkins University); and criteria set forth in the AMA's *Manual on Alcoholism*, first published in 1968.

Treatment for alcoholism can include attending AA; taking **Antabuse**, a drug that will make a person extremely sick if he or she drinks alcohol while on it; and counseling. A minority of addiction experts believe that people who are alcoholics can moderate their drinking; most say that complete abstinence is necessary. (*See also* addiction treatment)

Additional reading: Lender and Martin, *Drinking in America.*

alkylating agents

Alkylating agents are drugs that kill **cancer** cells by binding with their RNA or **DNA** and rendering the genetic material useless. These drugs were the first agents found to be effective against cancer. Like most cancer drugs, they are highly toxic because they attack the genetic material in normal cells as well. Alkylating agents, which include urea derivatives and the platinum-based drug cisplatin, work best against slow-growing cancers.

In 1942, Yale pharmacologists Louis Goodman (1906–) and Alfred Gilman (1908–) began studying **nitrogen mustard**, an alkylating agent. They convinced a surgeon to give the substance to a patient with advanced lymphatic cancer. The patient's tumors shrank dramatically, but grew back when the drug was stopped and ultimately became resistant to the drug.

Nitrogen mustards remain the most clinically useful drugs in this class; others commonly used today include cyclophosphamide, chlorambucil, and melphalan.

Additional reading: Sneader, *Drug Discovery*, pp. 335–52.

allergy

An allergy is a hypersensitivity to a particular substance that produces what is known as an allergic reaction. Allergy symptoms strike immediately, as opposed to delayed-type hypersensitivity, in which a reaction may occur a day or two after exposure to the allergen.

An allergy can produce itching, watery eyes, sneezing, coughing, wheezing, and nasal congestion if the allergen is inhaled (for example, pollen in hay fever). Allergic reactions of the skin include redness, itching, and hives. A severe reaction can produce **anaphylaxis**, a potentially fatal condition in which the respiratory passages close down and **blood pressure** drops dramatically.

Antihistamines can ease allergy-related congestion. They work by blocking the effects of **histamines**, chemicals that the body releases during an allergic reaction. **Cortisone**-like drugs may be given to patients with allergies to reduce swelling of the nasal and bronchial passages.

The ancient Greeks described hay fever and **asthma**. The Greek physician and writer Claudius Galen (129–c. 199) believed a person's individual constitution and "antipathies" were responsible for allergic reactions.

In the 1800s, because the immune system was thought to have evolved along Darwinian lines to protect humans and to thus be completely benign, the idea that the immune system was responsible for hay fever and other unpleasant conditions seemed absurd. But Paul Portier (1866–1962) and Charles Richet's (1850–1935) observation of anaphylaxis in 1902 provided the first evidence that the immune system could in fact be harmful.

In 1903, Maurice Arthus (1862–1945) observed that repeatedly injecting certain **antigens** into the skin caused the tissue to bleed and die, basically a local version of anaphylaxis. This came to be called the Arthus reaction.

Clemens von Pirquet (1874–1929) and Bela Schick (1877–1967), in 1906, investigated the phenomenon of serum sickness, which occurs in some people after they receive **diphtheria** or **tetanus** antitoxin to treat or prevent these infectious diseases. They decided that the immune system was responsible for serum sickness, and coined the word "allergy" to refer to this and similar phenomena. The term comes from the Greek words "allos ergos," or "altered reactivity."

In 1906, Alfred Wolff-Eisner connected hay fever to allergy, and four years later Samuel J. Meltzer (1851–1920) linked asthma and allergy. In 1921, Carl Prausnitz (1876–1963) and Heinz Kustner (1897–1963) showed that a person's particular allergy could be transferred to another person with an injection of his or her serum (the cell-free liquid in the blood). This phenomenon, called the **Prausnitz-Kustner reaction**, demonstrated that something in the blood—which we now know to be **antibodies**—are responsible for allergic responses.

The exact reason certain people are allergic to certain things is still unknown. It is known, however, that people who suffer from allergies tend to have large amounts of **immunoglobulin** E (IgE) in their blood, while people who don't have allergies have much smaller quantities of this antibody. Also, allergies appear to be inherited. IgE, discovered in the 1960s, is responsible for the allergic reaction, but scientists still aren't sure what purpose IgE serves in health.

Additional reading: Silverstein, *A History of Immunology,* pp. 214–51; Clark, *At War Within,* pp. 87–100.

Alma Ata International Conference on Primary Health Care

Representatives from around the world met at this **World Health Organization (WHO)**-sponsored meeting in September 1978. The conference, named for the USSR city where it was held (now in Kazakhstan), put forth the idea that health is a fundamental human right. The conference's statement urged governments to ensure that all of their citizens had access to primary health care.

Primary health care involves working in partnership with communities to provide preventive services, health promotion, treatment, and rehabilitation for all citizens. The goal of the Alma Ata declaration was to attain an acceptable level of health for all people of the world by the year 2000. Twenty years later in 1998, according to WHO, infant mortality worldwide had dropped 34 percent, and immunization coverage had risen from 20 percent in 1980 to 80 percent in 1990. While at the time of the declaration 38 percent of people in developing countries had safe drinking water and 32 percent had adequate sanitation, the percentages in 1990 were 66 percent and 53 percent.

At the 1978 conference, attendees predicted that world peace and disarmament would free nations' resources for improving public health. WHO pointed out 20 years later that other forces— "economic instability, globalization, and the triumph of the free market credo"—have increased inequalities among nations, and called for stronger collaboration between government and society to ensure that the original goal of "Health for All" can be met.

Additional reading: *Primary Health Care,* Alma Ata Conference; Tarimo and Webster, *Primary Health Care.*

alternative medicine

Alternative medicine is a term for treatments that fall outside the realm of conventional allopathic medicine. Alternative medicine can include **herbal medicine, acupuncture, chiropractic, homeopathy,** naturopathy, and physical exercise such as yoga.

People frequently use alternative or unconventional therapies for difficult-to-treat, chronic conditions such as back pain, arthritis, anxiety, and depression. According to government statistics and medical studies, people with **cancer** and with **AIDS** also often resort to alternative medicine. These therapies are often used in conjunction with conventional medicine.

Acceptance of these alternative techniques in mainstream medicine is growing, and some doctors with positive views of these techniques prefer to call them "complementary medicine," because they believe they complement conventional medicine.

A frequently cited survey published in the *New England Journal of Medicine* in 1993 found that about one-third of Americans used "unconventional therapy" in the past year, and that Americans visited alternative practitioners more often than they saw primary care doctors.

Another sign of the growing acceptance of alternative medicine is the fact that leading teaching hospitals have begun to add divisions focusing on this discipline. For example, Columbia University's College of Physicians & Surgeons founded a Center for Alternative/Complementary Medicine in 1994, and the Harvard Medical School-affiliated Beth Israel-Deaconess Hospital in Boston founded its Center for Alternative Medicine Research and Education in 1995.

The **National Institutes of Health (NIH)** also formed an Office of Alternative Medicine at the behest of Congress in 1992, which in 1998 became the National Center for Complementary and Alternative Medicine.

Additional reading: Cassileth, *The Alternative Medicine Handbook.*

Alzheimer's disease

Alzheimer's disease is a degenerative brain disorder that causes dementia and eventual death.

The disease was first described by Alois Alzheimer (1864–1915) in 1906, when he presented, to a meeting of his colleagues, the case of a 51-year-old woman with dementia. During the **autopsy,** Alzheimer found neurofibrillary tangles and plaques in her brain.

Until the 1960s, Alzheimer's disease was known as presenile dementia and thought only to occur in people under the age of 65, while **atherosclerosis** was thought to be the major cause of senility in older people. But in 1968, the disease was shown to be the leading cause of dementia among the elderly.

Alzheimer's disease is now thought to account for about half of all dementia in people over 65. Currently, there is no treatment for Alzheimer's disease, although some medications and nutrients may slow mental deterioration. Two drugs, tacrine (approved by the **Food and Drug Administration** in 1993) and donepezil (approved in 1997), do not affect the underlying disease process of Alzheimer's but may help preserve mental function temporarily. Studies have also shown that the drug selegeline and the nutrient **vitamin E** delayed functional deterioration. Researchers currently are investigating whether **hormone replacement therapy** with **estrogen**, anti-inflammatory drugs, and nerve **growth factors** can help slow the progress of Alzheimer's as well.

Additional reading: Restak, *Brainscapes,* pp. 130–34.

ambulance

An ambulance is a vehicle designed to transport an injured person to the hospital and to provide medical care en route.

Dominique-Jean Larrey (1766–1842) coined the phrase *hopital ambulant*, or moving hospital, for the system he developed to treat battlefield casualties during the Napoleonic wars. Larrey also designed quick transportation for injured soldiers in the form of two- and four-wheeled horse-drawn vehicles, which followed the battle to provide emergency care and take wounded men off the battlefield. He called the carts "ambulances volantes"—flying ambulances. He perfected his system by 1796, and by the middle of the

nineteenth century nearly every European army was using ambulance wagons.

The United States did not use ambulances in wartime until the Civil War. During this war, four-wheeled wagons with springs as well as locomotives were employed to transport the wounded.

Ambulances for civilians became necessary with the advent of modern city traffic and city sprawl; more people were seriously hurt in traffic accidents, and since cities had grown larger it became necessary to find a means of transportation for injured people to sometimes faraway hospitals.

Edward B. Dalton (1834–1872) is credited with developing the nation's first urban ambulance system, for New York City's Bellevue Hospital, in 1866. Dalton's ambulances and the others that followed were basically horse-drawn wagons with pillows to make the ride more comfortable for patients. By 1883, 7 New York hospitals were running 19 ambulances in all. Washington, D.C., Philadelphia, Cleveland, and several other cities soon followed.

In 1973, funding provided by the federal Emergency Medical Services Systems Act made it possible for most U.S. cities to establish ambulance services.

Additional reading: Haller, *Farmcarts to Fords.*

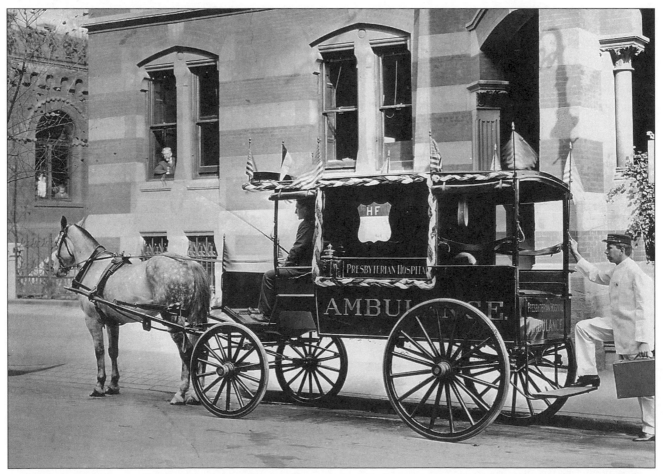

The New York Presbyterian Hospital's horse-drawn ambulance in a 1909 photo. (Courtesy of Archives and Special Collections, Columbia University Health Sciences Division.)

ambulatory surgery

Ambulatory or outpatient surgery is an operation that requires a short recovery time and no overnight hospital stay. This type of surgery arose in the 1970s and has become increasingly common for both financial and clinical reasons: a shorter stay is cheaper, improvements in the precision of **anesthesia** are making recovery easier and quicker, and more operations are performed with **minimally invasive surgery** methods.

The philosophy that returning to normal activity as quickly as possible makes for a better recovery arose in Scotland in 1890, when surgeons began requiring patients to get up and walk around after surgery, with excellent results. Some American physicians noticed and advocated this approach. The first recorded ambulatory surgeries in the United States were performed at the Downtown Anesthesia Clinic in Iowa.

In the 1960s, the first modern same-day surgery programs were opened in Michigan and California, and a freestanding center for ambulatory surgery opened its doors in Arizona in 1970. By 1996, according to the National Center for Health Statistics, 51 percent of surgical patients were not admitted to a hospital for their operations. By 2000, health care experts estimate that 75 percent of all surgeries in the United States will be performed on an outpatient basis.

Additional reading: Zuger, "Surgeons Leave OR for the Office."

amniocentesis

Amniocentesis is a technique for diagnosing fetal abnormalities in which fluid is sampled from the amniotic sac surrounding the fetus via a needle inserted through the pregnant woman's abdomen. The cells and liquid are then analyzed to detect birth defects and determine the maturity of the fetus. Amniocentesis can reveal genetic defects, metabolic disorders, and certain **birth defects** such as a paralyzing malformation of the spine known as spina bifida. Normally, the procedure is done between the 14th and 18th weeks of pregnancy.

Withdrawal of fluid from the amniotic sac has been common practice since the mid-1950s, when it was first used to drain excess fluid and also to check the blood type of a fetus if the mother was Rh-negative.

In 1955, four independent groups of researchers—two in the United States, one each in Israel and Denmark—found it was possible to predict the sex of a fetus by analyzing cells in amniotic fluid. This was useful because many genetic disorders, such as hemophilia, are sex-linked, meaning they occur in only one of the sexes. If parents had a history of a sex-linked genetic disease, this made it possible to determine if the child would be affected or would merely carry the trait.

Jerome LeJeune (1926–), a French researcher, found a genetic basis for a common form of **Down syndrome** in 1959. This cued researchers that it might be possible to karyotype fetal cells collected via amniocentesis to detect genetic abnormalities. In 1960, Danish researchers reported

performing an abortion on a hemophilia carrier because prenatal testing revealed the fetus was male.

The need to invent a culturing method to produce enough cells for analysis, as well as political considerations about **abortion**, prevented amniocentesis from immediately becoming available as a test for fetal abnormalities. Researchers found a way to culture the cells in 1966. Two years later, the first abortions performed after amniocentesis found abnormalities were reported.

The United States began a registry to determine the safety of amniocentesis in 1971, reporting the results in 1975 and publishing them in 1976.

After several lawsuits in the late 1970s were filed by parents of children with abnormalities detectable by amniocentesis whose gynecologists had not referred them for prenatal testing, amniocentesis became common practice for mothers over 35. By this time, the Supreme Court had made its 1973 decision *Roe vs. Wade*, which legalized first-term abortions. This meant parents could legally terminate a pregnancy if the tests revealed a serious birth defect.

Additional reading: Kolker and Burke, *Prenatal Testing.*

amphetamine

Amphetamines are stimulating drugs. The first amphetamine, Benzedrine, was introduced by Smith, Kline, and French in 1932 as an inhalant to treat nasal congestion. It was developed by University of California chemist Gordon Alles (1901–1963) as an artificial replacement for **ephedrine.**

Another amphetamine, desamphetamine (sold as Dexedrine) was introduced in 1935 to treat narcolepsy. This and other early amphetamines were available without a prescription, and people used them to treat depression, control appetite, and manage problem children. Long-haul truck drivers and students cramming for tests used them to stay awake. World War II soldiers took desamphetamine and the more potent methylamphetamine (Methedrine) to fight drowsiness. Amphetamine use and abuse soon became widespread.

Eventually, the dangers of amphetamine addiction became evident. The U.S. government began efforts to control these and other drugs by requiring prescriptions, but the Benzedrine inhaler remained available. People would break open the inhaler and swallow the amphetamine-impregnated paper inside.

Today, amphetamines are strictly controlled and are only used to treat narcolepsy and some cases of **depression**. Methylphenidate hydrochloride, better known as Ritalin, is chemically related to amphetamine and is used to treat **attention-deficit hyperactivity disorder (ADHD)**.

Additional reading: Sneader, *Drug Discovery*, pp. 100–02.

amputation

Amputation is the removal of an injured or diseased limb or other body part.

The first clinical description of a therapeutic amputation, aside from the ancient punishment of cutting off limbs, noses, or fingers, appears in the writings of Hippocrates (460–370 B.C.) as a treatment for gangrene.

To stop bleeding after amputation, surgeons in the Middle Ages would cauterize a wound with boiling oil or a hot iron, sometimes also using compression bandages or astringents.

In 1529, Ambrose Pare (c.1510–1590) was the first person to actually tie off blood vessels to stem bleeding after amputation. Pare, like many of his colleagues, honed his surgical skills on the battlefield. He also developed an alternative to hot oil for nongangrenous wounds, a mixture of egg yolk, rose oil, and turpentine that kept wound inflammation at bay, preserved tissue, and reduced pain.

Two centuries later, another French surgeon, Jean-Louis Petit (1674–1760), introduced a tourniquet that could be used to constrict blood vessels and control bleeding while the surgeon tied off blood vessels using Pare's method. Johann von Esmarch (1825–1908) invented a rubber bandage in 1873 that was more effective.

Patients were given whiskey or other spirits to deaden the pain of amputation, or "bit the bullet" when alcohol wasn't available, until the advent of **anesthesia** in the nineteenth century. Robert Liston (1794–1847) performed the first amputation using **ether** on the patient as an anesthetic in 1846.

Additional reading: Rutkow, *American Surgery,* pp. 132–43.

amyl nitrate

Amyl nitrate is a clear liquid that dilates the blood vessels and is useful for treating pain from **angina pectoris**, which occurs when the heart muscle isn't getting enough oxygen from the blood. Thomas Brunton (1844–1916) discovered this property of amyl nitrate in 1867. The drug is still used today for treating angina. It is taken by inhalation.

Additional reading: Fye, "T. Lauder Brunton and Amyl Nitrate."

analgesics

Analgesics are pain-killing drugs. There are two major classes of analgesics: opoids (**opium** and related drugs), which block pain receptors in the brain; and anti-inflammatory drugs, which interrupt the process leading to inflammation. Opoids, derived from the poppy plant, have been used for centuries.

Many of today's anti-inflammatory drugs come from three synthetic compounds formulated in the late nineteenth century: salicylic acid (**aspirin**'s precursor), pyrazolone, and phenaticin. The **nonsteroidal anti-inflammatory drugs** (**NSAID**s), such as **ibuprofen**, were introduced in the 1970s. They work by inhibiting the synthesis of **prostaglandin**, a substance produced by inflamed tissue.

Additional reading: Rey, *The History of Pain.*

anaphylaxis

Anaphylaxis is a severe allergic reaction that, when it leads to anaphylactic **shock**, can be fatal.

Paul Portier (1866–1962) and Charles Richet (1850–1935) discovered anaphylaxis in 1902 while testing animals' reactions to a sea anemone toxin. They found that a dog exposed to a small amount of the toxin suffered a severe immediate reaction and died within a half-hour after being reexposed. The two scientists named the phenomenon "anaphylaxis," from the Greek *ana* and *phylaxis*, meaning "not protection." The next year, another scientist discovered that the same reaction could be induced with nontoxic materials. Extensive experiments with guinea pigs, which are ideally suited to this research because they go into anaphylactic shock easily, confirmed this discovery. Richet won the 1913 Nobel Prize for this work.

Anaphylaxis occurs when a particular substance—which can be a drug such as **penicillin**, an insect sting, or a food—enters the bloodstream and begins to interact with **immunoglobulin** E (IgE) **antibodies**. People with allergies tend to produce large amounts of IgE, while nonallergic people only have small amounts in their blood. The reaction causes certain immune system cells to release **histamine**, which increases the permeability of the blood vessels, leading to swelling and rash. If this blood-vessel leakiness is widespread, it can lead to a life-threatening, severe drop in **blood pressure**. Histamine also causes smooth muscles to contract, which narrows airway passages and restricts breathing.

Anaphylactic shock is treated with drugs, such as **epinephrine**, that increase blood pressure and relax smooth muscle. It may be necessary to provide **artificial respiration** for a person in anaphylactic shock until he or she recovers the ability to breathe. (*See also* allergy)

Additional reading: Silverstein, *A History of Immunology,* pp. 332, 372–73.

anatomical theater

Anatomical theaters were arenas where surgeons and medical students performed dissections before an audience for entertainment and education. These theaters were popular in Europe during the Middle Ages.

Regulations for the performance of public human dissections date back to the early 1300s, while documents specifically addressing anatomical theaters first appear in the early sixteenth century. One common rule required that the person to be dissected must come from a different city, to spare the deceased's family and friends from what would have been an unpleasant experience. In some cities, anatomists had to agree to present an annual public dissection—usually around Christmas, when cold weather would help preserve the body—in order to receive a guaranteed supply of executed criminals' bodies for anatomical research.

Some historians argue that these public performances also served as a moral lesson to the audience and a "second death" for the criminal.

The first permanent anatomical theaters were built in Italy and the Netherlands around the turn of the fifteenth century. Dissected parts were passed around to the audience for their perusal, but the person's remains were to be buried with respect and care after the dissection was finished. Anatomical theaters also served as museums, containing biological and zoological specimens, books, and instruments.

Additional reading: Gonzalez-Crussi, *Suspended Animation.*

anatomy

Anatomy is the study of the structure of the body. Taboos against handling the dead in many cultures prevented people from learning much about anatomy until relatively recently. Even the ancient Egyptians, who removed organs from the body for mummification, contributed little anatomical knowledge to humanity; they believed that the blood vessels' two central points were the heart and the anus.

Anatomy was born in Alexandria around 300 B.C. At this center of Greek learning in what is now Egypt, on the Mediterranean Sea, the physicians Herophilus, Erasistratos, and their colleagues dissected animals and human corpses. Although no writings from the Alexandrian anatomists survive, they are credited by later authors with discovering many structures within the body, including the prostate and the duodenum, and also the concept of the heart as a pump.

In the first century A.D., Greek physician Claudius Galen (129–c.199) did not dissect humans, but he did dissect living animals. He performed experiments showing that kidneys produce urine, that arteries contain blood, and that severing the spinal cord produces paralysis. Galen's anatomical research on animals served as the basis for the understanding of human anatomy for centuries. To teach students anatomy in medieval medical schools, an instructor would read from Galen's works while a barber-surgeon did the actual cutting.

The first modern anatomist was Andreas Vesalius (1514–1564), a Belgian professor of anatomy at the medical school in Padua, Italy. Vesalius performed dissections himself and drew his descriptions from the body before him rather than from Galen's often incorrect accounts. Vesalius's great work of anatomy, *De humani corporis fabrica,* was published in 1543.

During the Renaissance, Italian physicians including Vesalius—as well as artists such as Michelangelo (1475–1564) and Leonardo da Vinci (1452–1519) —performed dissections to study anatomy.

Giovanni Battista Morgagni (1682–1771) performed thousands of **autopsies**, making careful observations of the changes in tissues and attempting to correlate these changes with symptoms. The next major advance in anatomy was the development of histopathology, in which the diseased tissues themselves were studied under a **microscope**. The leader in combining microscopic observations with gross anatomy was the German pathologist Rudolf Virchow (1821–1902). Virchow's technique for performing autopsies remains in use today.

Additional reading: Persaud, *Early History of Human Anatomy; A History of Anatomy.*

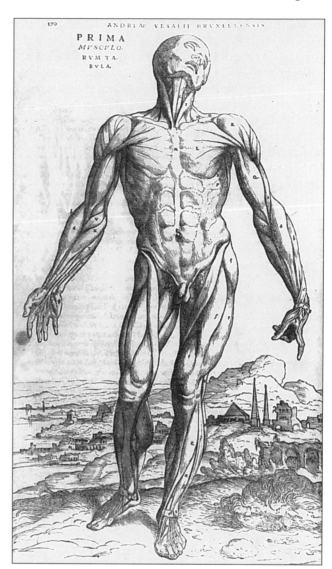

Plate from Andreas Vesalius's 1543 anatomical work, *De humani corporis fabrica.* (Courtesy of National Library of Medicine.)

androgens

Androgens are **hormones**, such as testosterone and androsterone, that stimulate the growth of male sexual characteristics and also help to maintain these characteristics.

Originally it was thought that physiological changes in males that occurred after castration came about via the nervous system. Arnold Adolf Berthold (1803–1861) demonstrated otherwise in 1849, when he showed that reimplanting the testes of a castrated rooster in its abdominal cavity resulted in a return of its comb and wattles, as well as of characteristic rooster-like behavior. He theorized that there must be some substance that traveled through the blood that was responsible for producing these characteristics. A number of similar experiments were performed in which extracts of testicles were given to animals—and to humans.

In 1931, Adolf Butenandt (1903–1995) isolated 50 milligrams of a substance he named androsterone from 25,000 liters of policemen's urine. In the summer of 1935, Ernst Laqueur (1901–1947) and his colleagues in

Amsterdam isolated pure male hormone from bulls' testicles, naming the substance "testosterone." At about the same time, Leopold Ruzicka (1887–1976) of Zurich announced that he had developed a technique for synthesizing testosterone from cholesterol, making it possible to produce large quantities of the hormone for therapeutic use. Butenandt and Ruzicka shared the 1939 Nobel Prize for Chemistry. **Clinical trials** of testosterone injections in humans for various purposes began two years later.

During the 1940s, researchers found testosterone stimulated the growth of muscle **tissue**, causing bodybuilders to begin experimenting with the hormone and other athletes to follow. In the early 1990s, studies began on giving testosterone to older men with low-to-normal testosterone levels, resulting in gains in muscle strength, increases in libido, and improvement in memory. The hormone also appears to be useful in restoring strength and energy to patients with **AIDS**. Testosterone may be given to women to improve the sex drive or treat hormone-dependent cancers of the breast and ovary.

Dehydroepiandrosterone, or DHEA, is a type of androgen hormone secreted by the cortex of the **adrenal gland** and also by the testicles. The hormone is believed to be a precursor for both testosterone and **estrogen** formed in the peripheral tissues (that is, beyond the gonads). Half of androgens in adult men derive from DHEA and the associated hormone DHEAS, while in women 75 percent of estrogens before menopause and up to 100 percent of estrogens after menopause are thought to come from DHEA and DHEAS.

In 1944, researchers from the University of Chicago led by Paul L. Munson (1910–) isolated DHEAS from urine. In 1957, Claude J. Migeon (1923–) of the Johns Hopkins University School of Medicine and his colleagues reported the results of their study on how DHEA levels vary with age and sex. They found that for both males and females, secretion accelerates during childhood (a period known as adrenarche that occurs at age 6 to 8) and reaches a maximum between the ages of 20 and 30. Levels of the hormone drop dramatically after about age 70 (a phenomenon known as andropause), to about 20 percent of peak levels. They continue to drop steadily afterwards.

No other adrenal hormones exhibit this pattern, so researchers theorized that low levels of the hormone might play a role in age-related conditions such as heart disease, insulin insensitivity, weakened immunity, and loss of muscle strength. Studies in which mice are given DHEA back up this theory, but this animal model is flawed because mice actually have virtually no circulating DHEA, while humans do.

Human studies so far have yielded little evidence that DHEA is the "anti-aging hormone" that nutrition supplement makers claim it is. However, in 1994, Stanford University Medical School researchers reported that the hormone is an effective treatment for an **autoimmune disease** that mainly strikes young women, systemic lupus erythematosus. A few studies in humans also have found that the

hormone increases muscle strength and improves immune-system function. In a 1999 clinical trial of DHEA in women who did not produce sufficient amounts of adrenal hormones, the drug improved sexual function as well as blood cholesterol levels.

In 1997, the National Institute on Aging, part of the **National Institutes of Health (NIH)**, warned consumers that there is little evidence for the anti-aging claims of DHEA makers, and that in fact the drug can cause liver damage and increase **cancer** risk. For this reason, doctors say the hormone should only be taken as part of a carefully supervised clinical trial. Today, researchers continue to investigate whether DHEA and DHEAS might one day be useful as hormone supplements.

Additional reading: Mainwaring, *The Mechanism of Action of Androgens;* Okie, "Can Hormones Stop Aging?"

anemia

In anemia, the number or volume of red blood cells, or red blood cells' hemoglobin content, is below normal, meaning the body cannot meet its oxygen demands. Red blood cells, with the help of the pigment hemoglobin, carry oxygen through the body to supply this vital gas to the tissues. The most common type of anemia is iron-deficiency anemia, which is caused by insufficient iron intake, blood loss, or a combination of both. Iron-deficiency anemia is common among adolescent girls, on whom growth and menstruation place a double iron demand.

In 1554, Johannes Lange (1485–1565) described anemia as "orbus virgineus," and theorized that it occurred when virgins retained menstrual blood. He advised patients with this disease to marry as quickly as possible, as did Hippocrates (460–370 B.C.).

Iron-deficiency anemia was also known as "greensickness" or "chlorosis," because the skin of iron-deficient white women can develop a yellowish-green tint. William Shakespeare (1564–1616) mentions greensickness several times in his writings.

Pierre Blaud recommended giving iron to women with chlorosis in 1832, and 13 years later Gabriel Andral (1797–1876) observed that the red blood cells of people with chlorosis were much smaller than normal. Blaud's prescription, although it worked, met with resistance; many physicians of the time believed chlorosis was a neurotic disease, and it was also difficult to show scientifically that the body would absorb iron from nonorganic sources.

Chlorosis became very common in nineteenth-century Europe, perhaps because so many young women who had moved to the cities to work in factories subsisted on iron-poor diets consisting mainly of bread.

The Scottish physician Ralph Stockman (1861–unknown) performed a series of experiments he reported in 1893 in which he showed that iron supplements increased hemoglobin levels in anemic women. Two years later, he wrote that young women became chlorotic because they ate little food, especially meat, while menstruation and growth were placing increased iron demands on their body.

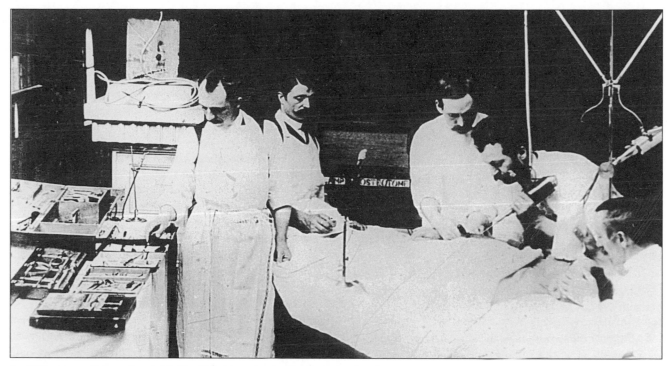

An 1895 surgery at Bellevue Hospital in New York. The patient is enjoying the benefits of anesthesia; however, surgeons are not using another relatively recent innovation to control contamination of the surgical field: asepsis. (Courtesy of New York University Medical Center Archives.)

Stockman's observations, though correct, were not generally accepted for more than 20 years because of the persistence of the belief in neurosis as the source of anemia.

Additional reading: Kiple, *The Cambridge World History of Human Disease,* pp. 571–76.

anesthesia

Anesthetics are drugs used to block the perception of pain, and anesthesia is the state produced by these drugs.

In local anesthesia, used for dental and minor surgical procedures, only the area to be operated upon is numbed. **Cocaine** was the first local anesthetic discovered, in 1860 by Albert Niemann (1834–1861). In general anesthesia, inhaled or injected substances make a person unconscious and unable to feel pain. There are also forms of anesthesia that only deaden feeling in some areas of the body, such as spinal and **epidural anesthesia**.

Painkillers have been known for thousands of years, but anesthesia has only been perfected in the late nineteenth and twentieth centuries. The ancient Greek author Homer mentioned a pain-deadening substance called "nepenthe" in his writings, which was probably cannabis or **opium**. Another Greek, the army surgeon Dioscorides (c.40–c.90), was the first person to use the word anesthesia. Arabian physicians gave their patients opium and henbane to ease pain, while British sailors got rum before **amputations**. All of these methods came with problems; the patient was not totally dead to the pain, and handling a drunk or otherwise intoxicated patient could be more difficult than dealing with a sober one. Surgeons of the days before anesthesia prided themselves on being quick. They also relied on colleagues to restrain and even gag patients during surgery.

Nitrous oxide, or laughing gas, was one of the first agents investigated for anesthesia, and is still in common use as an anesthetic today. Crawford Long (1815–1878) is credited with performing surgery under anesthesia for the first time, using **ether,** in 1842, although William Morton (1819–1868) became more famous for performing the first public demonstration of ether anesthesia in 1846. The amphitheater at Massachusetts General Hospital, where Morton anesthetized the patient who was having a tumor removed from his arm, is now known as the "Ether Dome." The demonstration was written up in the *Boston Medical Journal.* Although Long discovered ether anesthesia, the article was responsible for popularizing it. By the following year, hospitals in Europe, South Africa, and South America were using ether anesthesia based on this report.

University of Edinburgh professor James Simpson (1811–1870), who was also Queen Victoria's doctor, used **chloroform** to ease the labor pains of his niece and subsequently recommended the gas for the queen. She delivered her eighth child with the help of chloroform, administered by John Snow (1813–1858).

Early anesthetics were given via sponges soaked in the anesthetizing substance, a messy and sometimes dangerous technique. The early anesthetics themselves were not ideal, either; ether could cause vomiting and irritated the patient's airways, while chloroform caused liver damage.

The next new anesthetic to be introduced was ethylene, which had actually been tested in 1849 and entered clinical use in the 1920s. The gas was phased out in the 1950s because of concerns about its flammability. Cyclopropane was also investigated by researchers in Toronto and found to be safe and effective in the 1930s, and is still in use today.

The next advance was the discovery of a group of related chemicals, fluorocarbon anesthetics, which were derived from chemicals developed by U.S. scientists during wartime as uranium solvents. The safest and most effective of these was halothane, synthesized at the British company ICI in 1953. Clinical trials began at a Manchester hospital in 1956. Halothane remains the most widely used anesthetic today.

Other advances in surgical anesthesia include **endotracheal intubation,** which came into general surgical use in the late 1920s. Intubation made it possible for anesthetists to regulate breathing. Anesthetists began giving patients the muscle relaxant **curare** during the 1940s.

Machines to provide a flow of anesthetic gas were invented in the late 1800s. E.I. McKesson (1881–1935), an Ohio anesthetist, invented a machine that he described in 1926. This was a demand flow machine. Henry Boyle (1875–1941) of London developed a continuous flow machine in 1917. A portable version was developed for use by the British Army during World War I. "Boyle machines" are still used today, although the original has undergone many modifications and additions.

The first device to measure gas flow, the rotameter, was invented in Germany and patented in 1908.

Today, patients usually are first given an injection of sodium thiopental, and then receive inhalation anesthetics such as trichloroethylene or halothane mixed with nitrous oxide and oxygen, administered by an anesthetic machine.

Additional reading: Friedman and Friedland, *Medicine's 10 Greatest Discoveries,* pp. 94–114.

aneurysm

An aneurysm occurs when the wall of a blood vessel weakens and begins to bulge, which means the vessel is in danger of bursting and causing a hemorrhage.

Physicians in the late eighteenth and early nineteenth century tied off one of the carotid arteries, which are the main blood vessels leading to the head, in order to treat aneurysms in the brain. This would cause the blood to form a clot in the aneurysm, reducing the threat that the vessel would burst. Victor Horsely (1857–1916) performed one of these operations in 1885.

Norman Dott (1897–1973) performed the first planned—rather than emergency—operation on an aneurysm within the brain in 1931 in Edinburgh. The surgery was performed on the chairman of his hospital board. Dott also developed a technique for reinforcing the weakened walls of aneurysms by packing muscle around the vessel. Walter Dandy (1886–1946) treated several aneurysms surgically with great success. He was the first to use a clip to close off the neck of an aneurysm, in a 1938 operation. Dandy also first "trapped" the aneurysm, tying it off at either end, in a 1942 operation.

By 1955, 278 operations for aneurysms within the brain had been performed, with nearly 30 percent mortality. During this decade, techniques were introduced for lowering blood pressure during surgery, which made the operation easier and less hazardous because it caused the blood to exert less force on the vessel walls. The first method was to remove large quantities of blood from the body; later it was found that blocking certain nerves with drugs could achieve the same results.

The surgical microscope began to be used for aneurysm operations in the early 1970s. Now, better anesthesia and strategies for interrupting blood flow have made aneurysm surgery much safer.

Additional reading: "Abdominal Aortic Aneurysms Run in the Family," *Harvard Heart Letter.*

angina pectoris

Angina pectoris can be a moderate-to-crushing constricting pain over the heart and breastbone areas of the chest caused by obstructed heart-muscle blood flow. The pain can also spread along the inside of the left arm to the fingers, and may be felt on the left side of the neck. Pain may occasionally be felt in the jaws and teeth.

William Heberden (1710–1801), a British physician, provided a detailed description of angina pectoris in a 1768 paper and named the condition, although cases had been described since the seventeenth century. Heberden did not link angina pectoris to the heart but just to the chest.

John Johnstone, in the *Memoirs of the Medical Society of London,* wrote in 1787 that angina pectoris resulted from heart disease, because the heart was "unfit for its office of carrying on the circulation of the blood." After performing an **autopsy** on a patient who suffered from angina, Edward Jenner (1749–1823), was convinced that the pain was caused by obstruction in the coronary arteries, because the arteries had become "bony canals." His colleague and friend Caleb Parry (1775–1822) agreed.

John Hunter (1728–1793), Jenner's friend and mentor, suffered from angina, so Jenner decided not to publish his findings, which illustrated how life-threatening the condition was, while Hunter was still alive. Hunter died in 1793, and an autopsy confirmed that his coronary arteries were indeed blocked. Parry finally reported on the link between angina pectoris and blood-vessel blockage in 1799.

Nitroglycerin has long been an effective treatment for angina, but surgical procedures such as **bypass surgery** and **angioplasty** can also eliminate angina in most patients. In 1998, doctors at St. Elizabeth's Hospital in Boston began using **vascular endothelial growth factor**, a natural protein that stimulates blood vessel growth, to treat patients with severe angina, with good results. Another new technique for treating angina is a surgical procedure called **transmyocardial revascularization.**

Additional reading: Acierno, *The History of Cardiology,* pp. 291–97, 302–12.

angiography

Angiography is a technique for imaging blood vessels.

Werner Forssmann (1904–1979), a German physician, made the first angiograms in 1931. Forssmann, who invented **cardiac catheterization** and proved it would work by catheterizing his own heart, theorized that it would be possible to "see" the interior spaces of the heart, arteries, and veins by injecting a contrast agent into the bloodstream and taking a series of **X-ray** images of the area. A contrast agent is opaque to X-rays, which makes structures containing the agent appear solid on an X-ray image. The agent had to be injected near the area to be examined, which was accomplished by passing a rubber tube or catheter into the circulatory system, usually through a vein.

Portuguese, French, and Argentine scientists followed up on Forssman's work by making angiograms of blood vessels in the lungs and brain. In 1937, the technique was used to diagnose a heart defect in a living patient. In 1945, a team at Johns Hopkins University in Baltimore set up the first catheterization lab. It was dedicated to diagnosing congenital heart defects in children.

While performing a cardiac catheterization in 1958, Frank Mason Sones (1919–1985) and his colleagues accidentally allowed the catheter to pass into one of the patient's coronary arteries (vessels serving the heart muscle itself). The patient suffered no ill effects. That same year, Sones began performing angiograms of the coronary arteries and observing the images using a **fluoroscope**. He pioneered the technique of "cine-angiography," taking a series of images of the arteries to provide a "motion picture" of arterial function.

Now, technicians are able to create angiograms of arterial systems virtually anywhere in the body.

Additional reading: Acierno, *The History of Cardiology*, pp. 564–71.

angioplasty

Angioplasty is a method for opening up arteries narrowed by disease. Coronary angioplasty can be life-saving, because blocked vessels in the heart are the leading cause of heart attacks.

In the late 1960s, Charles Dotter (1920–1985) pioneered a method for opening up arteries elsewhere in the body by pushing a series of successively larger catheters through the blocked vessel. Andreas Gruentzig (1939–1985), a Swiss surgeon living in Germany, learned the technique and decided to apply it to the heart. With colleagues he developed a catheter with a balloon attached. Once it reached the occlusion, the balloon could be inflated to push back the arterial walls.

Gruentzig performed the first coronary angioplasty in Zurich in 1977, on a 38–year-old man. The operation was a success. In the 1980s, surgeons proved that angioplasty could be performed safely in an emergency, while the patient was having a heart attack.

Throughout the 1980s, other developments such as rotary ablation for arteries obstructed with hard material and **stents** placed within arteries to keep them open added to the effectiveness of the procedure. Several techniques are now being investigated for keeping blood vessels open after angioplasty, including radiation and medication.

Additional reading: Acierno, *The History of Cardiology*, pp. 669–70.

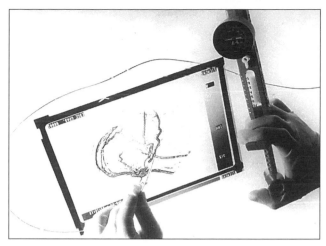

Dr. Frederick Feit with balloon catheter used to perform balloon angioplasty and an angiogram of the blood vessels of the heart. (Courtesy of New York University Medical Center Archives.)

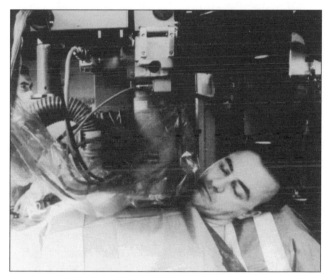

A patient receiving angioplasty to clear blocked blood vessels. (Courtesy of New York University Medical Center Archives.)

anorexia nervosa

Anorexia nervosa is a form of mental illness in which a person obsessively restricts their food intake. People with anorexia nervosa may lose up to 25 percent of their body weight, which results in profound metabolic and systemic physical changes and can ultimately be fatal.

About 90 percent of those with the disease are women between the ages of 13 and 25. Anorexia nervosa appears almost exclusively in developed nations and among the middle and upper classes. While about 70 percent of people treated for anorexia nervosa recover, as many as 5 to 18 percent die within 10 years, usually from suicide or from complications related to anorexia.

Some historians argue that Richard Morton (1637–1698) provided the first detailed description of anorexia in 1694, and others point to older stories of self-starvation by female saints as cases of anorexia. Others believe that anorexia nervosa is a uniquely modern condition, created by media images of fashionably thin women.

In 1859, an American asylum doctor described a condition he called "sitomania," in which a person became disgusted by and afraid of food. He also discussed a unique form of the condition that occurred in adolescent girls. Sir William Gull (1816–1890) proposed the name anorexia nervosa for the condition in 1868, and in 1873, he and Charles Lasegue (1816–1883) described treatment. Gull argued that anorexia nervosa was different from appetite loss related to disease or another type of mental illness, and was in fact the primary characteristic of the disease. Lasegue suggested that a patient's family environment was related to anorexia. However, most doctors of the time rejected Gull's and Lasegue's relatively sophisticated construction of the disease, instead attributing anorexia to imaginary conditions such as hysteria of the gastrointestinal tract.

In the early 1900s in the United States, the idea emerged that anorexia was due to endocrine problems, either with the **pituitary** or **thyroid gland**, and attempts were made to treat the condition with supplements of hormones in the 1920s and 1930s.

Sigmund Freud (1856–1939) and Pierre Janet (1859–1947) went in the other direction and investigated psychological reasons for anorexia. They suggested that it occurred because a girl was attempting to suppress her sexual drive and forestall puberty.

Hilde Bruch (1904–1984) developed a more well-rounded theory of the causes of anorexia, suggesting that while girls who developed anorexia were indeed not prepared for sexual maturity, dynamics within the family were also responsible. She suggested anorexia was an effort by a young girl to retain control of her life.

People with anorexia nervosa often must begin treatment in the hospital so their weight can be brought back to normal with intravenous feeding. Treatment also requires intense psychiatric counseling, to restore a normal body image to the victim and also to help her relearn how to eat. Family therapy also is important. Anorexia nervosa has recently been linked to a type of **anxiety disorder** known as obsessive-compulsive disorder (OCD). Anorexia, like **bulimia nervosa,** is closely associated with **depression** and treatment with **antidepressant drugs** can be helpful as well.

Additional reading: Brumberg, *Fasting Girls.*

Antabuse

Antabuse, or disulfram, is a drug used to treat alcoholism. Usually, the body converts alcohol to acetaldehyde and then quickly oxidizes this substance into acetic acid. Antabuse hampers this process. If a person drinks alcohol while taking Antabuse, acetaldehyde will collect in the body, progressively poisoning the drinker. Illness—and sometimes even death—will result.

Antabuse was discovered by accident. During World War II, Danish researchers were investigating disulfram, which had been used topically for treating scabies, to see if it would kill intestinal parasites. The scientists tested disulfram pills by giving them to rabbits, and then tried them on themselves. Several of the researchers taking disulfram became ill after drinking wine at lunch. They compared notes and concluded that alcohol and disulfram made a sickening combination. One of the scientists spoke on the unexpected properties of disulfram at a public meeting in 1947. Newspapers reported on the meeting, and alcoholics wrote to the researchers seeking to try the pills.

Today, some abstinent alcoholics take disulfram to discourage themselves from impulse drinking.

Additional reading: Altman, *Who Goes First,* pp. 98–104.

anthrax vaccine

Anthrax **vaccine** was one of the first vaccines developed by the pioneering French bacteriologist Louis Pasteur (1822–1895). Pasteur investigated anthrax and other diseases of farm animals, and he developed vaccines—a term he coined—to prevent costly illnesses in these animals. These vaccines paved the way for human immunization against disease.

Pasteur had to fight the skepticism conservative doctors and many veterinarians felt toward his **germ theory**, which they said had no application in the real world. His dramatic public demonstration of his anthrax vaccine helped convince them of its value, and opened the door to public acceptance that bacteria caused disease and that vaccines could protect animals, and people, from infection.

Anthrax is an extremely contagious disease transmitted by spores of the anthrax bacillus. It is fatal in cattle and sheep, and can be passed to humans. In the 1860s and 1870s, epidemics of anthrax struck many European cattle herds.

To make his vaccine, Pasteur used nonvirulent strains of anthrax grown in chicken broth. In an 1881 demonstration, he gave 24 sheep, six cows, and one goat five drops each of the weakened bacillus. Two weeks later his colleagues inoculated the animals with a more virulent culture. After another two weeks, Pasteur injected these animals and a control group of unvaccinated animals with three rounds of live anthrax bacilli. A few weeks later, the vaccinated animals were healthy but the unvaccinated ones were dead or dying.

Most of Pasteur's critics were convinced of the vaccine's effectiveness by this demonstration. By 1894, more than three million sheep and about half a million cattle had been vaccinated against anthrax.

Additional reading: Geison, *The Private Science of Louis Pasteur,* pp. 145–76.

anti-anxiety drugs

Anti-anxiety drugs are used to treat patients with **anxiety disorders**.

The first anti-anxiety drugs were discovered by a Czech pharmacologist named Frank Berger (1913–) working at London's British Drug House. He was testing potential antiseptic drugs in mice to determine the chemicals' toxicity and found that some substances caused the animals' limbs to become paralyzed. With smaller doses, Berger and his colleagues found the animals were calmed, not paralyzed.

They published their findings in 1946, and called this effect "tranquilization." The best of these compounds was found to be a drug named mephenisin.

Berger subsequently emigrated to the United States to work at the Wallace Laboratories in New Jersey. He began looking for an alternative to mephenesin, which was very short-acting. He ultimately found meprobamate, which was longer-acting and had sedative and muscle relaxant properties. Marketing of meprobamate as Miltown or Equanil began in the early 1950s. The drug was extremely popular, especially as it became available when concerns were arising over the safety of **barbiturates**.

The next class of anti-anxiety drugs to be discovered were the benzodiazepenes. In 1954, Leo Sternbach (1908–), a chemist at the pharmaceutical company Hoffmann-La Roche in New Jersey, decided to re-examine the drug potential of compounds that he had investigated as a doctoral student in Cracow, Poland, 30 years before. He found one that appeared to be an effective muscle relaxant and tranquilizer, and applied for a patent on the drug in 1958. The drug, chlordiazepoxide (to be sold as Librium) was approved by the **Food and Drug Administration** in 1960. A number of related drugs soon became available. Diazepam (Valium), synthesized in 1959, went on the market in 1963.

Suspicions arose in the early 1970s that benzodiazepines also produced dependence, but this was not confirmed scientifically until the 1980s. Sales of benzodiazepines peaked in 1975, although they are still widely prescribed. Alprazolam, or Xanax, the benzodiazepine used most widely today, was introduced in 1983.

Additional reading: Smith, *Small Comfort*.

antibiotic

Antibiotics are products of one organism that are capable of killing other organisms. Bacteria, fungi, and other microorganisms produce antibiotics, which usually kill by stopping infectious microbes from forming cell walls or making the proteins they need to survive.

Alexander Fleming (1881–1955) discovered the antibiotic properties of penicillium by accident, in 1928. Fleming named the substance **penicillin**. The next major breakthrough was **streptomycin**, which Selman Waksman (1888–1973) isolated in 1943 from a soil microbe. The new drug killed tuberculosis and typhoid fever bacilli. Waksman also coined the word "antibiotic." Other breakthroughs by pharmaceutical companies included Lederle Laboratories' Aureomycin (1948), Pfizer's Terramycin (1950), and Chloramphenicol, the first completely synthetic antibiotic, introduced by Parke-Davis in 1949.

The macrolide antibiotics, which include erythromycin, were introduced in the 1990s. Vancomycin, which was introduced in 1958 and fell out of favor in the 1960s and 1970s, has come back into use recently because it is useful against bacteria that resist other commonly used antibiotics.

Rifampin, released in 1965, is used to treat **tuberculosis** and meningitis. The newest class of antibiotics are the fluoroquinolones, which are based on a quinolone antibi-

otic called nalidixic acid. Synthetic versions were released in the late 1980s and early 1990s, including ciprofloxacin.

Although drug manufacturers have been making increasingly powerful antibiotics, the rise of infectious agents resistant to many antibiotic drugs has become a major public health problem. Campaigns are underway to discourage antibiotic overuse, which has been a significant factor in the development of resistance. (*See also* cephalosporin)

Additional reading: Friedman and Friedland, *Medicine's 10 Greatest Discoveries,* pp. 168–91; Sneader, *Drug Discovery,* pp. 296–330.

antibody

Antibodies are substances produced by the immune system—also known as **immunoglobulins**—that seek out and attach themselves to foreign invaders, such as viruses and bacteria, thus initiating an immune system response.

Emil von Behring (1854–1917) and Shibasaburo Kitasato (1852–1931) discovered the existence of antibodies, although they called them antitoxins, in 1890. They injected a rabbit with a small dose of **tetanus** and then collected the animal's blood. This blood, they found, contained a substance capable of neutralizing tetanus toxin.

Ten years later, Paul Ehrlich (1854–1915) proposed that cells had a wide variety of receptor molecules for nutrients on their surface, some of which could bond with toxins to render them harmless. Stimulation by a specific **antigen**, he hypothesized, would cause the body to produce extra copies of the antibody capable of destroying the invader. Ehrlich was close to the truth.

The work of Karl Landsteiner (1868–1943), who discovered human **blood groups/types**, led to the abandonment of the nutrient part of Ehrlich's theory. Landsteiner, Linus Pauling (1901–1994), and others assumed that antibodies molded themselves to antigens so they could match and thus fight them. By the 1930s, it was understood that antibodies were proteins, which aren't capable of altering shape by using other molecules as a template, and Landsteiner's theory fell out of favor.

In 1955, Nils Jerne (1911–1994), a Danish immunologist, suggested that the instructions for making antibodies were encoded in **DNA**. Humans already have all of the thousands of possible antibodies circulating in their blood at low levels, Jerne proposed, where they waited for stimulation by a specific antigen to manufacture more of themselves, but he did not offer an explanation about how these antigens reproduced.

F. Macfarlane Burnet (1899–1985) put forth the theory of clonal selection in 1957, arguing for the existence of antibody-forming cells that were dedicated to making a single antibody, and that displayed a copy of this antibody on their surface. When such a cell met an antigen that bound to this marker, the cell would begin churning out copies of itself that would make the antibody. His idea still holds, and he received the 1960 Nobel Prize for his work. Jerne shared the prize that year for his own work on antibodies.

These antibody-making cells turned out to be B cells, each of which inherits a series of protein fragments that it uses to make antibodies from scratch. From 300 of these Lego-like pieces, more than 20,000 different antibodies can be produced, so all of the B cells in concert can produce hundreds of millions of different antibodies. Each cell waits for the stimulus to make a particular antibody. Ehrlich was correct when he proposed that all of the antibodies existed in an organism before stimulation.

Antibodies are made in quantity about three days after the antigen is first encountered. These chemicals then begin patrolling the blood stream looking for more antigens. Once an antibody finds an antigen, it binds to it tightly and then triggers the rest of the immune system to attack. Since the development of **monoclonal antibodies** and genetic engineering, it is now possible to make an antibody to nearly any substance, and researchers are currently investigating the possibilities of this technology in treating cancer and other diseases.

Additional reading: Silverstein, *A History of Immunology,* pp. 59–86; Clark, *At War Within,* pp. 243–65.

anticholinesterase

Anticholinesterase drugs inhibit the breakdown of **acetylcholine** into acetic acid and choline. In the body, acetylcholine helps transmit nerve impulses to muscles, so slowing its breakdown increases the strength and tone of skeletal muscles and speeds motions vital for digestion known as intestinal peristalsis.

Acetylcholinesterase drugs, including **physostigmine**, were first introduced in 1934. They are used to treat myasthenia gravis (a disease in which muscles progressively weaken), **tetanus**, and as an antidote to strychnine poisoning.

Additional reading: Karczmar, "Anticholinesterase Agents."

anticoagulant

An anticoagulant is a substance that stops the blood from clotting, or "thins" it. Scientists began searching for anticoagulants so they could keep blood liquid outside the body. This would allow them to transfuse blood more easily and would also make it possible to pass blood through machines that could take over organ function during illness or surgery.

Hirudin, a substance leeches produce to keep blood flowing from their hosts, was the first anticoagulant used medically in the late 1800s. Other agents such as dicumarol and **heparin** became available in the twentieth century.

Now, highly sophisticated, short-acting anticoagulants known as thrombolytic drugs are used with dramatic life-saving effect. These "clot busters" can help patients survive a heart attack by preventing the formation of dangerous blood clots and can prevent deadly embolisms—clots that can block blood flow in the brain and lung—from forming. They may also lessen the damaging effects of **stroke**, but their use for this purpose is more controversial because the drugs also can promote bleeding in the brain.

These anticoagulants, often given in combination, allow doctors to precisely control the clotting of blood, but their effects must be closely monitored to prevent hemorrhage. (*See also* thrombolysis)

Additional reading: Sneader, *Drug Discovery,* pp. 160–64.

antidepressant drugs

Antidepressant drugs are medications used to treat **depression**.

Iproniazid was the first antidepressant drug discovered. It was used to treat **tuberculosis (TB)** in the early 1950s. Several New York state doctors began using it to treat depression after noticing that it elevated patients' moods. At the 1957 meeting of the American Psychiatric Association, Nathan Kline (1916–1983) reported that iproniazid helped chronically depressed psychotic patients. The drug was soon used for several hundred thousand depressed patients, but was withdrawn from the market in 1961 because it could damage the liver. Other similar and safer drugs were soon introduced.

Iproniazid and its relatives inhibit the action of monoamine oxidase, an enzyme that "cleans up" impulse-transmitting chemicals in the brain, thus lengthening the amount of time that brain chemicals including dopamine and **serotonin** are active. Low levels of these chemicals are believed to be connected with depression. Consuming food or drink containing tyramine, such as cheese or red wine, while taking MAO inhibitors can cause a dramatic increase in blood pressure leading to headaches or even brain hemorrhage. This is because monoamine oxidase normally inactivates tyramine, which boosts blood pressure.

MAO inhibitors fell out of favor because of their potential toxicity in the early 1960s, but today new, more selective, and less toxic versions of the drug have been found to be useful. Also, people with certain types of depression appear to respond better to MAO inhibitors than to other antidepressants.

Swiss researcher Ronald Kuhn discovered imipramine, a second type of antidepressant drug. He had been investigating chemicals structurally similar to the **antipsychotic drug** chlorpromazine (Thorazine), which was somewhat helpful for depressed people. The maker of that drug, Geigy, sent Kuhn a sample of a similar drug, which he used on depressed patients in 1955, with dramatic results. Two years later, he announced his findings. The drug went on the market as Tofranil and other manufacturers soon introduced similar drugs.

Imipramine belongs to a class of drugs known as tricyclics, because their chemical structure contains three carbon rings. Imipramine and its relatives, including Elavil (amitriptyline) and Norpramin (desipramine), slow the reabsorption of the neurotransmitters serotonin and norepinephrine, so there are more of these chemicals present in the brain. A side effect of this class of drug is that it induces a mild version of the fight-or-flight response. This means body functions related to the neurotransmitter **acetylcholine** are slowed so a person can handle the perceived emergency. This can cause dry mouth, sweating, and constipation.

The newest class of antidepressant drugs are the selective serotonin reuptake inhibitors (SSRIs). SSRIs are antidepressant drugs that prevent the reabsorption of the neurotransmitter serotonin, thus boosting the level of this chemical in the brain and increasing a person's sense of well-being. MAO inhibitors and tricyclics have "dirty" effects, meaning they affect several neurotransmitters; the SSRIs are the first drugs to limit their effects to a single neurotransmitter. Efforts to develop the SSRIs were motivated as evidence mounted that serotonin played an important role in regulating mood.

Research in the late 1960s and early 1970s linked low serotonin levels to depression. In 1968, Swedish researcher Arvid Carllson (1923–) developed a serotonin hypothesis of depression, after he and other researchers observed that imipramine reduced blood levels of the neurotransmitter. He also reported that part of the effectiveness of the tricyclic antidepressants was due to the fact that they slowed the "reuptake" of serotonin, thus increasing levels of the **hormone** in the brain.

In 1971, Eli Lilly pharmaceuticals researcher David Wong (1935–) and his colleagues began investigating chemicals that slowed the reuptake of serotonin. They used a pioneering technique, testing chemical preparations of rat brain tissue known as synaptosomes that made measuring neurotransmitter uptake relatively simple. In 1974, Wong and his team reported that they had synthesized fluoxetine, and predicted that the chemical would have antidepressant effects. Animal tests found that the drug decreased animals' appetite and reduced aggression. In monkeys, the drug was found to promote social dominance without increasing aggression. Human studies in the 1980s found that the drug was an effective antidepressant medication with relatively few side effects, and the **Food and Drug Administration (FDA)** approved Prozac on December 29, 1987. The drug is now the most prescribed antidepressant drug worldwide.

The FDA approved second and third indications for Prozac in 1994, for treating obsessive-compulsive disorder (OCD) and **bulimia nervosa.** Although other drugs in this class have been introduced, Prozac remains the most popular and no studies to date have found that the newer drugs are more effective.

SSRIs do not make patients feel "drugged." They appear to be more effective than other antidepressants for people with chronic, low-level depression, but not as effective for patients with severe depression that requires hospitalization. They also have been used successfully in patients with certain types of **anxiety disorder,** such as obsessive-compulsive disorder.

Recently some SSRIs, such as Effexor (venlafaxine hydrochloride), have been introduced that also increase brain levels of **norepinephrine.** Despite the manufacturers' claims, **clinical trials** so far have found these drugs to be no more effective than the other SSRIs.

In the 1990s, St. John's wort became an increasingly popular treatment for depression. Several studies have found that this **herbal medicine,** also known by the Latin name *Hypericum perforatum,* is as effective or even more effective than the pre-SSRI antidepressant drugs. The herb also has few side effects. Although many physicians believe the herb to be an effective treatment for mild depression, it is currently not recommended for treating major depression.

St. John's wort is a plant (*Hypericum perforatum*). This herbal medicine contains several chemicals, and it is not clear which are responsible for the herb's antidepressant effects. These chemicals include flavonoids, xanthones, bioflavonoids, and naphthodianthrons.

The herb has been used in herbal preparations for more than 2,000 years. Dioscorides, in the first century A.D., described the herb, as did the Roman physician Claudius Galen (130–c.199). Ancient Anglo-Saxon peoples believed the herb should be gathered in midsummer, when it flowers, which is around the time that St. John's Day is observed.

The herb's popularity increased after a 1996 report in the *British Medical Journal,* an analysis of more than 20 studies, that found the herb to be as effective as antidepressant drugs for treating mild depression, with fewer side effects. The main side effect of St. John's wort is that it increases sensitivity to the sun, so that people who take the herb may become suntanned or sunburned more quickly than they would if they were not taking the medication.

St. John's wort is frequently prescribed in Germany, where herbal medications are more widely accepted by the medical establishment than they are in the United States. It may also be useful as an antibacterial preparation.

Additional reading: Gorman. *The Essential Guide to Psychiatric Drugs,* pp. 47–119; Kramer, *Listening to Prozac.*

antidiabetes drugs

Antidiabetes drugs are given to people with Type 2 **diabetes mellitus,** to help them metabolize sugar more easily.

Early oral drugs developed to bring down blood sugar, based on extracts from the *Galega officinalis* plant, were tested in the 1920s, but pulled off the market by the 1940s because they were toxic to the liver.

A French physician in 1942 accidentally discovered the potential of a sulfonamide drug for treating diabetes when he tested it in patients with **typhoid.** Some patients became extremely sick and died, but intravenous glucose brought on a dramatic recovery. Further research on the drug ultimately found it was too toxic to use, but a related drug called tolbutamide, which had been synthesized in 1956, was found in large-scale trials to be effective and safe. This and other related drugs, known as sulfonylureas, trigger more insulin production in the pancreas.

Two other drugs, phenformin and metformin, were discovered by researchers at the U.S. Vitamin Corporation in Yonkers, New York, and marketed in 1957. These drugs, which are still in use, appear to target the body's absorption and use of glucose.

Newer forms of antidiabetes drugs include alpha glucoside inhibitors, which delay the digestion of carbohydrates, and thiazolidinedions, which reduce the body's resistance to insulin's effects. The first of these drugs to become available is called troglitazone. However, these drugs are ineffective in Type 1 diabetes mellitus, also known as juvenile diabetes.

Additional reading: "Oral Antidiabetes Drugs," *Patient Care.*

antigen

An antigen is a marker a cell carries on its surface in order to show the immune system that it is "self." The immune system uses these markers to recognize foreign invaders as "nonself."

The discovery of antigens has made a number of medical advances possible. For example, knowledge about antigens helped make safe **blood transfusions** possible. Also, physicians can check the tissue type of an organ donor (basically, by categorizing what types of tissue antigens he or she has) and match it with the recipient, decreasing the chances that the organ will be rejected.

In 1937, British researcher Peter Gorer (1907–1961) was the first to observe that structures on the cell surface were responsible for giving away the "foreignness" of transplanted tissue. For example, a person's **blood type** is determined by the antigens on his or her blood cells.

The chromosome region that controls the expression of these identifying fragments in animals is called the **major histocompatibility complex**, and in humans these antigens are called histocompatibility locus antigens.

Additional reading: Hall, *A Commotion in the Blood,* pp. 403–05.

antigen-presenting cell

Antigen-presenting cells bring foreign invaders to the attention of the immune system's **T cells**, which will then seek out and destroy the foreigners while recruiting the help of the rest of the immune system.

Macrophages are one type of antigen-presenting cell. They engulf the foreign cell, chop its components into protein fragments called peptides, and "show them" to helper T cells. Macrophages move through the body. Another type of antigen-presenting cell remains stationary in certain body tissues. These cells are called dendritic cells, because their long snare-like extensions make them look like nerve cell extensions called dendrites.

Rolf Zinkernagel (1944–) and Peter Doherty (1940–), working in Australia, were the first to show that these "packaging" molecules are essential in the antigen-presentation process, and won the 1996 Nobel Prize for their work.

Additional reading: Hall, *A Commotion in the Blood,* pp. 270–74.

antihistamine

Antihistamines are drugs that block the action of **histamines**, substances that play a role in inflammatory and allergic reactions and many other physiological processes.

Daniele Bovet (1907–1992), a Swiss physiologist, began searching for chemicals that would block the action of histamine in order to understand the function of this chemical more clearly. Bovet and his colleagues developed several compounds with antihistamine properties during the 1930s, but all were too toxic for clinical use. Bovet won the 1957 Nobel Prize for this research.

A number of antihistamines suitable for human use were developed in the 1940s: phenbenzamine, synthesized at the drug company Rhone-Poulenc; tripelennamine, made by researchers at Ciba Pharmaceuticals in New Jersey; and diphenhydramine (Benadryl), developed by researchers at the University of Cincinnati. Parke-Davis bought the rights to diphenhydramine.

These drugs were effective for treating **allergy** symptoms, and soon became extremely popular. Their drawback was that they all caused drowsiness.

The compound dimenhydrinate (Dramamine), introduced by G.D. Searle as a antihistamine that wouldn't make people drowsy, was found accidentally to be an excellent treatment for motion sickness in the 1940s. But it still made people drowsy.

Most pharmaceutical researchers believed it would be impossible to develop a nonsedating antihistamine. But in 1973, researchers at Merrell National Laboratories in Cincinnati reported that a substance they had synthesized, terfenadine, had antihistamine properties but did not cause drowsiness. Subsequent studies proved the drug was indeed an effective antihistamine.

After this research was publicized, workers at the drug company Schering-Plough began searching for a drug that could compete with terfenadine. A team led by Frank J. Villani (1921–) found that a chemical, loratidine, that they had synthesized in 1972 was a good candidate. Tests of the drug in humans began in 1981. The **Food and Drug Administration (FDA)** approved the drug, which is sold under the name Claritin, in 1993.

Seldane, the commercial preparation of terfenadine, was introduced by the drug company Hoechst Marion Roussel in 1985. This company produced another nondrowsy antihistamine, fexofenadine hydrochloride (sold as Allegra), which the FDA approved in 1996. One year later, the FDA recommended that Hoechst withdraw Seldane from the market, after it was found that the drug could interact with other drugs to cause a potentialy fatal heart condition. Hoechst stopped making Seldane in 1998.

In the 1960s, scientists began looking for substances that would block histamine receptors in the stomach, known as H2 receptors, in order to halt the release of stomach acid. James W. Black (1924–) began investigating drugs for this purpose in 1964 at Smith, Kline, and French. The fruit of his research, the anti-ulcer drug **cimetidine** (Tagamet), went on the market in 1976. H3 receptors were discovered in 1983, and their possible role in regulating the nervous and cardiovascular systems is now being evaluated.

Additional reading: Sneader, *Drug Discovery,* pp.165–72.

anti-idiotype antibodies

Anti-idiotype antibodies are manufactured **monoclonal antibodies** designed to attack abnormal cells in order to defend the body against **cancer**.

Hybridoma technology, developed in 1975, made it possible to create large quantities of these "tailored" antibodies. The first custom-designed antibodies were used to treat a man with terminal lymphoma in 1981. The treatment worked; the man's cancer went into remission, although his disease relapsed twice. Anti-idiotype antibodies brought dozens of cancer patients into remission in similar experimental studies, but unfortunately this approach is too expensive to be commercially viable; it costs at least $500,000 per person.

A variation of this technology is being tested as a **cancer vaccine**; patients in remission from cancer receive an injection of their specific idiotype protein along with an immune system stimulant. About half the patients given the vaccine produce **antibody** against the cancer on their own, which appears to have kept them in remission.

Additional reading: Hall, *A Commotion in the Blood*, pp. 405–06.

antimetabolites

Antimetabolites are drugs for cancer **chemotherapy** that are structurally or functionally similar to natural chemicals called metabolites essential to the formation of **DNA** and RNA. Because cancer cells divide and grow more quickly than normal cells, their division can be inhibited by careful administration of these drugs without fatal harm to healthy tissue. These drugs include folic-acid antagonists, pyrimadine analogs, and purine analogs.

The first antimetabolite to be found useful was aminopterin, a drug with a structure similar to that of folic acid. In 1948, Dr. Sidney Farber (1903–1973) and his colleagues at Boston Children's Hospital found that the drug produced complete remissions in one-third of children with acute **leukemia**. The drug was produced by Dr. Yellapragada Subbarow (1896–1948) at Lederle Laboratories at Farber's suggestion. Early researchers had thought that folic acid, a B-vitamin essential to blood-cell formation, accelerated the progress of leukemia. Therefore, they believed, a chemical that blocked the action of folic acid would slow the disease. Although this assumption turned out to be false, the drug's antimetabolite properties made it an effective cancer treatment.

Methotrexate, a drug also developed by Subbarow during the 1940s that is similar to aminopterin but less toxic, succeeded the earlier drug and is still used in combination with other drugs to treat leukemia and other cancers. Methotrexate also is useful for treating **rheumatoid arthritis** and other autoimmune diseases and for suppressing the immune system after donated tissue is transplanted. It is the most commonly used member of the folic-acid antagonist class.

Antimetabolite drugs known as arabinose nucleosides, which are also useful for treating viral infection, were originally isolated from a type of sponge and are now made synthetically. They are considered to be pyrimadine analogs. A group of drugs known as fluorinated pyrimidines, which include 5–fluorouracil, were synthesized by researchers at the University of Wisconsin Medical School in Madison in the late 1950s, with assistance from scientists at Hoffman-LaRoche in Nutley, New Jersey.

The first purine analog was **six-mercaptopurine (6–MP)**, developed by Gertrude Belle Elion (1919–1998) and George H. Hitchings (1905–1988) in 1951. Elion and Hitchings, who were working at the Wellcome Research Laboratories in North Carolina when they discovered the drug, shared the 1988 Nobel Prize for their discovery. In 1953, Joseph Holland Burchenal (1912–) and his colleagues at the Memorial Hospital in New York reported that 6–MP produced remission in certain types of leukemia. This and related drugs, such as azathoprine, are also used for immunosuppression and to treat certain illnesses such as ulcerative colitis.

The newer antimetabolite drugs interrupt the synthesis of DNA by different pathways than methotrexate. The choice of which drug to use depends on the type of cancer and how far it has progressed, among other factors. Some, such as 5-fluorouracil, are highly effective for colon cancer, while methotrexate is used to treat acute lymphoblastic leukemia in children and choriocarcinoma.

Additional reading: Timmis, *Chemotherapy of Cancer*, Foye, ed., *Cancer Chemotherapeutic Agents*.

antiparasitics

Antiparasitic drugs are used to kill parasites that cause disease, such as one-celled organisms and worms. Infection with parasites can be extremely difficult to treat, because parasites often have complex lifecycles that allow them to evade eradication. Some of the most serious parasitic diseases include **malaria** and diseases caused by trypanosomes such as **Chagas' disease** and African sleeping sickness. Other common parasitic infections include amebiasis, which is an infection with a type of one-celled organism called an amoeba (especially Entamoeba histolytica); and leishmaniasis, an infection with protozoa of the Leishmania family. Amebiasis is usually contracted by consuming food or drink contaminated with the organism, while leishmaniasis is spread by the bite of sandflies infected with the parasite. Parasites are commonly spread either by contaminated material or insect or animal bites.

Historically, drugs used to treat parasitic infections have included mercury, arsenical drugs, and bismuth, all of which were extremely toxic. Peruvian tree bark, or cinchona, was found in the seventeenth century to be an effective and relatively nontoxic treatment for malaria.

Another development was Emetine, or **ipecac**, which was first used to treat amebiasis in 1912; tartar emetic was first used that same year to treat leishmaniasis and **schistosomiasis**. Emetine is still used today and can be toxic, although a less-toxic form called dehydroemetine may be used instead.

The first effective therapy for giardiasis, quinacrine (Atabrine), was introduced in the 1930s. Chloroquine was also first used in 1948 to treat amebiasis and malaria.

During the 1950s, scientists from French drug company Rhone-Poulenc isolated a substance from a *Streptomyces* bacteria that was active against Trichomonas vaginalis, an organism that frequently infects the vaginal area. They chemically modified the substance and produced the drug metronidazole (Flagyl), which has since been found to effectively treat many other types of parasites.

A nontoxic and effective drug for many types of parasitic infections called praziquantel, made by Bayer, became available in the 1980s and was approved for sale in the United States as biltricide in 1982. This drug remains the treatment of choice for infection with flukes and worms, including schistosomiasis. A drug for treating river blindness, ivermectin, was introduced in 1987. This disease, also called onchocerciasis, plagues tropical West Africa.

Additional reading: James, *Human Antiparasitic Drugs.*

antipsychotic drugs

Antipsychotic drugs are medications used to treat **schizophrenia**, as well as other conditions, such as mania, **depression**, and dementia, in which a person may have psychotic symptoms. Psychosis occurs when a person loses touch with reality.

There are two main classes of antipsychotic drugs: those that became available in the late 1950s and work chiefly by affecting levels of the neurotransmitter dopamine, and newer drugs introduced in the 1990s that have fewer neurological side effects. These newer drugs tend to have less of an effect on dopamine and more of an effect on **serotonin**, although their exact mechanism of function is unclear.

The first antipsychotic drug discovered was Thorazine (chlorpromazine). French surgeon Henri Laborit (1914–1995) had been experimenting with chemicals synthesized by the drug company Rhone-Poulenc that enhanced the effects of anesthetics. These chemicals had been synthesized as possible **antihistamines**.

One sample Laborit tested in surgical patients not only seemed to help make anesthesia safer and more effective, but it also seemed to calm patients down. He suggested in 1951 that this chemical, chlorpromazine, might be effective for treating some psychiatric symptoms. The drug was tried on manic and psychotic patients at the Val de Grace hospital, with dramatic success. Rhone-Poulenc named the drug chlorpromazine, and began marketing it in 1952. The drug is sold as Thorazine in the United States.

Heinz Lehmann (1911–1999) introduced chlorpromazine to North America, first giving it to patients in 1953. He and his colleagues also observed the drug's neurological side effects, which included a strange walk and a masklike grimace. Other "extrapyramidal" effects (so called because they acted on the extrapyramidal nervous system, which maintains equilibrium and muscle tone) included

Parkinson's disease-like tremors, abnormal muscle contractions, and involuntary twitches.

Janssen Laboratories synthesized a similar drug, haloperidol, in 1958, which was also effective on psychotic symptoms but also produced neurological side effects. Although the antipsychotic effects of both chlorpromazine and haloperidol were dramatic, their extrapyramidal side effects are so unpleasant that as many as 40 percent of people prescribed them stop taking them. This is the major drawback of the older antipsychotic drugs.

Clozapine, the first of the newer class of antipsychotic drugs, was synthesized in 1958, but it was not released in the United States until 1990 because of its potentially fatal side effect of agranulocytosis, a depression of formation of white blood cells. (This side effect occurs in fewer than 1 percent of the people who take the drug.) The drug is free from the neurological side effects associated with earlier drugs, and also works in a higher percentage of people. In the United States, patients taking clozapine must have their white blood cell count monitored weekly. The drug itself costs approximately $6,000 a year, with an additional $1,000 annually for blood tests.

A 1997 study found that the cost of putting people on clozapine was roughly the same as if they were on the less-expensive drug haloperidol, because people taking the newer drug tended to keep taking it and generally required less hospitalization.

A later drug, risperidone, does not cause agranulocytosis, but it does cause tremors and is somewhat less effective than clozapine. Olanzapine, a similar drug, was introduced in 1996. The relative effectiveness of risperidone, olanzapine, and clozapine is difficult to measure, because response to these drugs can vary from individual to individual. However, these newer antipsychotic drugs work in about 30 percent of patients who do not respond to the older class of drugs, which are still used, particularly in emergencies. The search continues for safer, more effective antipsychotic drugs.

Additional reading: Gorman, *The Essential Guide to Psychiatric Drugs,* pp. 197–254.

antisepsis

Antisepsis is the medical practice of fighting microorganisms that can cause infection.

The ancient Greeks and Egyptians used wine, vinegar, honey, and preparations of certain metals to treat wounds, all of which had antiseptic effects. Other antiseptics of antiquity, which probably were somewhat effective, include resins, herbs and spices, and fresh meat.

But from prehistory until the late nineteenth century, when physicians and surgeons generally adopted antiseptic methods, patients routinely died from infection—especially as surgery became more common, from the 1600s onward. Doctors actually hailed "laudable pus," which we now know is a symptom of infection, as a sign that the wound was healing properly. Also, the role of bacteria in

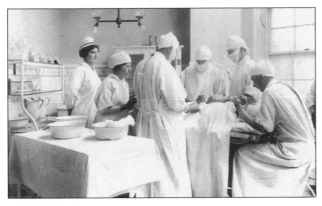

Surgery underway at the Hospital of the Good Shepherd in Syracuse, New York, early twentieth century. (Photo courtesy of the Department of Historical Collections, Health Sciences Library, SUNY Health Science Center at Syracuse.)

causing infection had to be understood before the importance of antisepsis could become clear.

The word "antiseptic" was first used by the British military surgeon Sir John Pringle (1707–1782) in a series of papers he presented to London's Royal Society from 1750 to 1752. In his studies, he reported on using salts to prevent beef from rotting.

In 1774, Swedish chemist Karl W. Scheele (1742–1786) discovered chlorine, now the basis of a number of antiseptic solutions. Claud Louis Berthollet (1748–1822) recommended chlorine as a disinfectant in 1788. A chloride preparation called Eau de Labarraque was produced by a Parisian pharmacy of the same name in 1825, and was used to disinfect wounds and for hand washing. These solutions were good skin disinfectants but were irritating to wounds.

In 1848, the Viennese physician Ignaz Semmelweis (1818–1865) demanded that surgeons in the hospital he ran wash their hands and their instruments after performing an **autopsy** and before touching patients in order to prevent **puerperal fever**. Semmelweis was the first administrator to require that antiseptic techniques be used in a hospital. The preparation he recommended was chloride of lime. Because the established belief of the time was that contagion came from nonhuman sources and was carried in the air, Semmelweis's colleagues scoffed at his theories.

One of the first effective antiseptics, carbolic acid (also known as phenol), was derived from coal tar waste in 1833 by Friedlieb Runge (1795–1867). French surgeons began investigating phenol for use in surgery as an antiseptic, with Jules Lemaire (1814–1886) publishing the first paper on carbolic acid in 1861.

The surgeon Joseph Lister (1827–1912), a professor at the University of Glasgow, became preoccupied with finding a way to treat infection after he took charge of the surgical wards at the Royal Infirmary. He noticed that many patients who had to come to the hospital after suffering accidents developed infections after surgery—a phenomenon that was at the time called "hospitalism." He read Louis Pasteur's (1822–1895) description of how microbes caused

rot, and became convinced that microbes must be at work in the patients' infections as well. After trying creosote on a patient with a compound fracture in 1865, who did not survive after being treated, he began using carbolic acid as a wound disinfectant, with excellent results. In an 1867 paper, he wrote of treating 11 patients with carbolic acid with only one death.

Other early treatments included iodine, which was first used as an antiseptic in 1836. Iodoform became widely popular after it was shown to kill anthrax bacteria in 1873.

An important advance in the development of antiseptic substances was Robert Koch's (1843–1910) discovery in 1881 of how to grow bacteria in culture, which made it possible to test these substances in the lab.

Henry Dakin (1880–1952), working at Rockefeller University in New York, developed less irritating solutions for wound disinfection called chloramine-T and chloramine-B, announcing his discovery in 1915.

As the **germ theory** gained acceptance, so did antisepsis, and methods for guarding against infection became more sophisticated. Today, mercury-based preparations, carbolic acid, alcohols, and iodine are used as antiseptics. Heat and ultraviolet light are also used to kill germs. However, washing the hands with simple soap and water remains one of the most important measures for controlling infection. (*See also* contagion theory; asepsis)

Additional reading: Majno, *The Healing Hand*, pp. 207–27; Bynum, *Science and the Practice of Medicine in the Nineteenth Century*, pp. 132–37.

anti-tumor antibiotics

Anti-tumor **antibiotics** are anticancer drugs that consist of, or are derived from, natural substances produced by living organisms. All of the anti-tumor antibiotics are derived from substances produced by cultured species of yeast from the Streptomyces family, and they all work by interfering with the normal function and synthesis of **DNA**.

The first anti-tumor antibiotic was Actinomycin D or dactinomycin. Selman A. Waksman (1888–1973) and his colleague Harold Boyd Woodruff (1917–) at the New Jersey Agricultural Experiment Station, a research unit of Rutgers University, isolated the species of Actinomyces that produced the substance in 1940. The drug entered clinical use in 1954, and has since been found to cure a number of **cancer**s including gestational choriocarcinoma, Wilms' tumor, and Ewing's sarcoma. Although the drug was originally discovered as a product of an Actinomyces species, it is now produced by the fermentation of Streptomyces.

The most useful and broadly acting class of anti-tumor antibiotics is the anthracyclines, of which doxorubicin and daunomycin are the most commonly used. Daunorubicin (also called daunomycin), isolated by scientists at the Milanese drug company Farmitalia in 1962 and first given to a **leukemia** patient in New York in 1963, was effective but had a limited use because it damaged the heart muscle. The related drug doxorubicin (or Adriamycin) was isolated by Farmitalia scientists in 1967 and turned out to be one of the most effective anti-tumor drugs ever discovered, although it is also toxic to the heart.

In 1966, researchers at the Institute of Microbiological Chemistry in Tokyo discovered several small molecules in a dish of cultured Streptomyces verticillis fungus that were found to be effective against several types of cancer. This family of anticancer antibiotics are called the bleomycins and are effective in treating head and neck cancer, testicular cancer, and non-Hodgkin's lymphoma and Hodgkin's disease. Bleomycins are unique among anticancer drugs in that they don't hamper bone marrow function, but they can damage the lungs. (*See also* Actinomycin)

Additional reading: Sneader, *Drug Discovery,* 352–56.

antiviral drugs

Antiviral drugs attack **viruses** while harming the cells they infect as little as possible. Some work by preventing viral infection from happening in the first place. There are only a handful of antiviral drugs. These medications also are difficult to use because viruses generally multiply very rapidly, often before an infection is identified.

The first antivirals were formulated to treat herpes virus infections topically. Idoxuridine was developed in the late 1950s and tested in the early 1960s on animals and humans whose eyes were infected with the virus. During this time, amantadine was tested for influenza infection prevention and found to be effective for high-risk populations.

The first oral drug to be used successfully to treat existing viral infection was vidarabine, tested in the late 1970s and early 1980s. Vidarabine wiped out herpes infections of the brain and in newborns, and also worked against varicella, the virus that causes chicken pox.

The debut of second-generation antivirals occurred with acyclovir, an antiherpes virus drug, which can be taken orally and given topically. This antiviral was introduced by the drug company Glaxo-Wellcome in the early 1980s. Acyclovir also is effective against cytomegalovirus and Epstein-Barr virus when given in higher doses. People with herpes infections can take it long-term to control outbreaks.

The demand for antivirals rose with the onset of AIDS. Pharmaceutical companies began scrambling to make drugs that would fight this lethal virus, as well as the viral infections that attack HIV-infected people with weakened immune systems. The first therapies for HIV infection were the dideoxynucleoside analogs, **AZT** (azidothymidine) and its cousins, followed by **protease inhibitors**.

A recent development in antiviral drugs are two new injectable drugs for cytomegalovirus, a common virus that can cause blindness in HIV-infected people. The two new drugs are foscarnet, approved by the **Food and Drug Administration (FDA)** in 1991, and ganciclovir, approved in 1989. Multiple-drug combinations for treating HIV infection have made it possible for people with AIDS to live years longer, but adhering to complex drug "cocktail" regimens is difficult and the drugs have troubling side effects, such as raising **cholesterol** levels.

Additional reading: Galasso, et al., eds., *Antiviral Agents and Human Viral Diseases*; Jeffries and DeClercq, eds., *Antiviral Chemotherapy*; Monroe, "Defenders Against the World's Smallest Attackers."

anxiety disorders

Anxiety disorders are a class of psychiatric problems characterized by abnormal anxiety and fear. They include panic disorder, obsessive-compulsive disorder (OCD), and post-traumatic stress disorder (PTSD). From 2 percent to 8 percent of the U.S. population suffer from anxiety disorders.

Anxiety disorders feature physical as well as psychological symptoms, including chest pain, pounding heart, and dizziness. The symptoms are basically identical to the "fight or flight" response. People with anxiety disorders may also suffer from panic attacks, characterized by chest pain, shortness of breath, sweating, dizziness, and a feeling of impending doom, which can last for minutes or for hours. Most people have experienced a panic attack at least once in their lives, but a person is thought to have a panic or anxiety disorder when such attacks begin to restrict normal activity.

Philadelphia physician Jacob Mendez DaCosta (1833–1900) is credited with first describing anxiety disorder, which he called "irritable heart," in 1871. The syndrome, common in soldiers who had seen combat, also became known as soldier's heart, effort syndrome, and neurocirculatory asthenia. Sigmund Freud (1856–1939) termed these symptoms "anxiety neurosis."

It had long been understood that warfare can lead to chronic anxiety, and the anxiety soldiers face has been called shell shock, battle fatigue, and traumatic war neurosis. This condition was determined to be a distinct disease and called post-traumatic stress disorder (PTSD) by the American Psychiatric Association in the third revision of the *Diagnostic and Statistical Manual of Mental Disorders*, or DSM-III, in the 1980s.

PTSD was the first psychiatric disorder defined as being due entirely to environmental causes, and not to internal factors. The main impetus for the development of the PTSD diagnosis was the commonness of these symptoms among veterans of the Vietnam War.

Obsessive-compulsive disorder, in which a person suffers from anxiety when he or she tries to resist compulsions, is another type of anxiety disorder. These compulsions tend to consist of ritualized activities such as washing the hands a certain number of times during the day.

In the first half of the twentieth century, anxiety disorders were treated with **barbiturates** and other tranquilizing medications. Unfortunately, these medications produced dependence in the people who took them and did little to improve their underlying condition. Today, psychiatrists believe that treating people with anxiety disorders with a combination of **behavior therapy** and medication, which can include **antidepressants** or benzodiazepines, is the most effective approach.

Additional reading: Leaman, *Healing the Anxiety Disorders.*

Apgar score

The Apgar score is a system used worldwide to gauge an infant's health and development at birth. Virginia Apgar (1909–1974), the first woman professor at the Columbia University's College of Physicians and Surgeons in New York, developed the system and published it in 1953.

The score requires assessing five signs: heart rate, respiratory effort, muscle tone, reflexes, and skin color. Each sign is scored 0, 1, or 2, with 0 being the lowest and 2 the highest. The infant is scored at one minute after birth, and again five minutes after birth. For example, a child with no heart rate scores 0; a child with a heart rate of less than 100 scores 1; and a child with a heart rate above 100 scores 2. For color, an indicator of how well a child's respiration and circulation are functioning, a child who is blue and pale gets a 0; babies with pink bodies and blue extremities score 1; and fully pink babies score 2.

A total score from 10 to 7 is excellent, 4 to 6 is fair, while a child with a score of less than 4 is considered to be in poor condition. If a child scores below 7 at five minutes after birth, he or she is assessed again five minutes later to determine if his or her condition has improved. At any time, if a child's score is less than 6, he or she may need assistance with breathing. An infant who scores less than 4 may need emergency help and may not survive.

Scoring helps physicians and nurses prepare for resuscitation if necessary, and also usually indicates the child's future neurological health.

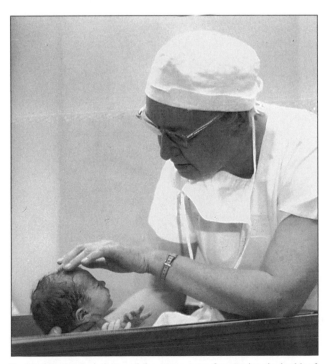

Dr. Virginia Apgar, inventor of the Apgar score for gauging the health of newborns. (Photo taken by Elizabeth Wilcox. Courtesy of Archives and Special Collections, Columbia University Health Sciences Division.)

Additional reading: Speert, *Obstetric & Gynecologic Milestones Illustrated,* pp. 274–78.

apoptosis

Apoptosis is the natural death of cells that occurs in embryonic development, adult tissue renewal, and other situations where cells must die in order to control growth or preserve the health of an organism. The cell breaks into membrane-bounded fragments, which are then consumed by adjacent cells.

In 1842, Carl Vogt (1817–1895) first reported observing this type of cell death during the metamorphosis of toads. A number of other nineteenth-century researchers reported on cell death during metamorphosis and development; they understood it to be the body's method for disposing of tissue that was no longer needed. Walther Flemming (1843–1905) described this type of cell death in ovarian follicles in 1885, calling it "chromatolysis."

Nearly a century later, the Australian pathologist John Kerr observed a phenomenon he called "shrinkage necrosis," to differentiate it from necrosis, which is cell death caused by disease or injury, and described this in 1970. Andrew Wyllie and Sir Alistair Currie (1921–1994), both working in Australia, had also observed this process, noting that it occurred in healthy as well as pathological cells. Kerr, Wyllie, and Currie proposed the term "apoptosis" to describe the phenomenon, and said it was a natural process that served to regulate tissue size.

Researchers are currently looking for ways to manipulate apoptosis to treat **cancer**, based on the theory that cancers are caused by failure of normal cell death.

Additional reading: Clark, *A Means to an End,* pp. 21–40.

appendectomy

Appendectomy is the surgical removal of the inflamed vermiform appendix, a vestigial structure attached to the beginning of the large intestine. The organ, first described in 1521 by anatomist Berengario DaCarpi (1470–1530), serves no known purpose, but when it becomes infected and inflamed, death can result from perforation and rupture.

Inflammation of the appendix as a cause of disease was understood by the 1700s, but surgical removal of the organ wasn't generally considered as a treatment, largely because anesthetic was unavailable and the possibility of infection made most surgery lethal. The first surgical removal of an appendix, from an 11–year-old boy, was performed in 1735. A handful of surgeons operated to remove the appendix or to drain abscesses in the lower abdomen in the 1800s, often successfully, but forgoing surgery and using opium to ease pain remained the standard treatment for an inflamed appendix.

The introduction of **antisepsis** around 1870 as well as **anesthesia** at the middle of the century made appendectomy more practical. At the first meeting of the Association of American Physicians in Washington, D.C., in 1886, Reginald Heber Fitz (1843–1913), a Harvard doctor, was the first person to recommend that the inflamed appendix be removed surgically as early as possible. Fitz's advice was controversial. The idea of surgery as a first resort was difficult for nonsurgeons to accept, but early appendectomy was widely accepted before the turn of the century.

Improved understanding of abdominal infections, as well as the introduction of antibiotics in the 1940s and 1950s, improved the success of the operation further.

The German gynecologist Kurt Semm (1927–) performed the first appendectomy using **laparoscopy** in 1981.

Additional reading: Rutkow, *American Surgery,* pp. 236–38, 402–03.

arsenic

Arsenic is a poison that has been used with some success in treating certain types of **leukemia**. The active form is arsenic trioxide, which Thomas Fowler (1736–1801) reported using in 1786 to treat fever and headache. The arsenic preparation he employed became known as Fowler's Solution.

Leukemia was described in 1845 by Rudolph Virchow (1821–1902). Two German physicians first tried to treat leukemia with Fowler's Solution 20 years later. Patients got better briefly, but their disease returned. This treatment was used until the 1940s in the United States. In 1998, researchers at Memorial Sloan Kettering Hospital reported producing remissions in leukemia patients with arsenic trioxide.

Ayurvedic physicians in India and Chinese practitioners have used arsenic to treat leukemia and other diseases for centuries. Unfortunately, several patients using Eastern medicines have been poisoned by arsenic preparations. (*See also* Ayurveda.)

Additional reading: Fackelmann, "Arsenic."

arthroscopy

Arthroscopy is a technique for visualizing the inside of a joint for diagnostic or surgical purposes. This technique has revolutionized joint surgery in recent years, making it possible to "clean up" and repair joints through very small incisions without an overnight stay in the hospital or long recovery time.

Kenji Takagi (1888–1963), a professor at Tokyo University Medical School, performed the first arthroscopic investigations in 1918, examining the knees of cadavers. By 1931, he had developed an arthroscope 3.5 millimeters in diameter that could be used to view the joints and other body cavities. Takagi went on to develop several other instruments for arthroscopy, as well as specific procedures for investigating various joints. In 1932, he took the first black-and-white photographs through the arthroscope and succeeded in taking color photographs and 16-millimeter films 4 years later.

Michael S. Burman (1901–1975) developed an arthroscope as well as instruments for performing arthroscopic surgery from 1931 to 1935, and used the devices to examine hip, knee, ankle, shoulder, elbow, and wrist joints.

Takagi's student Masaki Watanabe developed a special arthroscope in 1960 and used it to perform the first partial meniscectomy by arthroscopy in 1962. In a meniscectomy, damaged cartilage is removed from the menisci to improve the function of the joint. His American colleague Richard L. O'Connor (1933–1980) introduced the method to the United States, writing an arthroscopy textbook in 1977. The International Arthroscopy Association was founded in 1974.

In 1976, the operating arthroscope was introduced. Surgical instruments could be inserted through this device without obstructing view, so surgery could be performed under direct arthroscopic control. Today, many joint ailments can be repaired easily with arthroscopy, with less recovery time and expense than would be necessary for an open operation.

Additional reading: Galton, *Med Tech,* pp. 36–38.

artificial heart

Artificial hearts are mechanical pumps designed to replace the organ.

Today, they are used only as a bridge until a person can receive a human-heart transplant, but investigators had hoped at first that artificial hearts could serve as a permanent replacement for the organ.

American dentist Barney Clark (1921–1983) received the first artificial heart in 1982. Robert K. Jarvik (1946–) designed the heart, and the surgeon William DeVries (1943–) implanted it. Clark lived for 112 days after the operation.

In 1963, Texas heart surgeon Michael DeBakey (1908–) reported implanting a device into the chest of a patient to assist the heart in pumping blood. Although the patient died four days after the implantation, the device did help his heart to function more effectively.

In 1969, Dr. Denton Cooley (1920–) implanted an artificial heart in a patient who lived for 65 hours after the operation. He performed another operation in 1981 in which the patient lived with the artificial organ for 54 hours and then received a heart transplant, dying several days later. Experts in cardiology believe the device Cooley used was probably unable to keep a patient alive as long as Jarvik's design. Four people received the Jarvik-7 devices as a permanent heart substitute. The devices were later used to provide a temporary boost to heart function while a patient awaited a heart transplant. A moratorium on using the Jarvik heart was declared in 1991, because too many patients had developed life-threatening blood clots or severe infections while using the device.

Today, patients are usually implanted with left-ventricular assist device (LVAD) to bridge the gap until a donor heart is available. These devices supplement the function of this chamber of the heart, which pumps blood through the body. The **Food and Drug Administration (FDA)** approved LVADs as a bridge to heart transplant in 1994.

A number of LVADs were tested in the 1970s and 1980s, but all were attached to outside support systems.

New generations of these devices, with an outside control system the size of a deck of cards, entered clinical use in the early 1990s.

One such device, the Novacor Left-Ventricular Assist System (LVAS), was approved by the Food and Drug Administration (FDA) in 1998. A 1999 study, based on experiences at 22 transplant centers, found the LVAS was an effective "bridge to transplantation," helping patients with failing hearts to stay alive and relatively healthy as they waited for a new heart.

Jarvik is currently heading a research effort to develop left-ventricular assist devices for permanent use. The project is funded by several groups including the National Heart, Lung and Blood Institute, Bell Communications Laboratories, the Texas Heart Institute, and Transicoil, Inc., a Pennsylvania company that is developing its own heart-assist system. These devices, the researchers believe, could ultimately save 20,000 to 30,000 lives each year in the United States alone.

Additional reading: Acierno, *The History of Cardiology,* pp. 665–67.

artificial insemination

Artificial insemination is the introduction of sperm to egg for fertilization by mechanical rather than natural means.

Arab horse breeders used artificial insemination in the Middle Ages. Lazzaro Spallanzani (1729–1799) began performing artificial insemination of amphibians in the course of his experiments on fertilization and egg development, and successfully inseminated a dog in 1785. The world's first center for the artificial insemination of horses was founded in Russia in the early twentieth century, paving the way for large-scale use of the technique in cattle and sheep.

In the first reported case of human artificial insemination, John Hunter (1728–1793) assisted a couple in conceiving a child in 1785. The husband had a deformity of the penis that made it impossible for him to impregnate his wife naturally.

James Marion Sims (1813–1883), a British doctor, made 55 attempts at artificial insemination, with one successful pregnancy in 1866. By 1890 Dr. Robert Dickinson (1861–1950) was performing artificial insemination routinely. In 1949, Pope Pius XII (1876–1958) rejected artificial insemination on moral grounds.

The first child conceived through **in vitro fertilization (IVF)** was born in 1978, after her parents' egg and sperm were united in a glass dish and then implanted in her mother's uterus. Today, both IVF and the use of donor semen are nearly commonplace. About 60,000 children born in the United States each year are conceived with donated sperm.

Additional reading: O'Dowd and Philipp, *The History of Obstetrics and Gynaecology,* pp. 354–55, 367–69.

artificial respiration

Artificial respiration is the use of machines to "breathe" for people who cannot do so themselves.

In the 1500s, Flemish anatomist Andreas Vesalius (1514–1564) and physician Paracelsus (1493–1541) wrote about using a bellows inserted in the trachea to rhythmically inflate an animal's lungs while its chest was open, because cutting into an animal's chest makes normal lung function impossible. This is because the outer membrane of the lung and the inner wall of the chest are usually held together by a vacuum, which allows the diaphragm to power respiration; once this vacuum is lost, the lungs can no longer inflate or deflate normally.

Robert Hooke (1635–1703) and William Harvey (1578–1657) did similar experiments in the following century. In the eighteenth century, a few humans were resuscitated with bellows equipment, but this technique was abandoned in the early 1800s after it became clear that the elevated pressure severely damaged the lungs.

From 1840 to 1940, investigators worked on the principle of negative pressure on the thorax to build resuscitation devices. A jacket or a full-body tank surrounded the patient's chest, lowering pressure around the chest so that air would be inhaled, then squeezing the chest to increase pressure and expel the air. There was even a version for chest surgery that was large enough to contain both patient and surgeon, with the patient's head outside the tank and an airtight cuff surrounding his or her neck.

Following the opposite principle, a tank was built that surrounded only the head, exerting positive pressure rhythmically, pushing the air into the lungs and then lowering pressure for exhalation. A bellows version came back into use in the late nineteenth century, which surgeons modified themselves.

Demand increased for mechanical ventilation in the mid-twentieth century, with the **poliomyelitis** epidemic. Many polio victims suffered paralysis of the chest, so it was necessary to help them breathe until they recovered the ability to move. Many of these patients relied on the iron lung, or **Drinker respirator**, to stay alive.

In the mid-twentieth century, anesthetists began giving patients **curare** during surgery to paralyze patients' muscles and thus make operations easier. Curare halted normal breathing as well, making it necessary to develop better ventilation techniques. The use of positive-pressure ventilation during surgery came back into favor; many new modifications made it safer, such as the addition of water vapor to breathing gas, better techniques for inserting the ventilator through the trachea, and better control of pressure throughout the breathing cycle. The improved ventilators became available commercially in the United States in the late 1950s.

Since then, researchers have been working on refining mechanical "breathing" rhythms to ensure that oxygen gets into the body and carbon dioxide comes out. The introduction of blood gas electrodes in the 1960s have made it much easier to monitor the effectiveness of artificial respiration.

Additional reading: Emili, *Basics of Respiratory Mechanics and Artificial Ventilation.*

artificial skin

Artificial skin is used to replace natural skin lost to injury, usually skin damaged by a burn. A number of companies are developing artificial skin, because covering burn areas with the patient's own skin can be impossible if the patient has been burned extensively. Using skin from corpses is also problematic both because of the danger of infection and rejection and because donated skin is scarce.

In the early 1960s, James G. Rheinwald (1948–) and Howard Green (1925–) at the Massachusetts Institute of Technology developed techniques for culturing human epidermal cells in the laboratory. Subsequently, several research teams used these techniques to grow sheets of skin cells for use in grafting. The material was first used on a human patient by Nicholas O'Connor and his colleagues at Peter Bent Brigham Hospital in Boston in 1981. Now, lab-grown skin is used regularly to treat certain types of wounds. Only a small sample of skin from the patient is required.

The major drawback to this technique is that it takes three to four weeks for enough skin to grow for grafting. To solve this problem, researchers developed a way to grow skin grafts from infant foreskins discarded after circumcision. These grafts do not contain cells that produce an immune response, so they are not rejected. The patient's own skin will eventually replace the graft. Burn patients were first given this type of graft in 1983.

Researchers also developed artificial matrices of collagen that could be used as scaffolds for healing skin. The patients' own cultured skin cells were combined with later improved versions of these artificial skin materials for better results. The latest type of artificial skin uses immunogically inactive skin cells that are seeded into a mesh that the body will ultimately reabsorb.

Additional reading: Morrison, "Advances in the Skin Trade"; Stix, "Growing a New Field."

asepsis

Asepsis is the absence of microorganisms that can cause infection or rot. In medicine, aseptic technique is the creation of a sterile field for surgery by sterilizing instruments and other items used in the operating room. Operating-room personnel also wear gloves, masks, gowns, and caps so they will not carry microorganisms into the operating theater.

Asepsis, like **antisepsis**, was pioneered by German surgeons in the mid-1800s. Glove-wearing became a common practice in 1889, a few years after Dr. William Halsted (1852–1922) of Johns Hopkins University suggested that his nurse and fiancee Caroline Hampton wear **rubber gloves** to protect her hands from antiseptics, which she was allergic to.

Aseptic technique became generally accepted in the early 1900s.

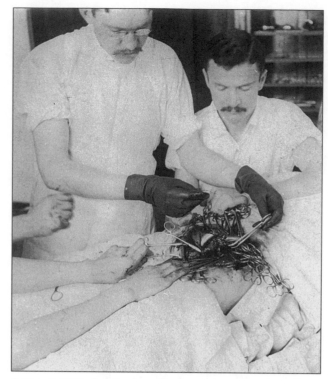

Dr. Joseph C. Bloodgood performs the first surgery using rubber gloves at Johns Hopkins, 1895. Another surgeon at Johns Hopkins, William Halsted, requested that Goodyear Rubber Company make gloves in 1889 to protect the hands of his operating-room nurse. (Photo courtesy of The Alan Mason Chesney Medical Archives of the Johns Hopkins Medical Institutions.)

Additional reading: Duffy, *From Humors to Medical Science,* pp. 189–90.

aspirin

Aspirin, which kills pain, eases inflammation, and cools fever, was one of the first drugs synthesized in a laboratory. It was introduced in 1899.

Aspirin is the world's most popular drug. In the United States alone, 50 billion aspirin tablets are consumed annually. The major drawback to aspirin and other **nonsteroidal anti-inflammatory drugs (NSAIDS)** is that they cause stomach irritation.

Also known as acetylsalicylic acid, aspirin descends from salicin, a substance found in willow bark. The Roman author Pliny (62–c. 113 A.D.) recommended willow bark for treating aches and fevers.

In 1763, Reverend Edmund Stone (unknown–1768) reported to the British Royal Society that he had tested powdered willow bark on 50 patients. He proposed that since the willow grew in damp areas, where people tended to suffer from aches in the joints, the plant preparation would be helpful in easing this type of pain.

Salicylic acid, the active ingredient in willow bark, was synthesized in 1838 and became a popular and effective treatment for fever and joint pain. In 1875, doctors working with the substance reported that it lowered body temperatures of patients with **typhoid fever**, although the drug did not cure the disease. The problem with salicylic acid, however, was that it was extremely unpalatable and often caused stomach irritation and vomiting.

In 1853, German chemist Charles Frederick von Gerhardt (1816–1856) synthesized the related drug acetylsalicylic acid, but it would be more than 40 years before its powers were discovered. The drug was eventually rediscovered by chemists at the Bayer Chemical Works in Elberfeld, Germany, who were looking for an alternative to salicylic acid for treating inflammation and pain. Clinical trials began in 1898 at two German hospitals. Bayer named the drug aspirin, patented the process for its manufacture, and began marketing it in 1899.

Patients with heart and blood vessel disease often are prescribed aspirin because the drug slows blood clotting and decreases the likelihood that a person will suffer a heart attack or stroke. Several large clinical trials to test whether aspirin could prevent heart attack and stroke began in the 1970s, and it was found that the drug indeed reduced the chances that a person would have a heart attack or stroke. In 1985, the **Food and Drug Administration (FDA)** sanctioned labeling that describes aspirin as approved treatment for patients who had suffered a heart attack or experienced heart pain.

Additional reading: Porter, *The Cambridge Illustrated History of Medicine*, pp. 134–35, 261; Podolsky, *Cures Out of Chaos*, pp. 375–90.

asthma

Asthma is a disease in which allergic reactions cause the airways to constrict, making breathing difficult.

The first description of an asthmatic attack is credited to Aretaeus of Cappadocia (c.30–90 A.D.) in the second century A.D. Moses Maimonides (1135–1204) wrote a "Treatise on Asthma" in the twelfth century that included recommendations for managing the disease with diet and lifestyle changes, as well as suggestions for air pollution control. Henry Hyde Salter (1823–1871) observed in 1860 that nervous excitement, fatigue, smoke, and "animal emanations" could bring on asthma attacks.

Morphine was a popular treatment for severe asthma in the early part of the twentieth century. Other early treatments involved inoculating the person with the substance to which he or she was allergic, based on the idea that the person would thus produce an antitoxin to neutralize the toxin. High-altitude treatment, in which asthmatics were sent to the mountains, was helpful because mountain air tends to contain fewer **allergy**-producing particles.

Aminophylline was introduced in 1938 for treating acute asthma attacks. In the 1940s, asthma "cigarettes" containing stramonium leaf and potassium nitrate were inhaled for short-term relief.

Antihistamines, introduced in 1942, were expected to provide great relief for people with asthma but have turned out to be useful for mild cases only because they can thicken mucus. Air flow meters were introduced in the 1950s to allow people with asthma to measure the amount of obstruction in their airways, which helped them to manage the disease. Treatment of asthma with **cortisone**-like drugs began in the 1950s. Steroids are effective in reducing asthma symptoms, but have serious side effects.

Drugs that dilate the bronchi by stimulating the sympathetic nerves, known as beta-2 agonists, have been available since 1950. A new generation of this type of drug was introduced in 1967. The new drugs, including salbutamol and terbutaline, have largely replaced the older ones. Longer-acting beta-2 agonists, including sametrol and formetrol, have also been introduced recently. The drug beclomethasone dipropionate, given by inhalation, was introduced to treat asthma in the 1970s.

Today, although treatment is good enough that patients seldom die from asthma or suffer a severe attack, the disease remains a serious problem. In fact, asthma is on the rise, particularly among inner-city children. During the past decade, the number of deaths and hospital visits due to asthma attacks has risen by more than 50 percent.

Public health efforts throughout the United States designed to help such children and their families treat and control the disease began in the 1990s.

Additional reading: Cook, editor, *Allergies Sourcebook*, pp. 77–94.

atherosclerosis

Atherosclerosis, or "hardening of the arteries," is a disease in which blood vessel walls grow less resilient and the interior of the vessels becomes blocked with fatty plaque. High fat consumption, cigarette smoking, and a sedentary lifestyle all can contribute to atherosclerosis, which can lead to heart disease.

Atherosclerosis has been found in the hearts of Egyptian mummies, but descriptions of the disease did not appear until the dawn of modern anatomy in the 1500s.

A number of different theories were set forth in the eighteenth century regarding the cause of atherosclerosis. Some thought the fatty lesions were hardened pus, or a result of malnourishment of the blood-vessel tissues. Others proposed injury, inflammation, or blood clots as the cause.

Johann Lobstein (1777–1835) introduced the term arteriosclerosis in 1833. In 1908, Russian scientists demonstrated that rabbits who were fed egg yolks and milk developed atherosclerosis. By the 1930s, it became clear that **cholesterol** was the responsible factor.

Today, high fat consumption is still considered a major cause of atherosclerosis, but other factors such as heredity and cigarette smoking are also thought to play a role. Blood clots and damage to the blood vessels are also considered factors that contribute to atherosclerosis.

Recent **autopsy** studies have found preliminary signs of atherosclerosis, such as plaque formation, in young children, suggesting that efforts to prevent the disease must begin early in life.

As a result of studying atherosclerosis, doctors have discovered a number of treatments for the disease. **Cholesterol-lowering drugs** have been used with some success to treat and even reverse atherosclerosis. Some nutrients, such as **vitamin E,** also appear to prevent and possibly treat hardening of the arteries.

Additional reading: Khan and Marriott, *The Heart Trouble Encyclopedia,* pp. 37–39.

atropine

Atropine is a drug that acts on the nervous system, widening the pupils and inhibiting salivation and secretion from the respiratory tract. It is derived from belladonna, found in the poisonous *Atropa belladonna* plant, also known as deadly nightshade. The botanist and classifier Carolus Linnaeus (1707–1778) named the plant family "Atropos," after the Fate of Greek mythology who cuts the thread of life.

Atropine was known as a poison to ancient Egyptian and Hindu civilizations. The drug's first medical uses, both in the 1800s, were in ophthalmology and to "dry up" the mouth and respiratory tract prior to receiving **anesthesia.** Today, atropine is used less frequently in preparation for anesthesia because less-irritating anesthetics are available.

Additional reading: Sneader, *Drug Discovery,* pp. 120–26.

attention-deficit hyperactivity disorder (ADHD)

Attention-deficit hyperactivity disorder is a condition marked by easy distractibility, low tolerance for frustration or boredom, impulsivity, and excess energy. People with ADHD have difficulty focusing on one task at a time, and thus have a hard time getting things done. They may also become depressed.

Experts on ADHD estimate that 15 million Americans have the condition, and that one-third of the people who have it as children will outgrow it. ADHD usually is treated with medication (**antidepressant drugs** or stimulants such as Ritalin), counseling, and behavior modification.

One ADHD expert suggested that the first description of a person with ADHD in literature was a poem printed in the British medical journal *The Lancet* in 1904, titled "Fidgety Philip."

In 1902, researcher George Frederic Still (1868–1941) described a group of 20 children, mostly boys, who had been raised in healthy circumstances but exhibited impulsive, defiant, and overly emotional behavior. The psychologist William James (1842–1910) also is reported to have identified a syndrome, marked by the inability to inhibit one's actions properly and difficulty in sustaining attention, that he thought may have had a biological cause.

A 1934 article in the *New England Journal of Medicine* suggested that a group of people exhibiting this type of behavior did so because they had been infected with encephalitis. This was the first attempt to link the syndrome that became known as ADHD to a physical disease.

Researchers began using the **amphetamine** Benzedrine to treat children with behavior problems in the late 1930s. These problems were eventually called "hyperkinetic syndrome," and were treated with the stimulant drugs Ritalin

and Cylert. The disorder also was known as "minimal brain dysfunction."

During the 1970s, psychologists linked distractibility and impulsivity to the familiar "hyperactivity" syndrome. Researchers found the condition appeared to be hereditary in some cases.

The syndrome has long been controversial, with opponents of the ADHD theory arguing that there is no such thing, and that inability to concentrate, hyperactivity, and impulsivity may be normal or they may be the result of parents' (or schools') failure to teach children to behave properly. The use of Ritalin for children is also controversial, since it may produce such side effects as nervousness and insomnia, dizziness, drowsiness, and other side effects. Some people believe that some physicians may be too quick to prescribe it.

Strong evidence for a biological basis for the disease has come with the advent of positron emission tomography (PET) scans, which allow researchers to observe brain function in real time by seeing how quickly glucose is metabolized (*see* **PET scanning**). In a 1990 study of adults, researchers at the National Institute of Mental Health found that people with ADHD used less glucose than those without the condition, suggesting that their brain activity was lower. Other research has found similar differences in the brain function of people with ADHD. New theories on the source of ADHD include improper function of the neurotransmitter **serotonin.** Although these discoveries have not yet resulted in new treatments for ADHD, they have improved psychologists' understanding of the disorder.

In early 2000, a study published in the *Journal of the American Medical Assoc*iation found that the administration of Ritalin and other psychoactive drugs to children from two to four years old had tripled from 1991 to 1995. The report raised serious concerns about whether medicating children that young for ADHD and other conditions is safe, and whether the prescription of psychiatric medications for young children is being regulated adequately. Ritalin is not approved for use in children younger than six.

Shortly after the release of the JAMA report, First Lady Hillary Rodham Clinton called for a major effort to investigate the use of Ritalin and other drugs in young children. The effort will recommend new warning labels for these medications and a national study on the prescription of psychoactive drugs to young children.

Additional reading: Hallowell and Ratey, *Driven to Distraction.*

auscultation

Auscultation is a technique for listening to the sounds of the heart, lungs, and digestive system to detect abnormalities. This medical method is ancient, dating back at least to the time of Hippocrates (c.460–375 B.C.).

The invention of the **stethoscope** by French doctor Rene Laennec (1781–1826), as well as Laennec's careful analysis of the significance of sounds heard through auscultation documented in his two-volume work *De* *l'Auscultation mediate* (1816–1819), made auscultation more precise as a diagnostic tool.

Auscultation is often used along with **percussion**, in which the chest is thumped and the resulting sound analyzed.

Additional reading: Callahan, et al., *Classics of Cardiology,* Vol., 1, pp. 323–82; Bynum, *Science and the Practice of Medicine in the Nineteenth Century,* pp. 37–40.

autoimmune disease

Autoimmune disease occurs when the immune system attacks the body's own tissues. Normally, the body "tolerates" all of its own cells, as the B cells and **T cells** of the immune system are programmed to ignore them. But in autoimmune disease this tolerance is lost, and the B cells begin producing **antibodies**, called autoantibodies, that attack "self" tissues.

The cause of autoimmune disease remains a mystery. Scientists have shown that the body naturally contains B cells designed to make anti-self antibodies. One theory proposes that in autoimmune disease these cells grow out of control or produce too much self-**antigen**. Other explanations include the idea that the immune system is responding to a tiny, no-longer-infectious fragment of a bacterium or virus remaining in the body, or that the body is producing antigens to a bacteria or **virus** that contains a protein mimicking the body's own protein, a phenomenon called antigenic mimicry.

Ernest Witebsky (1901–1969) and Noel Rose (1927–) produced the first experimental autoimmune disease in an animal in 1956 by injecting it with protein from the **thyroid gland** along with an immune stimulant. The animal developed autoimmune thyroiditis.

Insulin-dependent **diabetes**, **multiple sclerosis**, systemic lupus erythematosus, and **rheumatoid arthritis** are just a few diseases caused by autoimmunity. Acceptance of the autoimmune origin of many of these diseases came slowly. Still other diseases are suspected to have an autoimmune origin, such as ulcerative colitis, while the destruction caused by some infectious diseases, such as **tuberculosis (TB)** and **hepatitis** B, is largely due to the body's immune system overzealously attacking foreign protein in the lungs and liver, respectively.

Women are more prone to develop some types of autoimmune disease; some scientists have suggested that this is because they have stronger immune systems so they can keep a fetus safe from infection during pregnancy.

Additional reading: Clark, *At War Within,* pp. 107–33.

autopsy

Autopsy is the dissection and examination of the body to determine the cause of a person's death.

Taboos about human dissection prevented the ancient Muslims, Chinese, and Romans from performing autopsies. Physicians from Alexandria, including Herophilus (335–280 B.C.) and Erasistratus (c. 310–250 B.C.), performed the first dissections to study disease.

Reports of autopsies to determine the cause of death appear in European sources in the 1100s and 1200s. One of the first autopsies performed for legal reasons was requested by a Bolognese magistrate in 1302, after a nobleman named Azzolino died under circumstances suggesting poisoning. The report of the autopsy survives, but the court's conclusion has not.

The practice of autopsy was sanctioned by the Roman Catholic Church when Pope Sixtus IV (1471–1484) permitted autopsies at the medical schools in Bologna and Padua.

Antonio Benivieni (1443–1502), a physician who practiced in Florence, described 111 cases in his book "The Hidden Causes of Disease," including the results of 15 autopsies. The book was published in 1507, after his death, and suggests that by this point autopsies had become relatively common.

Giovanni Morgagni (1682–1771) collected life and post-mortem observations on 700 patients in his landmark work "On the Seats and Causes of Disease as Investigated by Anatomy," published in 1751. Morgagni argued that correlating symptoms observed during a person's life with anatomical findings from autopsy would allow physicians to understand how structural changes in the body produce abnormal function. His belief is now a central tenet of medicine.

After Morgagni, physicans worldwide began to recognize the importance of the autopsy in advancing medical knowledge.

Rene Laennec (1781–1826), who popularized **auscultation** and invented the **stethoscope**, based much of his work in chest disease on careful study of autopsy findings. Rudolf Virchow (1821–1902), who pioneered the idea that the understanding of disease should be based on the study of changes within the cell, is the father of the modern autopsy, in which gross (naked-eye) observation is combined with the study of tissue samples under a **microscope**. The autopsy procedure used today is basically the same as Virchow's.

Additional reading: King and Meehan, "A History of the Autopsy."

Ayurveda

Ayurveda is an ancient Hindu philosophy of health based on harmonizing mind and body that employs herbal medicine, massage, yoga, and pulse diagnosis. Ayurveda means "science of life" in Sanskrit.

In Ayurveda, there are three doshas, or humors, that must be in balance. They are called vata (motion), pitta (metabolism), and kapha (fluid). Disease is caused by an imbalance in these humors, usually resulting from unhealthy habits. Patients are said to heal themselves.

Susrutha and Charaka, who both lived before 500 B.C., are considered the fathers of Ayurveda. Susrutha advocated cleanliness during surgery and anesthesia with wine and hemp, and urged surgeons to have clean-shaven heads. He wrote a textbook of obstetrics and recommended closing wounds with the heads of large black ants. Charaka recommended that physicians use interrogation, palpation, auscultation, and inspection to come up with a diagnosis, and he compiled a list of 1,120 diseases.

Although Ayurvedic medicine faded by the nineteenth century, it was revived with the Indian nationalism movement of the twentieth century, and remains popular throughout Asia today.

Additional reading: Porter, *Medicine,* pp. 98–101.

AZT (Azidothymidine)

AZT, synthesized in 1964 as a possible **cancer** therapy, was the first drug found to be effective in treating infection with the human immunodeficiency virus (HIV).

AZT is the first and best-understood of a group of drugs called nucleoside analogs or nucleoside reverse transcriptase inhibitors, which work by stopping the step by which HIV's RNA is converted to **DNA**.

Although AZT cannot cure **AIDS**, it can bring down levels of the HIV **virus** in the blood temporarily, which can lengthen the life of AIDS patients. If a pregnant woman takes AZT after her third month of pregnancy, and the child receives the drug for the first six weeks of life, the child's chances of being infected with HIV drop from 25 percent to 8 percent. Other drugs similar to AZT include didanosine, approved by the **Food and Drug Administration (FDA)** in 1991; and zalcitabine, approved the following year.

The **Public Health** Service discovered AZT's effectiveness against the AIDS virus in the laboratory in 1985, and gave it to a patient two months later. In 1986, after a trial in 280 patients showed that AZT worked, the drug was distributed free of charge to 5,000 AIDS patients and licensed for general distribution in 1987.

AZT has serious side effects, including bone marrow suppression, and the HIV virus can develop resistance to it. Other drugs such as **protease inhibitors** have become available to fight HIV, but AZT remains a vital part of AIDS treatment, often used with newer drugs to make a "cocktail" that can bring HIV down to undetectable levels in patients' blood.

Additional reading: Arno and Feiden, *Against the Odds,* pp. 37–59.

B

barbiturates

Barbiturates are powerful sedative drugs that are now rarely used.

The original compound that formed the basis of these drugs was barbituric acid, which was synthesized by Adolf von Baeyer (1835–1917) in 1864. Emil Fischer (1852–1919) and Josef von Mering (1849–1908) developed a hypnotic drug based on barbituric acid that they called Veronal and patented in 1903. The drug was sold by the German drug company Bayer A.G. Fischer synthesized a related drug, luminal, in 1911. The drug is still used today to treat some types of **epilepsy**. More than 2,000 barbiturate compounds were eventually synthesized and about 50 went on the market.

Barbiturates are strongly addictive and were often abused, so only about a dozen drugs of this type remain in use today. Barbiturates still on the market include Seconal, Amytal, and Phenobarbitol. Benzodiazepenes were introduced beginning in the 1960s to replace barbiturates, but the newer drugs turned out to be addictive as well.

Additional reading: Lickey and Gordon, *Drugs for Mental Illness,* pp. 186–87, 230–32.

barium

Barium is a substance used to help image the digestive tract. A person consumes barium orally, or takes a barium enema, and then an **X-ray** can reveal the shape of the intestine or stomach because barium is opaque to X-rays.

Researchers in the United States and Germany had tried using a number of other substances as contrast agents that occasionally poisoned and even killed patients.

Dr. Paul Krause (1871–1934), a Bonn internist, promoted barium in 1910 as a safe alternative to bismuth, one of the early and often poisonous contrast agents. Because some late nineteenth-century bakers used barium sulfate as a flour additive (it was heavy, cheap, and had a flour-like color), it was known to be nontoxic.

Additional reading: Kevles, *Naked to the Bone,* pp. 70, 99.

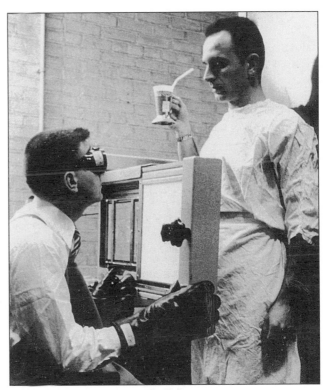

Patient at Johns Hopkins prepares for a fluoroscopic exam of his gastrointestinal tract in 1956. The technician, who wears red goggles to help him see the image, will follow the path of barium sulfate through the digestive system after the patient drinks the radio-opaque substance from the cup he is holding. (Reproduced with permission of *Johns Hopkins Magazine.*)

Barr body

The Barr body is a mass found inside the nucleus of body cells in most female animals—including humans—that does not appear in males.

Dr. Murray L. Barr (1908–1995) of Ontario discovered this object, which he called the sex chromatin body, in cat nerve cells while studying fatigue in 1949. Barr and his colleagues subsequently studied the cells of several other animals, including humans, and found that in most cases female animals' cells had the chromatin while male cells didn't. The Barr body was subsequently proven to be an inactivated X **chromosome**.

Discovery of the Barr body made it possible to determine the sex of a fetus before birth, because cells obtained from **amniocentesis** could be searched for the Barr body. In the course of his research, Barr developed a cell-collecting method called the buccal smear that involved gently scraping the inside of the cheek. Today this simple non-invasive procedure has hundreds of uses; before Barr introduced the buccal smear, it was necessary to collect cells by cutting tiny swatches from the skin or other body tissue.

Additional reading: Speert, *Obstetric & Gynecologic Milestones Illustrated,* pp. 262–64.

BCG vaccine

The Bacillus Calmette-Guerin (BCG) **vaccine** protects against **tuberculosis (TB)**, and has also been used at various times in **cancer** treatment with varied results.

The French bacteriologists Leon Charles Albert Calmette (1863–1933) and Jean Marie Camille Guerin (1872–1961) began studying tuberculosis in 1900. They had observed that adding ox bile to the tuberculus bacilli that infects cows made the bacterium less virulent. Since vaccines expose people to a weak or dead form of the bacteria so that they will be protected from the living, dangerous form, Calmette and Guerin used this strategy to produce the vaccine.

The first human to receive the BCG vaccine, in 1921, was a baby whose mother had died of tuberculosis. By 1924, the Pasteur Institute in France was producing large amounts of the vaccine. Disaster struck six years later, when several children died after accidentally being inoculated with virulent human tuberculosis bacilli.

When properly prepared, however, the BCG vaccine is safe, relatively effective, and inexpensive. The **World Health Organization (WHO)** endorsed the BCG vaccine in 1973.

BCG vaccine is also being used along with **cancer vaccines** as an immune-system stimulant.

Additional reading: Day, "Poor Vaccine Ruled Out in TB Puzzle."

behavior therapy

In behavior therapy, the therapist seeks to improve patients' mental health by directly modifying their behavior rather than by analyzing their thoughts or feelings, as is done in **psychoanalysis**.

B.F. Skinner (1904–1990) was the chief founder of behavior therapy. After studying learning in animals, he believed that a similar strategy of rewarding good behavior could encourage proper behavior in humans. The idea was to "shape" a person's behavior.

An important behavior therapy technique is desensitization, in which a person learns to overcome a phobia or anxiety by confronting it. Assertiveness training is another form of behavior therapy.

Behavioral therapy has also been used successfully to treat bedwetting, obsessive-compulsive disorder (OCD), drug **addiction**, and other problems. Psychologists have also tried using negative reinforcement such as electric shock to discourage inappropriate or deviant behavior, with much less success. (*See also* anxiety disorders.)

Additional reading: Plaud and Eifert, *From Behavior Theory to Behavior Therapy;* Cautela and Ishaq, *Contemporary Issues in Behavior Therapy.*

behaviorism

Behaviorism is a system of psychology in which all behavior, normal and abnormal, is seen as a set of conditioned reflexes separate from individual will.

American psychologist John B. Watson (1878–1958) launched behaviorism, partly in reaction to the Freudian school of **psychoanalysis**. He hoped to establish a new psychology that didn't depend on the idea of consciousness, was free from introspection, and could be evaluated with experimental methods.

Watson based his ideas, spelled out in his 1913 manifesto, on Ivan Petrovich Pavlov's (1849–1936) research on the conditioned **reflex**, which is an automatic response to a stimulus that has been induced by training and repetition. Pavlov's famous dogs, which salivated in response to the bell that signaled their mealtime, were exhibiting a conditioned reflex. Watson believed it would be possible to see all human behavior as conditioned reflex and break down all actions in terms of such stimuli and responses.

From the 1920s to the middle of the twentieth century, behaviorism dominated psychology. Neobehaviorism reigned from 1930 through the late 1940s. B.F. Skinner (1904–1990) and Clark L. Hull (1884–1952), who developed theories of learning, were the major figures in this era.

Although behaviorism is now basically defunct, **behavior therapy** is still used with success to treat a variety of psychological problems, including **anxiety disorders**.

Additional reading: Leahey, *A History of Psychology.* pp. 324–28.

beriberi

Beriberi is a nervous-system disease caused by a deficiency in thiamin, which is in the **vitamin B** family. Understanding of the cause of the disease in the early twentieth century led to the discovery of **vitamins** and to enrichment of food with these nutrients as a **public health** measure.

The name of the disease comes from the Singhalese word "beri," meaning "weakness." Symptoms include fatigue, memory and sleep disturbances, swelling of the extremities and face, extremely low **blood pressure**, and enlargement of the heart. The disease is common in Asia and some Pacific islands.

Descriptions of the disease appear in ancient Japanese and Chinese medical texts. The first European description of beriberi appears in the writings of Jacobus Bontius (1598–

1631), who worked in the East Indies as a medical inspector, in his *De medicina Indorum* of 1642.

People who rely on rice for nutrition, as well as people living on certain types of limited diets, are susceptible to beriberi. While traditional home preparation of rice, in which the husk is removed with mortar and pestle, leaves a sufficient amount of thiamin on the grain, machine milling or polishing of rice completely removes the nutrient. A person consuming a diet based on milled rice is thus at risk for developing beriberi.

Alcoholics face an increased risk of beriberi, as chronic alcohol consumption reduces the ability of the body to absorb thiamin while increasing the need for it. People on kidney **dialysis** are also at risk for beriberi.

Christian Eijkman (1858–1930), a Dutch scientist who was part of a team sent to Indonesia to investigate beriberi among soldiers and prisoners in Java, found that giving pigeons and chickens rice husks prevented beriberi. He theorized that people and animals would develop the disease if they were deprived of the substance contained in these husks. He and his colleague Gerrit Grijns (1865–unknown) determined in 1901 that this substance, also found in meat and vegetables, was necessary for proper nervous system function. Grijns prepared an extract of the factor and used it to treat people with beriberi. Grijns and Eijkman were the first to experimentally identify nutritional deficiencies, and Eijkman shared the 1929 Nobel Prize with fellow vitamin researcher Frederick Gowland Hopkins (1861–1947).

Working in the Philippines in 1910, U.S. Army captain Edward B. Vedder (1878–unknown) began treating beriberi with rice bran extract, and sought the help of the scientist Robert R. Williams (1886–1965) in isolating the beriberi-preventing substance from this extract.

In 1926, Barend Coenrad Petrus Jansen (1884–unknown) and W.F. Donath isolated the substance, but were not able to characterize its chemical structure correctly. Williams, who continued to work on isolating the substance on his own time, succeeded in doing so in 1933 and synthesized it three years later. The drug manufacturer Merck & Company worked with Williams to develop a commercial process for producing the vitamin. By the 1960s, artificially prepared thiamin was cheaper than that obtainable from natural sources. Williams continued to work to fight beriberi, contributing funds from his patent royalties and traveling to Asia to increase people's awareness of how to fight the disease.

Beriberi is easily treated by ensuring that a person gets adequate amounts of thiamin, through food or supplements. In the United States, white bread is now enriched with thiamin, which has virtually eliminated the disease. In Asia, efforts to reduce the milling of rice to leave some thiamin on the grain were successful in Japan and Indonesia, while in other parts of the continent efforts to enrich the grain with artificial vitamin preparations have been successful.

Additional reading: Kiple, *The Cambridge World History of Human Disease,* pp. 606–12.

beta-adrenergic blocking agents (beta blockers)

Beta-adrenergic blocking agents are drugs used to treat high **blood pressure**, **angina pectoris**, and some heart arrythmias. They interfere with the release of renin, a substance produced by the kidney that initiates a series of events leading to increased blood pressure. This mechanism is known as the **renin-angiotensin system.**

Sir James W. Black (1924–) developed the first beta blocker, propranolol, in the 1960s. In a series of clinical trials in the 1980s, he showed that the drug improved survival after a heart attack. He won the 1988 Nobel Prize for developing the drug, which the Nobel Committee called the greatest breakthrough in treating heart disease since **digitalis.**

Additional reading: Khan and Marriott, *The Heart Trouble Encyclopedia,* pp. 40–43.

biochips

Biochips are computer chip–like devices that contain miniature **DNA** sequencing and analysis components, making it possible to run several different genetic tests at one time in a very small space and to provide genetic analyses quickly and cheaply.

The chip is a piece of glass covered with gel, with several different sensor elements attached. A chip one-centimeter square can hold as many as 400,000 different sensors, which are strips of DNA. The chip is placed in contact with the substance to be analyzed, and some fragments of DNA will bind to these sensor strips. A computer will then interpret the results.

Biochips currently are used to detect disease markers in patients' tissue, such as the p53 mutation, which is linked to **cancer.** Chips can also detect viral mutations, making it possible to determine whether a strain of **virus** will resist certain drugs. This is particularly useful in treating HIV infection. Biochips can also detect levels of gene expression.

The Argonne National Labs in the United States and the Russian Academy of Science collaborated to build the world's first biochip, which is called the MAGIChip. In 1998, the electronics company Motorola announced it would work with the laboratory to mass produce the biochips. Other companies developing biochips include Affymetrix, Hewlett Packard, IBM, and Texas Instruments. The biochips are expected to be commercially available some time in the first decade of the twenty-first century.

Additional reading: Fisher, "Biology Meets High Technology."

biofeedback

Biofeedback is the use of instruments to measure pulse, temperature, **blood pressure**, muscle tension, and other physiological phenomena, so people can see these measurements and attempt to control their body processes.

The mathematician Norbert Weiner (1894–1964) coined the term "feedback" in 1961 to describe a method for controlling a system, such as a computer, by "reinserting into it the results of its past performance."

Biofeedback is an offshoot of **behaviorism** and **behavioral therapy**, which use conditioning to shape behavior. During the 1960s, psychologists and others began studying the possibilities of using biofeedback to control high blood pressure, headaches, and other physical problems. By the early 1970s, biofeedback was being touted as a cure-all, which further testing revealed it was not. However, biofeedback is useful for treating headache and anxiety, as well as for helping people to manage stress.

Additional reading: Birk, *Biofeedback.*

biopsy

A biopsy is a **tissue** sample from the body that is examined in the laboratory for the presence of cancerous or precancerous cells. The word "biopsy" comes from the Greek words for "life" and "view."

For biopsy to become useful, microscopy needed to be developed so that individual cells could be examined; techniques were also needed for making tissue sections and staining them so that these cells could be seen clearly.

Doctors began using **microscopes** to examine diseased tissue in the mid-nineteenth century. John Hughes Bennett (1812–1875), a professor of medicine in Edinburgh, and Scottish pathologist Robert Donaldson (1877–1933) were leaders in the new science, demonstrating that tissue smears could yield important information. In 1845, Bennett described examining tissue from an ulcer in a woman's breast, determining that it was not malignant and that surgery was not necessary. Donaldson sampled tissue by "nipping off little projecting points on the ulcerated surfaces."

In 1879, Berlin gynecologist Carl Ruge (1846–1926) reported that he could diagnose **cancer** of the cervix and uterine lining with tissue samples. Despite opposition from some pathologists, who required that more invasive cancer be observed for a cancer diagnosis, Ruge argued that doctors should sample this tissue themselves to make the diagnosis. Ruge's technique could be considered a forerunner of the **Pap smear**.

Paraffin wax embedding, in which tissue is enclosed in wax and then cut into thin slices, making it possible to see individual cells, was developed in the 1880s.

In the United States in the 1890s, surgeons including William Henry Welch (1850–1934) developed techniques for performing biopsies during operations with rapid frozen sections. This method made it possible to determine, during surgery, whether a lesion was cancerous and should be removed.

At the beginning of the twentieth century, biopsy had become an accepted practice. In 1918, the American College of Surgeons set standards for hospital clinical laboratories, where biopsies were examined.

Techniques for taking tissue samples for biopsy with a needle were developed in the 1930s. Studies established aspiration needle biopsy as an effective method for diagnosing **breast cancer** in the 1950s.

Donald L. Morton (1934–), a thoracic surgeon, and his colleagues at the John Wayne Institute for Cancer Treatment Research in Santa Monica, California, developed a system for tracking the lymph drainage of a tumor with dye that became known as the sentinel lymph node biopsy. Morton first reported on this technique in 1992.

Today, sentinel-node biopsy is used in patients with breast cancer and melanoma. Radioactive dye is injected into the tumor, and then its path is followed to the lymph nodes that drain the tumor. These nodes are checked for the presence of cancerous cells and removed if necessary. This technique allows patients whose cancer has not spread to avoid extensive lymph node removal, which is disfiguring and disabling.

Additional reading: Christopherson, "Cytologic Detection and Diagnosis of Cancer"; Wright, "The Development of the Frozen Technique, the Evolution of Surgical Biopsy, and the Origins of Surgical Pathology."

birth control pill

Birth control pills contain artificial **estrogen** and **progesterone** and suppress ovulation by mimicking the hormonal environment of pregnancy.

In the early twentieth century, researchers in Austria and Scotland, financed by the Rockefeller Foundation and birth control pioneer Margaret Sanger (1833–1966), respectively, began investigating the use of artificial hormones to prevent ovulation in animals.

Gregory Pincus (1903–1967) began working on synthetic hormones in the late 1930s, at the Worcester Foundation for Experimental Biology in Massachusetts. He found that ovulation could be blocked by stimulating the parts of the brain controlling this process and proved in 1951 that giving a woman the **hormone** progesterone could inhibit ovulation. With John Rock (1890–1984), a Harvard gynecologist, Pincus began testing an active form of progesterone, norethynodrel, in **clinical trials** in Puerto Rico, Haiti and Los Angeles. The drug was found to be nearly 100–percent effective, and was sold in combination with ethynyl estradiol as "Enovid" beginning in 1957 to treat menstrual problems.

The Food and Drug Administration approved the drug, which was made by the pharmaceutical company G.D. Searle and Company, as a contraceptive in 1960. Today, dozens of different formulations of birth control pills are on the market.

Additional reading: Watkins, *On the Pill.*

birth defects

Birth defects are malformations that a child has at birth. Birth defects are now known to be genetic, meaning they are caused by flaws in the **chromosomes**, and often are due to maternal exposure to a teratogen, such as alcohol or certain chemicals. They may also be inherited.

During the Middle Ages, birth defects were thought to be caused by the sins of a child's parents. Since ancient times, malformations have also been seen as omens of the future. Ambrose Pare (1510–1590) wrote that malformations could occur if an infant was conceived during menstruation, if the parents had copulated like beasts, if there was too much seed or too little, or if a woman saw frogs or was exposed to other disturbing images early in her pregnancy. This idea of maternal exposure to such influences as a cause of birth defects persisted, at least in folk wisdom, into the nineteenth century.

The effects of a pregnant woman's consumption of alcohol on fetal development have long been known and were described in the nineteenth century and earlier. Etienne Geoffrey St. Hilaire (1772–1884) said that birth defects occurred due to chemical and physical changes in the fetal environment, and suggested that this was how new species arose. He coined the word "teratology."

In 1904, John William Ballantyne (1861–1923) of Edinburgh said that infections, as well as substances given to the mother such as alcohol, lead, and **morphine**, could harm the developing fetus. But despite evidence to the contrary, the prevailing medical view was that the placenta was a "perfect barrier," protecting the fetus against any toxic substance, unless the mother was exposed to so much poison that she died. This idea persisted until the mid-twentieth century.

Research on teratology in experimental animals began in the 1920s. By 1929, researchers knew that maternal exposure to large doses of **X-rays** could cause birth defects. In the 1940s, Norman McAlister Gregg (1892–1966), an Australian ophthalmologist, reported that women infected with **rubella** gave birth to children with characteristic birth defects. Around this time, infection with the Toxoplasma gondii protozoa was found to cause eye problems as well as **hydrocephalus** and macrocephalus.

With these discoveries, and also as better nutrition and vaccination began to wipe out deficiency diseases and infectious illnesses as causes of childrens' death, congenital defects began to be studied more intensely. In 1959, chromosomal abnormalities were determined to be the cause of many birth defects.

After the thalidomide episode, in which thousands of women gave birth to deformed children after taking this drug to combat symptoms of morning sickness in the late 1950s and early 1960s, it became clear that certain drugs could be harmful to the fetus. Drug companies began testing their products for potential teratogenic effects. Such tests had been done in the past, but the connection wasn't made between effects on laboratory animals and possible damage to humans. In 1966 the **Food and Drug Administration (FDA)** began to require drug companies to test new products for teratogenic effects. Guidelines for radiation exposure for pregnant women also were developed at this time.

Additional reading: Moore, *Before We Are Born.*

birthing centers

Birthing centers provide a home-like environment for women in labor.

Since Colonial times, most American women delivered their children at home with the help of **midwives** or doctors, but this practice changed quickly in the twentieth century. At the beginning of the 1900s, more than 95 percent of women delivered their babies at home. This changed with the introduction of **twilight sleep** in 1915, a type of sedation given to women during labor that required hospital supervision. Also, giving birth at the hospital became a status symbol. By the end of World War II, nearly 80 percent of births in the United States took place in hospitals.

The natural childbirth movement came about in response to what many women saw as the medical establishment's impersonal way of handling labor and delivery. A move toward local **anesthesia** and childbirth preparation such as the **Lamaze method** began in the 1940s. "Rooming-in," keeping the mother and infant in the same room, also became more popular. With the rise of feminism and consumerism in the 1960s and 1970s, women increasingly demanded more control over the environment in which they gave birth.

In the mid-1970s, hospitals began to respond to the demand for a more home-like, warmer environment for labor and delivery. In 1975, the first free-standing birthing center, the Maternity Center Association, was established in New York. Birthing centers could provide care at about half the price of hospitals, and several studies have shown that they are as safe as hospitals for women with low-risk pregnancies.

There are currently about 145 freestanding birthing centers in the United States. Many hospitals have set up birthing centers on their own premises.

Additional reading: Harper, *Gentle Birth Choices.*

Blalock-Taussig procedure

This procedure is a technique for repairing the hearts of "blue babies," children born with heart defects that prevent their blood from being properly oxygenated.

Performed for the first time in 1944, this was also the first surgical operation on the heart. The procedure is named for Dr. Helen Taussig (1898–1986), an expert on congenital heart malformations, and cardiac surgeon Dr. Alfred Blalock (1899–1964), both of whom were working at Johns Hopkins Hospital in Baltimore.

Normally, blood flows from the right ventricle into the lungs, where it is oxygenated, returned to the heart, and then pumped through the body to provide cells with the oxygen they need to survive. In "blue" or cyanotic babies, a hole between the right and left ventricles allows blood to leak out to the left side before it can pass through the pulmonary artery to the lungs. The pulmonary artery also is quite narrow in these children. A passageway between the pulmonary artery and the aorta called the ductus arteriosis, which normally closes soon after birth, allows some blood flow to the lungs and keeps children with these defects alive. However, this temporary vessel closes off as the child grows, and children with this defect die young without surgical intervention.

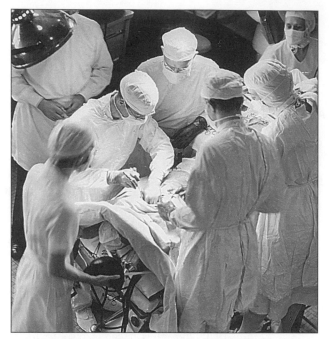

A team of surgeons at Johns Hopkins, led by Alfred Blalock, perform a "blue baby" operation to repair the birth defect that prevents the blood from being fully oxygenated, 1947. (Courtesy of The Alan Mason Chesney Medical Archives of the Johns Hopkins Medical Institutions.)

Taussig theorized that creating a more permanent duct by joining a branch of the aorta to the pulmonary artery would keep these children alive. Blalock agreed to try, and operated on the first child in 1944. Soon after, hundreds of "blue babies" had the operation. It wasn't a cure, but the surgery did keep the children alive and relatively healthy until a more complete repair was possible.

Once Dr. John Gibbon's (1903–1973) **heart-lung machine** had made open-heart surgery practical in 1953, blue babies' hearts could be fixed permanently.

Additional reading: Weisse, *Medical Odysseys*, pp. 51–57.

blood bank

Blood banks store blood and blood products for later transfusion to people in need.

In order for blood to be stored, scientists had to figure out a way to keep the blood a liquid and preserve blood cells outside the body. Around 1914, researchers discovered that adding citrate to the blood would keep it in liquid form. The substance binds with **calcium** in the blood, inactivating this mineral and thus preventing clotting. Adding citrate to blood eventually became the standard means of preservation.

The world's first organized blood donation system was established in London in 1922. In the Soviet Union, doctors began storing blood collected from cadavers, placentas, and live donors in the early 1930s. Soon the country had 60 large centers for storing and shipping preserved blood. In 1937, doctors gave patients more than ten thousand quarts of stored blood. Patients were often given blood that had been stored for several weeks and more than half of patients suffered severe reactions.

In 1937, Bernard Fantus (1874–1940) established a Blood Preservation Laboratory at Cook County Hospital in Chicago, which he soon dubbed a "blood bank," the first such facility in the United States. Patients who received the blood were much less likely than the Soviet patients to de-

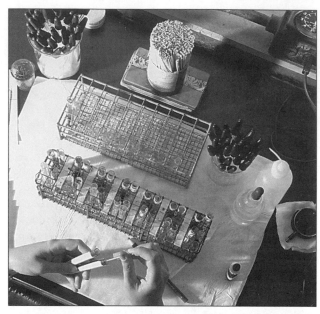

A blood-bank technician at Johns Hopkins prepares samples. (Courtesy of The Alan Mason Chesney Medical Archives of the Johns Hopkins Medical Institutions.)

velop transfusion reactions, possibly because Fantus made efforts to keep his equipment sterile.

Stored blood was first used widely in combat medicine during the Spanish Civil War (1936–1939), with Canadian doctor Norman Bethune (1890–1939) running Madrid's blood bank. A blood bank also was established in London during World War II that served victims of the Blitz. The American Red Cross began storing donated blood for soldiers during World War II as well. Although the Red Cross stopped collecting and storing blood after the war was over, the group initiated a peacetime blood banking program in 1947.

Scandal rocked the blood banking system worldwide during the 1980s, as thousands developed **AIDS** from contaminated blood products. Systems for screening blood donors (and donated blood) for HIV infection, **hepatitis**, and other transmissible diseases are now in place.

Additional reading: Starr, *Blood.*

blood cell separation

In blood cell separation, blood is divided into its various components, such as red cells, white cells, platelets, and plasma.

Harvard chemist Edwin J. Cohn (1892–1953) began searching for methods to separate fractions of the blood in 1940. Plasma—the liquid portion of blood—was known to be an effective treatment for **shock**, but he theorized that one of the proteins contained in plasma might be equally effective and easier to store. He began working on separating blood by centrifuging it and adding alcohol under a variety of different chemical conditions. Cohn and his colleagues had separated blood into five fractions by the close of the year and found that the plasma protein albumin could be used alone to protect against shock.

U.S. military forces used albumin to treat soldiers in shock. Although the protein helped them out of crisis, it became clear that the soldiers needed **red blood cells** as well to stay alive.

Cohn later designed a machine for dividing donor blood into various components. Allen Latham, Jr. (1908–), an engineer with the Cambridge, Massachusetts company Arthur D. Little, Inc., worked with Cohn and carried the project on after his death. Several Cohn-ADL machines were built and sold to blood research centers in the mid to late 1950s. Throughout that decade and into the 1960s, researchers developed methods for collecting, separating, and storing various blood components. In 1973, Latham founded his own company, Haemonetics Corporation, and began building and selling disposable blood-cell separation containers and machines.

Additional reading: Starr, *Blood,* pp. 103–04, 177–78.

blood group/type

There are four basic human blood groups or types: A, B, AB, and O, named for the **antigens** found on a person's **red blood cells**.

Dr. Karl Landsteiner (1868–1943) discovered the ABO system in 1900 while running tests on blood he collected from himself and five colleagues. He found that certain people's blood clumped up when mixed with another person's blood, while some combinations mixed without clumping. Landsteiner determined that people had antigens he called A or B—or no antigens—on the surface of their red blood cells. If people are exposed to a foreign antigen, they will produce antibodies that attack the strange substance, resulting in the clumping that Landsteiner observed, and illness and possibly death if the wrong blood type is transfused. Agglutination is the term devised for this "clumping" reaction between antigens and antibodies.

Type A blood has antibodies against Type B blood, for example, so mixing the two causes red cells to agglutinate, while Type A from one person can be safely mixed with Type A from another person. Landsteiner called the antigenless blood type "O." Further research found that some people have both A and B antigens, a type called "AB."

People with Type O blood are called "universal donors," because anyone can tolerate the antigenless blood. Type AB people are called "universal recipients," because they can tolerate any type of blood.

Landsteiner's research made blood transfusion possible. As long as the recipient had no antibodies to the donor's blood, transfusion would be safe—unless, of course, the blood had pathogens (bacteria or a virus) in it.

Landsteiner won the 1930 Nobel Prize for his discovery. (*See also* antibody)

Additional reading: Starr, *Blood,* pp. 38–40.

blood pressure

Blood pressure is the force that blood exerts on vessel walls. It is measured as systolic pressure over diastolic pressure, in millimeters of mercury. Systolic pressure is the strongest force exerted by the left ventricle as it contracts, while diastolic pressure is the force exerted between heartbeats.

British clergyman Stephen Hales (1677–1761) made the first measurements of blood pressure in the early 1700s. He checked the height to which various animals' hearts could pump blood by attaching a brass tube to an incision in the animal's artery. A glass tube, through which Hales could see the blood rise, was connected to the brass tube with a goose's windpipe. He observed that the blood pressure changed with the beat of the heart.

In 1828, Jean Leonard Marie Poiseulle (1799–1869) adapted Hales's cumbersome system (which required about nine feet of tubing) into a U-tube mercury manometer only eight inches high. This method still required that a needle or tube be inserted into the artery to measure blood pressure.

In 1896, Italian physician Scipione Riva-Rocci (1863–1939) developed an inflatable cuff called the **sphygmomanometer** that measured systolic blood pressure without puncturing blood vessels. Then, in 1905, Russian vascular surgeon Nikolai Korotkoff described how to measure both systolic and diastolic pressure with Riva-Rocci's cuff. Physicians continue to use his method today. This discovery has made it possible for physicians to study and treat high blood pressure, or **hypertension**, which puts a person at risk of heart disease, **stroke**, and other maladies. The first physician to make regular blood pressure measurements a part of clinical treatment was Frederick Mahomed (1849–1884).

Instruments are now available that provide automatic blood pressure readings, along with continuous printouts.

Additional reading: Acierno, *The History of Cardiology,* pp. 493–502.

blood transfusion

In a blood transfusion, a patient receives blood or blood products to replace blood lost to illness or injury. Certain blood products also may be given to supplement deficiencies in the patient's own blood.

Early transfusions weren't done to make up for blood loss, but in belief that the blood (even of animals) carried personality traits and that the donor could thus pass along desirable qualities (health, youth, strength) to the recipient. In fact, one recommended marital therapy was for spouses to exchange blood.

The first recorded blood transfusions in humans were performed in Europe in 1667, using animal blood. In one famous case from this series, Jean-Baptiste Denis (1643–

1704) gave a local madman an infusion of blood from a calf. The exchange was performed via a silver tube inserted into the animal's artery and the man's vein. Although the man suffered a severe reaction, he was extremely calm after he recovered, leading Denis and his colleagues to believe that the transfusion cured his insanity. The practice fell out of favor throughout Europe after an early experimenter killed one of his patients.

London obstetrician James Blundell (1790–1878) experimented with animals for several years in the 1800s before trying a human transfusion. He concluded that transfusions should only be given after hemorrhage (his interest was blood loss after childbirth), and that humans should not be given animal blood. But experimental animal-to-human transfusions continued. In 1898, Jules Bordet (1870–1961) showed why animal blood often killed humans. He proved that an individual injected with cells of any kind from another species would react to them by producing antibodies, which formed large molecules known as "immune complexes" that clogged blood vessels and organs.

It remained unclear why human-to-human transfusions didn't always work until Karl Landsteiner (1868–1943) discovered **blood types** in 1900. This discovery made safe transfusions possible, but the transfusion process was expensive and cumbersome. The preferred method—known as direct transfusion—was to stitch the donor's artery to the recipient's vein.

In 1914, researchers found a way to keep blood from clotting outside the body and thus made indirect blood transfusion and **blood banks** possible.

Additional reading: Acierno, *The History of Cardiology,* pp. 622–25.

bloodletting

Bloodletting, in which blood is drained from the body by cutting blood vessels with a lancet or applying leeches to the skin, is one of the most ancient medical treatments. Since ancient times, bloodletting—along with a suction method called **cupping**—was used to treat just about every type of illness. Today bloodletting is only used in two rare disorders: hemochromatosis, in which the blood and liver store too much iron; and polycthemia vera, in which a person has too many red blood cells.

Bloodletting as therapy was originally a corollary of **humoralism**, a concept of health developed in ancient Greece that held sway into the nineteenth century. Blood was thought to be one of four humors that had to be in balance for proper health. The condition of having too much blood was called "plethora," and symptoms included heaviness in the body, sluggishness, and lassitude.

Claudius Galen (129–c.199) called bloodletting the "essential remedy" and recommended it for treating insanity, melancholy, fractures, and even hemorrhage.

By the Middle Ages, people thought having their blood drained regularly was a healthy habit that would make them stronger. Barber-surgeons provided the service. Even Wil-

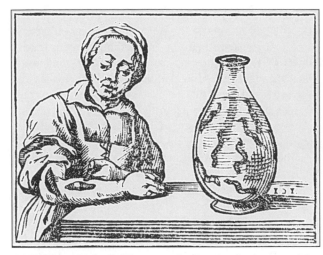
A 1639 illustration by Guilliaume van den Bossche of a woman applying leeches to her arm. (Courtesy of National Library of Medicine.)

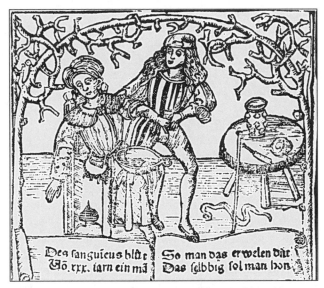
Woodcut illustrating bloodletting, from a book published around 1500 by Hieronymous Brunschwig. (Courtesy of National Library of Medicine.)

liam Harvey (1578–1657), who discovered **circulation** of the blood, supported bloodletting as therapy.

Beginning in the 1830s, Pierre-Charles-Alexandre Louis (1787–1872) gathered and analyzed information on patients' diseases, symptoms, and treatment. His statistical methods showed that bloodletting was not an effective treatment for certain diseases. When the **germ theory** of disease gained acceptance in the late nineteenth century, bloodletting began to fall out of favor.

Additional reading: Starr, *Blood,* pp. 17–30.

bone graft

Bone grafting is used to replace bone lost to disease or injury, or to correct skeletal deformities.

In the 1800s, several attempts were made to perform bone grafts both from patients themselves and from animals.

Two New York surgeons, Fred Albee (1876–1945) and Russell Hibbs (1869–1932), used bone grafting with some success to treat deterioration of the spine caused by **tuberculosis (TB)** infection (also known as Pott's disease) in 1911. They used different methods, but Albee's was the most influential at the time. He also used grafts to treat fractures, using material from the tibia or from the fractured bone itself. In the early twentieth century, treated beef and human bones were also used as grafts.

The first bone bank was founded in Cuba in the early 1940s. Healthy bone collected from patients during surgery was preserved by refrigeration in saline solution or citrated blood.

In the 1970s, surgeons began working with a person's own bone, removing the vascular attachments and reattaching the blood vessel system to the area.

Today, a number of different materials may be used for bone grafting, including fresh, freeze-dried, or frozen bone and demineralized bone matrix. The bone may be taken from sites in a person's own body, such as the hip bone or rib, or from a bank of stored, donated material. Depending on the type of material used, bone grafts can serve to stimulate a patient's own healing.

Additional reading: Albee, *Bone Graft Surgery in Disease, Injury and Deformity*.

bone marrow transplant

A patient may receive bone marrow transplants from a donor—or from themselves—to treat blood diseases. Bone marrow transplants are also used in conjunction with high-dose **chemotherapy** as a last-resort treatment for **cancer**.

Blood cells form in the bone marrow, so replacing diseased marrow with healthy material can restore its function. Bone-marrow transplants are used to treat aplastic **anemia**, immunodeficiency, and some types of **leukemia**. These transplants are given after a person has had heavy doses of chemotherapy or radiation treatment for cancer because these therapies can destroy bone marrow. In this case, patients may have their bone marrow cells removed and stored before the cancer treatment so they can be replaced afterwards, which is known as an autologous transplant. Transplant of material from another person is referred to as allogenic.

In the 1950s and 1960s, researchers began attempting bone marrow transplants in humans to treat leukemia after scientists learned in the early 1950s that shielding a mouse's spleen or injecting the animal with genetically identical marrow cells allowed it to survive lethal doses of radiation.

Using bone marrow transplants, George Mathe (1922–) successfully treated five patients who stopped producing new blood cells after being exposed to radiation in an accident in Yugoslavia in 1958. But most early bone marrow transplant attempts failed due to graft-versus-host-disease (GVHD); Mathe's attempt probably worked because the radiation had weakened the patients' immune systems.

E. Donnall Thomas (1920–), who conducted extensive animal research on bone marrow transplants and began a human bone marrow transplant program in 1955, won the 1990 Nobel Prize for his work.

When the human leukocyte **antigen** (HLA) system was discovered in the 1960s, this made transplants much easier because donors and recipients could be matched by **tissue** typing, thus avoiding GVHD. The first matched bone marrow transplant to a child with immune deficiency was reported in 1968. By the 1970s, people with aplastic anemia and leukemia were receiving bone marrow transplants from HLA-matched siblings.

One-quarter to one third of people have an HLA-matched sibling. Registries of potential tissue-typed volunteer donors have been created for those who do not.

Methods to fight GVHD, including immunosuppressant drugs and donor blood treatment, have made bone marrow transplants from less closely matched donors possible but still risky. **Cyclosporine**, introduced in 1980, was found to be very helpful when used with the older drug **methotrexate** for staving off GVHD.

Today, bone marrow transplants have become an accepted treatment for leukemia and other blood disorders, and some patients have survived after the transplants for more than 20 years. Researchers are also working on using transplants of **stem cells**—immature blood cells that are precursors of every type of mature blood cell—for the same purpose. The usefulness of bone marrow transplants in concert with high-dose radiation or chemotherapy is still somewhat controversial, but people still receive it, particularly for **breast cancer** that has not responded to other types of treatment. (*See also* immunosuppression)

Additional reading: Shaffer, *Bone Marrow Transplants*.

botulism toxin

Botulism toxin is a nerve poison released by the *Clostridium botulinium* bacterium. The toxin, which can be lethal when people consume it in spoiled food, is used therapeutically in patients with nerve spasms and also, cosmetically, to prevent wrinkles and eliminate excessive sweating.

The drug works by inhibiting the release of the neurotransmitter **acetylcholine**. Justinius Kerner (1786–1862) described the process of botulism poisoning from food in 1817, and later suggested that the toxin could be used to treat excessive muscular contractions, excessive sweating, and excessive salivation. But the therapy was not actually attempted until the late twentieth century.

Alan B. Scott (1932–), an ophthalmologist at Presbyterian Hospital in San Francisco, pioneered the use of botulism toxin in 1981 for people with strabismus, a condition in which the muscles around the eye contract abnormally and interfere with vision. Dermatologists first used botulism toxin injections to treat excessive sweating of the palms and armpits in 1996, with good results. The injections stop sweating for several months. Botulism toxin also has been used to treat vaginisimus, a condition in which the vagina is held closed by involuntary muscle spasms. The toxin has also been used to treat muscle spasms caused by cerebral palsy.

Botulism toxins (called "botox" for short) now are also given routinely in certain U.S. cities to men and women seeking to avoid wrinkles; the injections paralyze part of the face, for example the space between the eyebrows, preventing wrinkle-producing facial movements such as squinting.

Additional reading: Galton, *Med Tech,* pp. 97–99.

brain death

Brain death occurs when this organ has completely ceased functioning, even though other organs may be functioning with or without assistance. During the late 1950s, several groups of French neurophysiologists studying patients in extremely deep coma noted that these patients had virtually no brain function as measured by an electroencephalogram. Pierre Mollaret (1898–unknown) and Maurice Goulon described this condition as *coma depasse*—a state beyond coma.

The question of brain death became important as organ donation became possible. It is much more difficult to harvest organs from a donor whose heart has stopped, because the organs may have degraded, but the definition of death at the time was the point at which the heart stopped beating, no matter what state the brain was in.

In 1964, a Swedish team of surgeons transplanted a kidney from a donor with massive bleeding in the brain who was being kept alive on a mechanical ventilator. Thomas Starzl (1926–) in Philadelphia and Christiaan Barnard (1922–) in South Africa transplanted kidneys and a heart, respectively, from patients with no measurable brain activity who had been removed from mechanical ventilation. Both surgeons waited until the patient's heart had stopped beating before removing the organs.

In 1968 at Harvard University, a committee developed criteria for judging brain death that most doctors soon accepted. Patients had to be observed for an hour, have no reflexes, to stop breathing after being taken off a respirator, and be completely unresponsive to painful stimuli. All of these criteria had to be reconfirmed 24 hours later.

The concept of brain death became widely known and understood with the case of Karen Ann Quinlan (1954–1985). The parents of this New Jersey woman, who was comatose and brain dead, sued for permission to remove her from the mechanical ventilator that was keeping her alive. They argued that the patients have a right to refuse medical treatment and that they were acting on her behalf. They won the case in 1976 but Quinlan survived in a coma for nearly 10 more years. (*See also* electroencephalography)

Additional reading: Caplan and Coelho, *The Ethics of Organ Transplants.*

brain tumor/spinal cord tumor

Brain or spinal cord tumors are abnormal growths, malignant or benign, in the brain or spine or the meninges that surround and protect these organs. Although brain tumors usually do not spread to other parts of the body, they can be deadly even when they are benign because they can damage the brain. They usually are treated with surgery, radia-

tion, and **chemotherapy**. Approximately 17,400 people in the United States were diagnosed with some type of brain tumor in 1998, and 13,300 died of the disease that year.

The first reported case of surgery to remove a tumor was in 927, when the King of Dhar was operated on by two brothers, who used one drug to anesthetize the king and another to revive him.

Francois Quesnay (1694–1774), a French surgeon, removed tumors of the meninges of the brain. He observed that the brain itself did not feel pain. His countryman Antoine Louis (1723–1792) wrote an essay on removing brain tumors and likely operated on tumors inside the brain itself.

Toward the end of the nineteenth century, thanks to advances in **cerebral localization**, surgeons were able to determine where a tumor might be located in the brain by observing a patient's neurological symptoms. Sir William Macewen (1848–1924) is considered to be the first surgeon who used a "functional map" of the cortex to direct his scalpel. In 1876, he recommended operating on a boy with a brain abscess, but the boy's doctor objected to the surgery. When the boy died, he was found to have an abscess exactly where Macewen had predicted it would be. Three years later he predicted that a patient was suffering from a tumor in the motor region; he operated to remove the tumor, and the patient lived for several more years.

Richmond Godlee (1849–1925) operated on another patient in 1884, after predicting the location of the tumor. The 25-year-old patient lived and his symptoms improved, but he subsequently died from an infection of the meninges. The surgery received considerable coverage in the medical press, increasing acceptance of brain surgery.

Growing understanding of the nervous system anatomy allowed surgeons to develop a similar approach to localizing and removing tumors on the spine; Victor Horsley (1857–1916) performed the first such operation in 1887. The patient survived the surgery and regained full mobility.

Even with the development of **anesthesia** and **antisepsis**, however, surgery on the brain and spine remained rare. Harvey Cushing (1869–1939) decided to develop a system for performing the surgery on a regular basis. He became director of neurosurgery at Johns Hopkins University in 1901, and in 1908 wrote a comprehensive treatise on neurosurgery that was published in a surgery textbook. Cushing introduced silver clips in 1911 and electrocoagulation in 1926 to stop bleeding in the brain.

Cushing also developed a classification for different types of brain tumors that was published in 1932. In 1936, W. Grey Walter (1910–1977) showed that brain tumors could be detected by **electroencephalography (EEG)** because they produced abnormally slow waves in the surrounding **tissue**.

Lars Lekskell (1907–1986), a Swedish neurosurgeon, invented the **gamma knife** for treating brain tumors with highly concentrated doses of radiation.

The most common type of brain tumor is glioblastoma multiforme. Patients diagnosed with this type of **cancer** survive for a year, on average, a rate that has not improved for 30 years. Recent attempts at treating brain tumors with **gene therapy** have shown some promise. Investigators are also working on developing new ways to deliver chemotherapy to the brain, because the blood-brain barrier makes it impossible for many drugs to reach the brain when administered orally or into the bloodstream.

Additional reading: Roloff, *Moving Through a Strange Land.*

BRCA1, 2

BRCA1 and 2 are genetic mutations that have been found to increase a woman's risk of developing **breast** and **ovarian cancer**. They are most common in women of Eastern European Jewish, or Ashkenazi, heritage, and are associated with breast **cancer** that runs in families and appears at a relatively early age. About 1 in 50 Ashkenazi women is believed to have one of the mutations; the mutations also appear relatively frequently in Icelanders and Swedes.

Both genes are believed to be **tumor-suppressor genes** when they are not mutated and fully functional. Other possible breast cancer-linked genes have been found, including HRAS1 and p53.

Mary-Claire King (1946–) of the University of California at Berkeley and her colleagues located a breast cancer gene mutation on **chromosome** 17 in 1990, and Yoshio Miki of the Utah Medical Center and colleagues cloned the gene—named BRCA1—in 1994. That year, Richard Wooster and colleagues from the Institute of Cancer Research in Surrey found another breast-cancer susceptibility mutation on chromosome 13, which they cloned and named BRCA2.

Roughly 10 percent of women with ovarian cancer and 7 percent of women with breast cancer carry one or both of these genes. While women with one of the genes have 15 times the risk of ovarian cancer that other women do, this by no means guarantees that they will develop cancer. Women with a mutation of the BRCA1 gene who develop breast cancer may actually have a better chance of survival and less likelihood of recurrence than women without the mutation.

The discovery of the breast cancer genes mean that women with a history of early-onset breast cancer in their family can be screened for one of these mutations; however, this procedure also has created a great deal of anxiety among these women. Some who have no sign of cancer decide to have their breasts and ovaries removed to protect themselves against the disease.

Additional reading: Waldholz, *Curing Cancer,* pp. 211–32, 255–75.

breast cancer

Breast **cancer** is one of the most common cancers. There are an estimated 175,000 new cases of breast cancer in the United States each year, with roughly 43,700 deaths from the disease annually.

An Egyptian papyrus of 1600 B.C. recommends burning breast cancers with fire or removing them with a sharp instrument. Leonides, a Greek physician of the first century A.D. who worked at the great center of learning in Alexandria, is believed to have been the first person to surgically remove the breast, a procedure that is called mastectomy. He also used **cauterization** to treat breast tumors.

The surgeon Ambrose Pare (c.1510–1590) excised breast tumors, but he thought total mastectomy was too mutilating to the patient. Instead, he tried crushing tumors with a lead plate, with little success. Michael Servetus (1509–1553) recommended removing glandules (probably lymph nodes) as well as the underlying muscle. Guilhelmus Fabricus Hildanus (1560–1624) described a technique for mastectomy and dissection of the armpit, and he believed that he had cured a patient with the surgery. All of these early operations, done long before **anesthesia** and **antisepsis**, killed more often than they cured. Major advances in breast cancer surgery weren't made until these surgical aids became available in the late nineteenth century.

In 1890, William Steward Halsted (1852–1922) performed an operation in which he removed the breast, the underlying muscle, and the surrounding lymph nodes in order to eradicate any cancer that had spread from the breast. The surgery was much like radical mastectomies performed today, although simple mastectomy, modified radical mastectomy, and lumpectomy have largely replaced this more drastic procedure. In modified radical mastectomy, the lining covering the chest muscle is removed, but the muscles themselves are left in place. In simple mastectomy, the breast and nearby lymph nodes are removed. It was around this time that the first attempts at reconstruction after mastectomy were made.

Attempts to treat breast cancer with **radiation therapy** followed soon after the invention of **X-rays**. In Chicago in 1895, Emil H. Grubbe (1875–1960) reported treating a breast cancer patient with X-rays, shielding the skin around the tumor with tin foil.

In 1896, Glasgow surgeon George Beatson (1848–1933) removed a 33-year-old woman's ovaries, which resulted in a nearly four-year remission of her advanced breast cancer. He argued that ovarian secretions escalated cell growth and it is indeed true that **estrogen** speeds the growth of certain breast cancers. In 1907, Albert Ochsner (1858–1925) reported using radiation therapy after mastectomy to destroy the ovaries, and within 10 years radiation had replaced surgical removal of the ovaries, although the new technique turned out to be less effective.

The first breast **prosthesis** was produced in 1930. During this decade the American Cancer Society began urging women to perform breast self-examinations and promoting early cancer detection.

Hormonal therapies, including giving women testosterone or synthetic estrogen, were developed in the late 1930s and 1940s. Hormone therapy today remains a vital part of the armamentarium against breast cancer.

In 1948, researchers reported that simple mastectomy with radiation for breast cancer produced better results than radical mastectomy. The findings were called "retrogressive heresy" at the time, although decades later this recommendation would become the standard of treatment.

Several new chemotherapeutic agents were introduced in the 1950s, and in the 1960s it was discovered that combining these drugs made them more effective without producing too much extra toxicity.

In 1960, Elwood V. Jenson (1920–) reported the discovery of estrogen receptors, paving the way for the "designer estrogens" such as **tamoxifen** and raloxifene, also known as selective estrogen-receptor modulators (SERMS), that are now used to treat and prevent breast cancer. Estrogen receptor analysis of tumors has also proven to be a good technique for predicting whether a cancer will spread.

In the 1970s, doxorubicin, an **anti-tumor antibiotic**, was introduced and found to be very effective for treating breast cancer.

In 1976, V. Craig Jordan (1947–) proposed using tamoxifen as a preventive treatment for breast cancer; large-scale studies completed in 1998 found that tamoxifen can indeed prevent some high-risk women from developing breast cancer, although it also may increase a woman's chances of developing blood clots and cancers of the uterine lining.

During the 1970s, Dr. Bernard Fisher (1918–), chairman of the National Surgical Adjuvent Breast Project, concluded—in line with findings decades earlier—that modified radical mastectomy with radiation was as effective as radical mastectomy for treating breast cancer. By the late 1970s, modified radical mastectomy had virtually replaced radical mastectomy for breast cancer.

Fisher instituted ongoing clinical trials of breast cancer treatment in 1980. Soon afterwards, the taxane drugs such as paclitaxel (**Taxol**) and docetaxel, based on a substance found in the Pacific yew tree, were introduced and found to be effective in treating breast cancer.

The **BRCA1, 2** genes, mutations of which are implicated in 7 percent of breast cancers, were cloned in 1994. Now one of the most pressing questions in breast cancer treatment is whether women should be screened for these genes.

Although breast cancer is a common disease, for most of the twentieth century it was a taboo subject. First Lady Betty Ford's (1918–) public acknowledgment of her struggle with breast cancer in 1974 raised awareness of the disease and began to eliminate its taboo status. In 1989, a group of 11 medical organizations joined the force in raising awareness by urging women to begin having breast cancer screening after age 40. Millions of dollars are now spent annually to remind women to get screened. However, awareness among women in minority groups lags behind.

Recent advances in breast cancer diagnosis include better mammography and **biopsy** techniques. For example, if a woman 20 years ago was suspected of having breast cancer, tissue from the suspicious lump had to be sampled using traditional surgical techniques. Today doctors use fine-needle aspiration or core needle biopsy, sometimes guided by **ultrasound**, **magnetic resonance imaging,** or **stereotactic surgery** techniques, which is much more precise and leaves little or no scarring.

Another important development is the use of sentinel-node biopsy to gauge how far a cancer has spread. Dye is injected near the tumor and nearby lymph nodes that have taken up the dye are removed and checked. If these nodes show no cancer, the rest of the nodes are almost certainly negative as well, and a woman will not have to have the lymph nodes surrounding her breasts removed, which is a major and debilitating surgery.

However, sentinel node biopsy must be performed by extremely skilled physicians; otherwise it may provide a false-negative result when more treatment is necessary.

Lumpectomy—in which the lump itself is removed and the rest of the breast is preserved—along with radiation therapy, and hormonal and **chemotherapy** if necessary, is now the standard of breast cancer treatment in the United States.

Additional reading: de Moulin, *A Short History of Breast Cancer.*

Bright's disease

Bright's disease, a type of kidney inflammation now called acute or chronic glomerulonephritis, is named for the British physician who first described it, Richard Bright (1789–1858). His 1827 "Reports of Medical Cases," which contained several full-color illustrations of diseased organs, was a landmark because it linked clinical and chemical findings with **autopsy** reports.

Bright attributed the disease that would carry his name to overconsumption of alcohol and suppression of sweat, but it is now known to be due to disordered immune response. Bright was the first to suggest that urine containing abnormally high amounts of the protein albumin was linked to granular degeneration of the kidney. He also introduced the concept that cardiovascular disease might begin in the kidney, and he connected dropsy (fluid retention), albuminous urine, and a hard pulse (high **blood pressure**, or **hypertension**) with damage to the kidneys and heart. Bright suggested that some altered quality of the blood might mean more force was required to propel it through the circulation. The term "Bright's disease" is seldom used in the medical literature today.

Additional reading: Kiple, *The Cambridge World History of Human Disease,* pp. 746–49.

bubonic plague

The bubonic plague is a deadly infectious disease that killed millions throughout history.

The disease is caused by the bacterium *Yersinia pestis*, and is spread from rats and squirrels to humans by the bite of infected fleas. Bubonic plague's symptoms include inflamed and swollen lymph nodes, known as "buboes," and pneumonia.

Humans have little immunity to the disease, developing severe symptoms within six days of infection. Roughly 60 percent of people infected with the disease die a week after symptoms appear. When virulent strains of the bacterium are spread from human to human, fatality rates can approach 100 percent.

The first known epidemic of plague occurred in ancient Greece. There was a subsequent cycle of plague from roughly 500 to 700 A.D. in the Near East and Europe. A second cycle began in 1300 and lasted through 1800, striking Europe, the Middle East, and Asia. A seven-year period within this second cycle, in the mid-fourteenth century, is known as the "Black Death." The first **quarantines** were enacted in Italy during this time to prevent plague from spreading. Other public health measures of the time included street cleaning and regulation of burial.

A third plague cycle is believed to have begun in Asia in the mid-1800s, but Europe protected itself against the disease with the world's longest "cordon sanitaire" between Turkey and Austria. This third cycle was the first to strike the Americas.

Alexandre Yersin (1863–1943), a French physician and microbiologist working in southeast Asia, was the first person to culture the plague bacteria. The bug, originally called *Pasturella pestis*, was renamed in his honor in 1971.

The U.S. Marine Hospital Service, a precursor of the **Public Health** Service, led efforts to control plague by inspecting ships and controlling rat populations. The last major rat-borne plague outbreak in the United States occurred in 1924 and 1925 in Los Angeles. During this epidemic, the last reported U.S. case of human-to-human plague transmission also occurred.

The **antibiotics** tetracycline and **streptomycin** are effective treatments for bubonic plague. Today, roughly a dozen cases of the plague appear in North America annually.

Additional reading: Kiple, *The Cambridge World History of Human Disease*, pp. 628–31.

bulimia nervosa

Bulimia nervosa is a disease in which people ingest large quantities of food, and then either purge themselves of the food by inducing vomiting or taking laxatives, or exercise compulsively to work off the calories consumed. Bulimia has serious health consequences, ranging from tooth decay caused by exposure to stomach acids to heart arrhythmias to **osteoporosis**. Recognition of this disease has made treatment possible, and has also helped alert physicians to potential underlying causes of the disease, such as **depression**.

Bulimia was first described as a disease by Gerald Russell of London's Royal Free Hospital in 1979. The characteristics of the disease had been noted by Stunkard, who in 1959 described a binge-eating syndrome, and by Hilde Bruch (1904–1984), who in 1974 described people with these symptoms as "thin fat people."

People with bulimia also often suffer from depression and may abuse drugs and alcohol. Treatment for bulimia involves counseling, and medication with **antidepressant drugs** can also be helpful. (*See also* anorexia nervosa)

Additional reading: Friedman, *Encyclopedia of Mental Health*, pp. 111–18.

Burkitt's lymphoma

Burkitt's lymphoma is caused by an infection with the Epstein-Barr **virus** originating in the B cells of the immune system and is common in central Africa. The disease is named for its discoverer, Denis Burkitt (1911–1993).

While working in Uganda in 1957, Burkitt noticed a child with large tumors on his face and he saw a child with similar growths a few weeks later. He observed that these tumors frequently spread to the abdomen. Burkitt's pathologist colleagues reviewed **tissue** samples from children with the tumors and concluded that the disease was a type of lymphoma, or lymphatic system **cancer**. Burkitt then surveyed his colleagues throughout Africa on whether they had seen such a disease, and found the sickness occurred in a strip across the center of the continent and did not occur in places where the mean temperature fell below 15 degrees C.

Burkitt reported his findings in a 1961 article, after which Dr. Michael Anthony Epstein (1921–) asked him if he could review tissue samples from children with the disease to look for an infectious agent. Three years later, Epstein found the virus responsible, which was named the Epstein-Barr virus for himself and his colleague Yvonne Barr. The disease itself was dubbed Burkitt's lymphoma in 1963.

Burkitt and his colleagues found that about 80 percent of patients with early stages of the disease could be cured successfully with methotrexate, cyclophosphamide, or vincristin. Burkitt's lymphoma was the second tumor found to be curable with **chemotherapy**—the first was choriocarcinoma. (*See also* lymph system)

Additional reading: Radetsky, *The Invisible Invaders*, pp. 164–73.

burn treatment

Treatment of severe burns is among the most difficult medical challenges.

The major impetus for recent strides in burn treatment was a fire at the Cocoanut Grove nightclub in Boston in 1942, which killed 491 people. Physicians at the Massachusetts General Hospital made careful observations of the treatment of these patients. These observations provided the basis of further study and research into burn treatment.

Skin grafts, from patients themselves or from cadavers, came into use to repair burned flesh in the late 1940s.

The first burn center in the United States opened at the Medical College of Virginia in 1947, and the Army established another center that year at Fort Sam Houston in Texas.

In the 1950s, burn specialists began to realize the crucial role of infection in burn mortality, and Curtis Price

Artz (1915–) and Eric Reiss (1924–) reported in 1957 that as many as half of the deaths from severe burns could be attributed to infection.

Very toxic agents such as tannic acid had long been used to treat burns, often hastening the patient's death. In the mid-1960s silver nitrate solution, an old wound remedy, was found to be an excellent and relatively nontoxic antiseptic for burns. Also at this time researchers discovered the importance of giving burn patients massive amounts of sodium solution to replace fluid and minerals lost through their wounds. Once this treatment became prevalent, death from burn **shock** basically disappeared.

The Shriners of North America, a charitable organization, established burn institutes beginning in the early 1960s in Galveston, Cincinnati, and Boston. Dr. Irving Feller (1925–) established the Institute for Burn Medicine in 1968, to train doctors and nurses in burn treatment and managing burn centers, and the American Burn Association was founded that year as well. (*See also* artificial skin)

Additional reading: Mannon, *Caring for the Burned.*

bypass surgery

In bypass surgery, blocked heart vessels are bypassed with a graft using an artery or vein from elsewhere in the body, restoring blood flow to the heart. Cardiopulmonary bypass is performed to prevent heart attacks and eliminate chest pain from **angina pectoris.**

The first reported bypass surgery was performed by the Argentinean surgeon Rene Favolaro (1923–) at the Cleveland Clinic in 1967; he bypassed the heart-vessel blockage with a graft from the saphenous vein in the leg. Michael DeBakey (1908–) and his colleagues in Texas had performed a similar operation, which they did not report, in 1964.

These surgeries were made possible by Frank Mason Sones's (1919–1985) work in 1958 on imaging blood flow in the heart. Sones used the "cine" method of **angiography**, in which several **X-rays** are taken in succession, making a moving picture of blood flow through a vessel.

Years later surgeons began using sections of nearby arteries, "borrowing" them to restore blood flow to the heart while they also carried out their original function. When Andreas Gruentzig (1939–1985) introduced coronary **angioplasty** in 1977, this less-invasive method gradually replaced bypass surgery for patients with blockage in only a single artery.

Today, angioplasty generally is considered the first-line treatment for the obstruction of blood vessels in the heart, with bypass surgery used only in cases of multiple-vessel blockage, or complications developing during angioplasty or **stent** placement. (*See also* heart-lung machine)

Additional reading: Acierno, *The History of Cardiology,* pp. 662–65.

calcium

Calcium is a mineral that is vital to the development of bones and teeth and the maintenance of bone strength. It also is essential for most forms of signaling between cells, so calcium is necessary for functions requiring coordinated action among systems, such as muscle contraction. In the body fluids, calcium is usually in ionic form. The ideal balance of calcium ions in the body depends on the interaction of many factors, such as adequate amounts of **vitamin D** and healthy levels of the **hormones** excreted by the **parathyroid** gland.

British physiologist Sydney Ringer (1835–1910) made one of the first observations of the role of calcium ions in the body. In a series of experiments at University College London, he bathed hearts in various solutions, eventually finding that the heart would only contract strongly in solutions that contained calcium. He published his observations in 1882 and 1883. During the 1890s, several researchers showed that calcium was necessary for the formation of thrombin, a protein involved in blood clotting.

In a 1908 report, Johns Hopkins University researchers William George MacCallum (1874-1944) and Carl Voegtlin (1879–unknown) demonstrated in animal experiments that removing the parathyroid gland would produce tetany, a condition characterized by abnormally rapid heartbeat, rigidity, twitching of the muscles, and tremors, but that these symptoms would immediately disappear when the animal was given an injection of calcium. They proposed that the gland somehow controlled calcium levels, and that removing it would cause all calcium stores to be rapidly excreted. Subsequent experiments confirmed that parathyroid hormones help to regulate calcium levels.

Researchers had been debating in what form calcium was found in the body since the early twentieth century. In a complex series of experiments reported in 1935, Franklin C. MacLean (1899–1968) and Albert Baird Hastings (1895–1987) demonstrated that the protein content of body fluids was the factor that regulated calcium levels. In a 1943 report, Takeo Kamada (1901–1946) and his student Haruo Kinosita, working in the laboratory of animal physiology at Tokyo Imperial University, showed in an experiment with frog muscle tissue that injecting calcium ions induced muscle contractions. Kamada suggested that this occurred because the ion was bound with some substance within the cell when the muscle was at rest, and that stimulating the cell resulted in muscle contraction. The first report on calciphylaxis, a process in which calcium is abnormally deposited in body tissues, was written by Hans Selye (1907–) and published in 1962. He reported that the process was something like anaphylaxis, because it required sensitization by certain factors and a latency period before the actual calcification took place. Selye noted that vitamin D and the thyroid and parathyroid hormones played an important role in calciphylaxis, and observed that the mast cells of the immune system also took part in the process. Calcergy was the term coined to describe the same process when it occurred without the sensitization period. The study of these pathological conditions paved the way for understanding how calcium is deposited on the bones in normal conditions, and for treating conditions in which the bones become fragile, such as **osteoporosis.**

Adequate calcium intake is now understood to be essential for preventing osteoporosis. Researchers are currently investigating whether taking calcium may also prevent colon **cancer.** A 1999 report by the Calcium Polyp Prevention Group, a consortium led by Dr. John Anthony Baron (1945–) of Dartmouth-Hitchcock Medical Center in Lebanon, New Hampshire, found that calcium supplements produced a moderate decrease in the risk of recurrent colorectal adenomas, which are precursors of cancerous growths. Other recent research suggests that adequate calcium intake may prevent tooth loss and gum disease, high **blood pressure**, and severe premenstrual discomfort.

Additional reading: Brody, "Calcium Takes Its Place as a Superstar of Nutrients."

calcium channel blockers (CCBs)/calcium antagonists

Calcium channel blockers, also known as calcium antagonists, are a group of drugs that block calcium ions from passing into the **tissue** of the heart and blood vessels. The circulatory system requires calcium to function properly, but when tissues become overloaded with calcium ions, blood vessels narrow and the heart beats too quickly. CCBs thus dilate blood vessels, protect the heart from overstimulation, and lessen the heart's oxygen requirements. They are useful for treating **hypertension,** easing **angina pectoris**, and preventing heart attacks. There are several different classes of CCBs, each with different properties.

The first group of CCBs were discovered from 1964 to 1969. The term "calcium antagonists" was coined in 1966.

Some recent evidence indicates that CCBs also may prevent cardiovascular disease from developing by slowing the formation of plaques that can block the arteries. However, some studies have found that people who take a certain type of CCB are more likely to have heart attacks, so the drugs are currently controversial.

Additional reading: Vos, *Drugs Looking for Diseases,* pp. 123–55.

cancer

Cancer is the uncontrolled growth of abnormal cells. There are more than 200 known types of cancer, and humans have had cancers since ancient times.

The Indian physician Ramayana, in about 2000 B.C., mentions treating tumors by surgical removal or with **arsenic** ointments. Ancient Egyptians also treated tumors with surgical removal under **anesthesia** using **opium** or the application of "chemicals from the earth." Hippocrates (c.460–c.377 B.C.) coined the terms "carcinos" for non-ulcerating tumor and "carcinoma" for ulcerating tumor, and classified tumors as benign or malignant. He observed that early treatment of tumors was more successful, and he recommended using ointments containing copper, lead, sulfur, and arsenic. Hippocrates and his contemporaries believed cancer was caused by an excess of black bile, one of the four humors described in the theory of **humoralism**. This idea survived until the late seventeenth century.

The Greek physician and writer Claudius Galen (129–c.199) was the first to recognize that tumors could metastasize, or spread, to other parts of the body. He also observed that patients with cancer were depressed, and patients who were depressed developed cancer.

The first new idea for the cause of cancer was proposed by Rene Descartes (1596–1650), who argued that leakage from the **lymph system**—which had been discovered by the Italian anatomist Gasparo Aselli (1581–1626) in 1622--was responsible. Simple leaks caused benign tumors, while malignant tumors developed when the lymph "fermented" or "degenerated." The lymph idea held sway for 150 years.

Henry Francois Le Dran (1685–1770), a prominent French physician, believed cancer was local in its early stages and that the only hope for treatment was early surgical removal. He proposed that cancer spread via the lymph nodes, which is true in some cases.

In 1775, Percival Pott (1714–1788) was the first person to describe an occupational **carcinogen**. He found that chimney sweeps had a high incidence of scrotal cancer in adulthood and proposed that this occurred because the skin

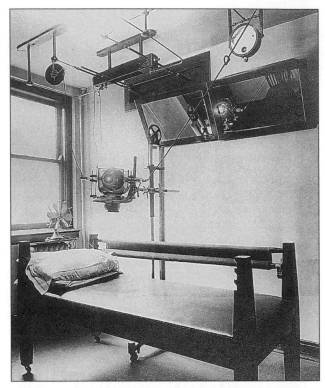

Cancer treatment room in Cleveland Clinic Building in 1921, with radiation apparatus. The clinic was among the first U.S. hospitals to begin offering radiation treatment for cancer. (Courtesy of Cleveland Clinic Archives.)

of the scrotum was constantly in contact with coal dust. This type of cancer nearly disappeared after the chimney sweeps' union recommended daily baths for its constituents.

In 1838, Johannes Muller (1801–1858) demonstrated that cancers were made of cells. He proposed that cancers developed from seed elements scattered in normal tissue. Rudolph Virchow's (1821–1902) theory that cells arise from other cells put this idea to rest. Virchow also believed that some people had a hereditary disposition toward cancer and that chronic irritation produced "granulation tissue" that could turn into tumors. Sir James Paget (1814–1899) added the idea of a "constitutional" disposition to cancer to Virchow's idea of hereditary tendencies.

In 1889, Paget suggested that the spread of tumors had something to do not just with the tumor itself but with the tissue where the metastasis occurred. He had observed that different types of tumors spread to different tissues: for example, cancer metastasized more frequently to the liver than to the spleen, and breast cancer frequently spread to the ovaries. His idea was called the "seed and soil" theory, and he recommended deeper study of the "soils."

Karl Thiersch (1822–1895) demonstrated that metastases arose from cells.

Theodor Boveri (1862–1915), a zoology professor, was the first person to suggest that chromosomal abnormalities caused cancer.

Surgical treatment for cancers advanced after the introduction of anesthesia and **antisepsis**, while **radiation therapy** was first used to treat cancer shortly after the discovery of **X-rays** in the late 1800s.

Early in the twentieth century, researchers also learned that **breast cancer**, **prostate cancer**, and a few other cancers could be controlled by reducing the natural supply of **hormones**, either by removing the organs that produced the hormones or by using drugs that fought the actions of these hormones.

Since the 1940s, a number of different chemotherapeutic agents have been introduced. The first agent found to be successful against cancer was **nitrogen mustard.**

Large-scale, cooperative clinical trials to test the effectiveness of cancer therapies were launched in the United States in the 1950s. This decade also saw the first cancer cure with **chemotherapy**. Dr. Roy Hertz (1909–) reported a cure of advanced metastatic gestational choriocarcinoma in 1956. This rare tumor develops in women during pregnancy.

In the 1960s, cancer experts found they could combine chemotherapeutic drugs for more effectiveness without too much more toxicity. In 1964, researchers worked out a dose-response system for chemotherapeutic drugs that maximized their effectiveness and established the importance of dosage and timing in administering these medications.

By the late 1960s, several cancers, including **Hodgkin's disease**, **Burkitt's lymphoma**, acute lymphocytic **leukemia** of children, and some cases of embryonal carcinoma of the testis could be cured by radiation oncology and chemotherapy.

Boveri's idea of a chromosomal basis of cancer was proved in the late twentieth century with many discoveries highlighting the role of genetic abnormalities in carcinogenesis, including the role of **oncogenes** and **tumor-suppressor genes** and the discovery of genetic mutations—some inherited—that predispose people to certain types of cancer. The Philadelphia **chromosome**, a genetic defect that causes people to develop a form of leukemia, was the first such gene discovered, in 1960. Genes known as **BRCA1, 2** that are linked to familial breast cancer were discovered in the early 1990s.

Additional reading: Shorter, *The Health Century,* pp. 179–211; Kiple, *The Cambridge World History of Human Disease,* pp. 102–10.

cancer center

Most **cancer** centers are hospitals devoted to caring for cancer patients that provide all the services these patients need in one place. Some conduct research only, not providing patient care.

The first cancer center in the United States was the Roswell Park Memorial Institute in Buffalo, New York, founded in 1898. The Memorial Hospital for the Treatment of Cancer and Allied Diseases was established in New York in 1906, and became the Memorial Sloan-Kettering Cancer Center in 1939. Two years later, an act of the Texas state legislature established the M.D. Anderson Cancer Center in Houston.

These early cancer centers were paid for with private and state funds, while the first federally funded cancer research lab began operating in 1922.

In 1937, Congress's National Cancer Act established the National Cancer Institute (NCI) as part of the **National Institutes of Health (NIH).**

In 1965, the NCI began funding regional medical programs at Congress's behest. The National Cancer Act of 1971 mandated that 15 new centers be established for diagnosing and treating cancer.

There are currently 58 NCI-designated cancer centers in the United States. Each has gone through a process of peer review, and each receives funding from the NCI to support scientific research. There are three types of cancer centers: those that conduct basic research only; clinical cancer centers that also conduct **clinical trials** of new treatments; and comprehensive cancer centers that do research and clinical work and also conduct epidemiological studies on cancer.

The National Comprehensive Cancer Network (NCCN), formed in 1995, is a nonprofit organization of 18 leading U.S. cancer centers. NCCN members collaborate by pooling their data on the effectiveness of treatment and also working together with **managed care** companies. The network also has a center for patient referral and has developed guidelines for treating **breast cancer** and **prostate cancer**.

Additional reading: Division of Cancer Research Sources and Centers, National Cancer Institute, *The Cancer Centers Program.*

cancer vaccine

Cancer vaccines are an attempt to treat cancer by priming immune-system cells to recognize tumor cells as abnormal, and thus find and destroy them. One advantage to this new treatment is that unlike **chemotherapy**, cancer **vaccines** have few side effects. Cancer vaccines are part of a group of new treatment approaches known as biological response modifiers, which include **tumor necrosis factor**, interleukins, and **interferons**.

Several types of cancer vaccines are being studied. Some use entire cells from tumors; others employ **monoclonal antibodies** targeted to attack tumor **antigens**; some introduce genetic material from a tumor and some use the antigens themselves. Vaccines are usually given along with an immune-system stimulant such as the **BCG vaccine** or interferon.

In the 1960s, research into transplants and the immune system showed scientists that some tumor cells had antigens different from normal cells that could be used as targets for immunotherapy. With some disappointing studies in the 1970s, the study of immunotherapy for cancer slowed down, but it was revitalized in 1975 with the discovery of monoclonal antibodies that could be used to identify these antigens specifically.

Monoclonal antibodies targeted at tumor antigens were found to induce remission in some patients with B-cell lymphoma and early stage colon cancer in the early 1990s.

Several trials of cancer vaccines are currently underway for **melanoma**, kidney cancer, **breast cancer**, **prostate cancer**, colorectal cancer, and lymphoma, including a large scale trial for a lymphoma vaccine announced by the National Cancer Institute in 1999. Vaccines for melanoma, for example, have not cured the disease but they have been shown to slow or reverse its progress.

Additional reading: Hall, *A Commotion in the Blood,* pp. 350–74.

capillaries

Capillaries are the tiny blood vessels that link the ends of the smallest arteries carrying blood away from the heart to the beginning of the smallest veins carrying blood toward the heart. Capillary walls are a single cell thick, allowing for gas exchange with body **tissues**.

Marcello Malpighi (1628–1694) discovered open channels from the arteries to the veins in frogs' lungs in 1661. Antoni van Leeuwenhoek (1632–1723) observed blood cells passing from arteries to veins in 1688, although he did not see that capillaries connected the two but instead saw a straightforward vessel-to-vessel connection.

August Krogh (1874–1949) and Marie Krogh (1874–1943), a Danish husband-and-wife team, discovered that the absorption of oxygen in the lungs and the elimination of carbon dioxide in these organs takes place when the gases diffuse across lung tissue, and published their work in 1909. August Krogh went on to discover the mechanism by which the body regulates capillary circulation. He had theorized that at rest only a few of the capillaries were open to let blood pass and supply oxygen to the tissues, but that with exercise and exertion more and more capillaries opened so that the tissues could take in more oxygen. August Krogh won the Nobel Prize for this work in 1920.

Additional reading: Acierno, *The History of Cardiology,* pp. 30–32.

carcinogens

Carcinogens are chemicals that stimulate the development and growth of malignant tumors.

In 1761, the British physician John Hill (1714–1775) observed that snuff could cause nasal **cancer**, and in 1775, Percival Pott (1714–1788) blamed coal dust for the high incidence of scrotal cancer among chimney sweeps. These were the first observations that a substance could cause cancer. In the 1870s, Richard von Volkmann (1830–1889) in Germany found that industrial workers exposed to tar and shale oil developed skin cancers. The German doctor

Ludwig Mettler Rehn (1849–1930) in 1895 suggested that chemicals known as aromatic amines caused bladder cancer, after finding three cases among workers exposed to aniline dyes. Several subsequent observations were made of cancers among workers exposed to aromatic amines.

In 1915, Japanese scientists demonstrated that repeatedly applying coal tar to the skin of rabbits caused cancer. The carcinogenicity of aromatic amines, coal tars, and soots was well established by the 1940s.

In the 1950s, evidence for a link between a dramatic increase in **lung cancer** during the twentieth century and a rise in cigarette smoking was building. Several substances produced by plants and microorganisms have also been found to be carcinogenic, including aflatoxin, which is produced by a fungus found on peanuts.

Certain environmental factors have been confirmed to contribute to cancer growth, such as exposure to ultraviolet rays and skin cancer and asbestos inhalation and lung cancer. There is evidence that cooking meat at extremely high heat may produce substances that are carcinogenic.

Before the discovery of genetic predispositions to cancer, some researchers believed that workplace exposure to carcinogenic chemicals caused most cancers, which is most likely not the case, although the role of these chemicals and environmental chemicals in cancer development remains unclear and may be significant.

Additional reading: Weinberg, *Racing to the Beginning of the Road,* pp. 16–31.

cardiac ablation

Radiofrequency catheter cardiac ablation is a technique for correcting abnormal heart rhythms by destroying the tissue within the heart responsible for setting the faulty pace. The procedure can be performed safely while a patient is under sedation.

The first type of arrhythmia to yield to surgical techniques was a condition called Wolff-Parkinson-White (WPW) syndrome, first described in 1930. The condition can strike healthy young people, and it is life-threatening.

In 1933, Charles Wolferth (1887–1965) and Francis Wood (1901–) suggested that "accessory pathways" between the right auricle and the right ventricle through which electrical current traveled might be responsible for the abnormal heart rhythm in the syndrome, which Wood and his colleagues confirmed in an **autopsy** study 10 years later. The idea followed that surgically interrupting these pathways could cure the arrhythmia. Will C. Sealy (1912–) and his colleagues first performed such an operation on a 32–year-old man in 1968. He was cured.

For this type of procedure to become safe and effective, surgeons had to devise a way to map all of the accessory pathways in a patient that are responsible for abnormal heart rhythm. The first such map was completed in 1967. The surgery was refined by several researchers in the 1970s and 1980s. **Cardiac catheterization** played a central role in mapping.

Various techniques for ablation have been studied, including chemicals, cryosurgery, laser, and electricity. Electricity in the form of radiofrequency, first used in 1987, has become the preeminent ablation technique, helped by the development of special catheters to deliver the energy. By 1991, WPW could almost always be safely cured, at little risk, with radiofrequency ablation.

Additional reading: Singer, ed., *Interventional Electrophysiology.*

cardiac catheterization

In cardiac catheterization, a tiny flexible tube is passed into the heart through a blood vessel, usually the main vein of the leg or arm. This technique can gauge how well the heart is working and diagnose malfunctions by sampling the oxygen level of blood within the heart and measuring blood pressure in each of the heart's four chambers.

Werner Forssmann (1904–1979) performed the first cardiac catheterization—on himself—as a medical student in 1929. He passed the catheter through an incision in an arm vein and along the vessel into the right side of his heart, after which he walked up a flight of stairs to an **X-ray** machine, where he had an image taken to show the position of the catheter. Forssmann catheterized himself six times, without any ill effects or pain. He thought the technique would be useful for injecting medicine directly into the heart.

In the 1940s, New York surgeons Dickinson Richards (1895–1973) and André Cournand (1895–1988) used cardiac catheterization to study how lung disease affected heart function. They used catheters to sample the oxygen and carbon dioxide content of venous blood within the heart, measure pressure within the heart, and for several other diagnostic tests. Richards, Cournand, and Forssmann shared the Nobel Prize for their work in 1956.

Now, cardiac catheterization labs are a vital diagnostic tool. In these labs, technicians record the chemical and electrical activity of the heart, deliver drugs and electrical impulses to the heart, and create images of the heart.

Additional reading: Franklin and Sutherland, *Guinea Pig Doctors*, pp. 227–54.

cardiopulmonary resuscitation. See CPR.

cardioversion

Cardioversion is a technique for restoring the normal beat of the heart with a carefully timed electric charge.

In 1960, Bernard Lown (1921–) at Harvard and his colleagues found a way to deliver a shock to a patient with a non-life-threatening heart rhythm disturbance without damaging the heart or bringing on more dangerous arrhythmias.

Alternating current (AC) electricity had been used for this purpose in patients who would otherwise die, but shocking relatively healthy patients this way was risky because it damaged heart fibers and could produce ventricular fibrillation, a type of heart arrhythmia that leads to death. Patients with cardiac arrhythmias usually were treated with anti-arrhythmic drugs, which weren't very effective and could actually cause other heart problems.

Working with animals, Lown investigated the possibility of shocking the heart with direct currents (DC), which are shorter and shaped differently than AC currents. The team also located the point in the heart's electrical cycle at which it was vulnerable to ventricular fibrillation: the T wave.

Lown found the DC technique, timed properly, was safer and often worked better than AC, and could be used on patients whose arrythmias were not life-threatening. Cardioversion is different from **defibrillation** in that it is timed to avoid the T wave, while defibrillation is not synchronized with the heart's electrical cycle. Cardioversion is delivered through electrodes placed on the patient's chest, and it may be necessary to give the patient sedatives before cardioversion.

Additional reading: Singer, ed., *Interventional Electrophysiology.*

carotid endarterectomy

Carotid endarterectomy is a surgery to prevent **stroke** in which blockage is cleared from the carotid arteries, the main blood vessels leading to the brain.

The operation was first performed in 1953 by Dr. Michael DeBakey (1908–) at Texas Medical Center in Houston and became more and more popular, reaching a peak of about 110,000 surgeries a year in the United States in 1985. The number of carotid endarterectomies fell off sharply after a report by the respected nonprofit think tank, Rand Corporation, found many were being performed unnecessarily, but since 1990 the popularity of the operation has been on the rise again thanks to favorable studies. Many experts believe the operation is still being done too frequently, because the risk of operation for some patients may be larger than their risk of stroke.

Numerous studies completed in 1998 refined medical understanding of the type of symptomatic carotid artery blockage that benefits most from carotid endarterectomy surgery; the operation is best and least risky for patients with blockage of 75 percent or more of one of the arteries that produces symptoms.

Additional reading: Squires, "Surgery to Prevent Strokes."

CAT scanning

CAT scanning (also CT scanning), or computerized axial tomography, is a technique for creating a cross-sectional, three-dimensional **X-ray** image of the body by combining multiple two-dimensional X-rays. CAT scans produce crisper pictures than X-rays and they are also capable of imaging soft **tissue** within the body, including organs such as the brain. X-rays can only capture clear images of bones and cartilage. Johann Radon (1887–1946), an Austrian mathematician, demonstrated that this was possible in 1917. But it was not until the 1950s and 1960s that Radon's theories were applied to imaging.

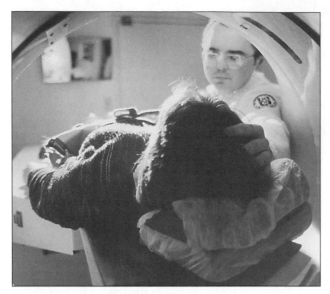

A technician prepares a patient for a CAT scan. (Courtesy of Archives and Special Collections, Columbia University Health Sciences Division.)

William Oldendorf (1925–), a neurologist at UCLA, began working on a machine for detecting the density of an object's interior—specifically the brain—in 1959. He had been inspired by an electrical engineer colleague's effort to develop a device that could detect frostbitten oranges, which are dehydrated but appear normal at the surface. Oldendorf patented his machine in 1963 and attempted to interest X-ray companies in the design, with no success. At this point, the computing technology necessary to make sense of the machine's readings was thought to be too cumbersome for practical use.

Allan MacLeod Cormack (1924–), a nuclear physicist, had observed that radiation was distributed differently throughout the body, and theorized that a device could provide an image of the body's composition based on this distribution. He built a test machine and used it in 1963 to image an asymmetrical object with good results, but his publication of his findings received little notice.

Around this time, Godfrey Hounsfield (1919–), an engineer at the British company EMI, began investigating image projection. Hounsfield, who had been a radar instructor in World War II, didn't know about Cormack or Radon's work. He built a prototype CT device and began experimenting with it in 1968. Once he had success imaging biological specimens, he constructed a brain-scanning prototype.

Hounsfield and neurosurgeon James Ambrose (1926–) used the machine on a living person, a woman with symptoms of a tumor in the frontal lobe of the brain, in 1971. The scan was recorded on magnetic tape and then processed by computer, revealing a tumor of the left frontal lobe, which Ambrose subsequently removed.

Ambrose and Hounsfield published the results of 70 human brain scans the following year, and EMI began producing the CT units commercially soon afterwards.

Robert Ledley (1926–), a professor at Georgetown University, conceived of the idea for a whole body scanner, which he and his colleagues built within two years. The machine was called the Automatic Computerized Transverse Axial, or ACTA, scanner. Ledley patented the device and licensed it to the drug company Pfizer.

A second-generation device invented by researchers at the Cleveland Clinic was particularly good for imaging the body, and Ohio Nuclear began selling this machine, the Delta scanner, in 1975. The third generation of machines used a fan-shaped X-ray beam that could sweep the whole body and perform a scan in seconds. With the help of computer simulations, a team of radioastronomers at American Science and Engineering were able to refine the computer algorithm for reading these third-generation images.

CT is also being used to guide surgical instruments, in some cases making it possible to drain infection or destroy tumors without surgery.

Spiral CT was introduced in 1989. This technique is faster and less cumbersome, and creates three-dimensional images that can be rotated on a computer and viewed from different angles. A spiral CT exam takes five to 10 minutes, versus 30 minutes to an hour for older techniques.

Hounsfield and Cormack shared the 1979 Nobel Prize for their work in developing CT scanning.

Additional reading: Kevles, *Naked to the Bone*, pp. 145–72.

cataract surgery

Cataract surgery is the removal of a lens that has clouded—usually due to age—in order to improve a person's eyesight. Nearly everyone 75 and older has cataracts to some degree. After the cataract is surgically removed, it is replaced with a permanent artificial lens.

Rufus of Ephesus paved the way for cataract surgery in about 100 A.D. when he described the correct location of the lens of the eye.

Couching, in which the clouded lens is pushed out of the way with a needle into the inside of the eyeball, was used for millennia to treat cataracts. The earliest record of this operation, whose name comes from the French word "coucher," to lie down, comes from a fifth-century B.C. Indian manuscript, which may have been written by the surgeon Susruta. Couching continued to be used into the middle of the twentieth century in some parts of the world, because it is easier to perform than cataract removal. When a person receives this operation, his or her vision will remain somewhat blurry because the clouded lens is not replaced.

Jacques Daviel (1696–1762) invented the operation that is used today to extract the lens, first performing it in 1747 or 1748. He got the idea for the operation when he was couching a patient's cataract and the operation failed. He left the exterior part of the lens in place. In 1753, Samuel Sharp (1700–1778) performed a version of the operation in which he squeezed the lens out through a slit in the cornea. Boston surgeon Henry Willard Williams (1821–1895) first described using sutures in cataract surgery, in 1867, with fine glovers silk and a short needle.

Early cataract surgeries were performed without **anesthesia** until general anesthesia was introduced in the

1840s; local anesthesia in the form of **cocaine** eyedrops became available in the 1880s and was more effective and less risky.

While cataract surgery became progressively safer, it was no better than couching in that it left the eye without a lens for focusing. Some patients used very thick glasses with good results, but the problem wasn't permanently solved until 1949 when British surgeon Harold Ridley implanted a permanent, plastic replacement lens after cataract surgery. Refinements in artificial lens technology developed in the 1950s and 1960s have greatly improved the results of the operation.

In the late 1960s, Charles Kelman (1930–) in New York developed a technique for dissolving the clouded lens using ultrasound. The broken-up lens material was then aspirated from the eye.

Today, cataract surgery is performed on an outpatient basis, with local anesthesia. It is the most common surgical procedure performed on Americans 65 and older.

Additional reading: Wangensteen and Wangensteen, *The Rise of Surgery,* pp. 526–29.

cauterization

Cauterization is the destruction of **tissue** with heat, cold, chemicals, or electricity.

Greek writings of the fifth and fourth centuries B.C. prescribed cautery for hemorrhoids and also to stop wounds from rotting. Ancient Islamic medicine recommended cauterizing wounds with a hot iron to stop bleeding and prevent infection, a practice common during the Middle Ages in Europe as well. Hot oil also was used for this purpose.

Today, cauterization is used to destroy abnormal tissue, for example to ablate the endometrium of the uterus when a woman is having irregular menstrual periods. Various methods are used, including **electrocautery**, heat, freezing (with liquid gases), and with caustic chemicals. Cauterization may also be used to prevent infection and to halt bleeding.

Additional reading: Wangensteen and Wangensteen, *The Rise of Surgery,* pp. 20–29.

CCBs. See Calcium channel blockers.

CDC. See Centers for Disease Control and Prevention

cell theory

Cell theory is the concept that all living things are made up of essential units called "cells" and is a central foundation of medical thought. The understanding of cells as the basic building block of life, as well as the way that cells function, has contributed to our knowledge of how conception occurs, how an embryo grows, and how the organs of the body function, among many other important topics.

In the late 1600s, Robert Hooke (1635–1703), was the first to see a cell, initially in a section of cork, and then in bones and plants. He suggested that cells were passages

through which fluid passed. Subsequent researchers saw cells, calling them "globules" or "bladders," and thought they were channels formed from fiber or smaller organisms. In 1824, Henri Dutrochet (1776–1847) proposed that animals and plants had similar cell structures.

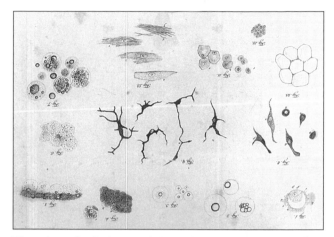

Illustrations of cells by one of the co-discoverers of the cell theory, Theodore Schwann, from an 1880 book. (Courtesy of New York Academy of Medicine)

Robert Brown (1773–1858) discovered the cell nucleus in 1831, and Matthias Schleiden (1804–1881) named the nucleolous (the structure within the nucleus now known to contain genetic material) around that time. Schleiden and Theodor Schwann (1810–1882) described a general cell theory in 1839, the former stating that cells were the basic unit of plants and Schwann extending the idea to animals. Both were mistaken about how cells were formed; they believed that they sprang from the nucleus, rather than from division of existing cells.

Robert Remak (1815–1865) was the first to describe cell division, in 1855, writing that "the cells of which the animal germ consists multiply by continuous division, which starts at the nucleus." Walther Flemming (1843–1905), working with salamanders (which have big cells and big nuclei), was the first to follow **chromosomes** through the entire process of cell division.

Additional reading: Harris, *The Birth of the Cell.*

Centers for Disease Control and Prevention (CDC)

The CDC is the arm of the **U.S. Public Health Service (PHS)** responsible for monitoring, investigating, controlling, and preventing disease.

The CDC sprang from a project launched during World War II to control **malaria** in the southern United States and the Caribbean. The Atlanta-based Malaria Control in War Areas (MCWA) program drained swamps and destroyed mosquito larvae to eradicate the disease in the region, where many military training camps were located. MCWA also worked on typhus control and trained doctors in recognizing and treating tropical disease.

The PHS's Joseph Mountin (1891–1952) and MCWA director Mark Hollis (1908–) suggested converting the program into a peacetime division for monitoring infectious disease, supporting local health units, and conducting field research. In 1946, the federal government took their advice. The MCWA became the Communicable Disease Center and Hollis was named its first director. Offices were established on land in Atlanta that had been bought for $10; the CDC is still located at this site.

In 1951, the Epidemic Intelligence Service (EIS) was founded within the CDC to train scientists to investigate epidemics. Then, as now, the division's appointees were on call at all times so they could respond immediately to disease outbreaks. **Poliomyelitis** was a major focus of the EIS's efforts. In 1955, a separate polio surveillance unit was established.

In 1957 and 1960, respectively, the Venereal Disease Division and the **Tuberculosis** Division of the PHS moved to Atlanta. In 1961, the CDC acquired the *Morbidity and Mortality Weekly Report*. This publication puts forth information on outbreaks of infectious disease around the world and continues to be published each week and distributed worldwide.

In 1966, the CDC launched a program to eradicate **smallpox.** Working closely with the **World Health Organization (WHO),** the CDC helped to wipe out the disease completely by 1980.

The Communicable Disease Center's name was changed to the Center for Disease Control in 1970, and pluralized to "Centers" in 1980.

The National Instutute for Occupational Safety and Health, in charge of overseeing **industrial hygiene** at U.S. workplaces, was incorporated into the CDC in 1973. A unit dedicated to studying violence as a public-health issue, the Violence Epidemiology Branch, was added to the CDC in 1983. Three years later, the Office of Smoking and Health became part of the Atlanta organization.

A Center for Chronic Disease and Health Promotion, dedicated to fighting heart disease, **cancer**, and **diabetes**, was established in 1988. The center launched a large-scale effort to detect **breast cancer** and **cervical cancer** early using **mammography** and **Pap smears** three years later. The following year, the CDC became the "Centers for Disease Control and Prevention." The National Childhood Immunization Program, to ensure that all children were inoculated with **vaccines** against infectious diseases such as **measles**, **mumps**, and **rubella**, began in 1993.

The CDC's recent efforts include the first annual report on pregnancy success rates at U.S. fertility clinics, released in 1997; and the first report on tobacco use among minority groups in the United States, published in 1998.

Additional reading: McCormick, *Level 4.*

cephalosporin

Cephalosporin was among the first natural **antibiotics** to be discovered, and now more than a dozen artificial variations of the original molecule are in use. This is the family of antibiotics most commonly used in hospitals.

Cephalosporin was isolated in 1945 from a fungus growing near a sewage outfall in Sardinia on the Mediterranean Sea. Howard Florey (1898–1968) tested a sample of the fungus, *Cephalosporium acremonium*, and found it produced a number of potentially useful compounds. In the mid-1950s, Edward Abraham (1913–1999) theorized that cephalosporin was structurally similar to **penicillin**, claiming that both shared a molecular structure called the beta-lactam ring. This was later found to be true.

Today several different derivatives of cephalosporin are used as broad-spectrum antibiotics.

Additional reading: Sneader, *Drug Discovery,* pp. 315–20.

cerebral localization

Cerebral localization is the creation of a functional map that pinpoints the part of the cerebral cortex that governs a certain activity, such as speech, sensation, or movement in a particular part of the body.

Identification of the roles played by sections of the brain has advanced neurology by allowing surgeons to avoid vital functional areas when removing **brain tumors/spinal cord tumors** or operating to treat **epilepsy**. Cerebral localization has also made it possible to identify where a brain tumor is located by observing the symptoms it causes. Finally, cerebral localization has contributed greatly to our understanding of how the brain works.

In his 1740 book, *Oeconomia regni animalis,* Emanuel Swedenborg (1688–1772) suggested that functions were located in discrete parts of the cerebral cortex, which he theorized were separated by fissures and gyri—the "wrinkles" of the cerebrum. The motor functions, Swedenborg proposed, were located at the front of the brain, with distinct regions corresponding to certain parts of the body. He believed that automatic motor functions were controlled by centers in the medulla and spinal cord.

Swedenborg went on to found the Swedenborg Church, and though his thoughts on cerebral location were largely correct, they were not widely known until neurologists already had discovered and accepted cerebral localization on their own.

Mainstream medical thought on cerebral localization sprang from phrenology, the pseudoscience of examining the shapes of people's skulls to determine their aptitudes and behaviors. Franz Joseph Gall (1758–1828) first suggested that brain development might be discernible by examining the shape of the skull.

Gall claimed that he conceived of his ideas as a child, when he noticed that students with good verbal memories tended to have bulging eyes. He began lecturing on his ideas in Vienna in 1796, but the Austrian government—driven by local church authorities—barred him from lecturing in 1802. He moved to Paris and began writing on phrenology in 1808. Gall pursued his ideas by examining the skulls of prominent men and women with special talents, as well as criminals and the insane. He collected 300 skulls and made more than 120 casts of living people's skulls. He ultimately came up with 27 characteristics that he thought could be localized, including acquisitiveness, destructiveness, and philoprogenitiveness (love of children).

Aside from this largely invalid information, Gall also collected relevant information on cases of patients who lost certain abilities after suffering injuries to a particular part of the brain.

French physiologist Marie-Jean-Pierre Flourens (1794–1864) rejected phrenology, and believed he had disproved the idea of cerebral localization in experiments he conducted with animals.

The first function to be firmly linked to a locus on the cortex was the function of speech, located on the frontal cortex by Paul Broca (1824–1880) and reported in 1861. Broca used the case of Monsieur Leborgne, who suffered epilepsy, paralysis of the right side of his body, and aphasia. Although others had argued for and against this idea before him, Broca's complete and detailed case history of this patient settled the question for many of his colleagues.

Edouard Hitzig (1838–1907) and Gustav Fritsch (1838–1927) discovered the motor area in the cortex of a dog in 1870. Using electrical stimulus they found areas on the animal's brain that when touched produced movement in a specific body part. They also noted that destroying the area of an animal's brain that controls the forepaw didn't impair sensation in the forepaw, but did produce abnormal motion in that part of the limb.

Sir David Farrier (1843–1928) continued these experiments, working with monkeys and other animals, and produced more detailed brain maps.

In the early 1900s, a number of anatomists observed that cell structure varied throughout the brain, supporting the theory of cerebral localization.

Today the idea of cerebral location for many functions is generally accepted, but only a small portion of the cerebrum has been mapped. General mental functions such as intellect and memory are thought to be located in the frontal lobe, but cannot be compartmentalized as can senses such as vision and hearing.

Additional reading: Kosslyn and Koenig, *Wet Mind*, pp. 4–15.

cerebrospinal fluid (CSF)

Cerebrospinal fluid (CSF) is the liquid that fills the spinal canal and cranium. For a long time, the examination of this fluid was the single tool available to doctors for assessing neurological health, and "spinal taps" remain an important technique for detecting certain diseases.

Claudius Galen (129–c.199) had observed fluid in the ventricles of the brain of living animals; he deduced that the brain produced the fluid, which he theorized provided energy for the whole body. In 1764, Domenico Cotugno (1736–1822) observed correctly that the fluid surrounding the brain and the fluid in the spine were continuous.

In 1825, French anatomist Francois Magendie (1783–1855) proved that spinal fluid was always present. His contemporaries had thought CSF only appeared in disease. Two years later, he suggested that changes in the pressure of this fluid might have something to do with apoplexy and **hydrocephalus**. He was wrong about the former, but correct about the latter.

Heinrich Quinke (1842–1922) developed the technique of lumbar puncture (or spinal tap), making it possible to sample and analyze CSF, perfecting his technique in 1891. William Mestrezat (1883–1928) provided the first comprehensive description of the chemical composition of CSF in 1911.

Additional reading: Spillane, *The Doctrine of the Nerves,* pp. 120–23.

cervical cancer

Cervical **cancer** is cancer of the neck of the uterus, which links this organ to the vagina. In the United States and other developed countries, cervical cancer is rarely fatal because most women receive regular **Pap smears** to screen for precancerous cells, which can then be removed before invasive cancer develops. However, in nations where women do not receive regular screening, cervical cancer remains a leading killer.

The cellular changes that may herald early cancer growth, also called dysplasia, were first described in 1900. In 1962, because of confusion over what constituted severe dysplasia and what was cancer in situ, the First International Congress on Exfoliated Cytology defined both terms. "Cervical intraepithelial neoplasia" is now the preferred term for describing the range of cellular changes.

Treatment for cervical cancer until quite recently had been to remove a cone-shaped section of the cervix (conization) for diagnostic purposes and then perform a hysterectomy if cancer was found. Research by Norwegian gynecologist Per Kolstadt (1925–) during the 1970s showed that conization was enough. Today, treatment of early-stage cervical cancer can include conization, **electrocautery**, **cryosurgery**, or **laser surgery** to remove abnormal **tissue.**

In 1995, a panel convened by the **World Health Organization (WHO)** concluded that there is compelling evidence for a connection between infection with human papilloma **virus** (HPV), the agent that causes genital warts, and cervical cancer. There are more than 70 known HPV types, and some are more strongly associated with cervical cancer and with more severe disease. Several studies completed in 2000 found that HPV screening is helpful in detecting cervical cancer.

Additional reading: Rosenthal, *The Gynecological Sourcebook,* pp. 239–64.

cesarean section (c-section)

In a cesarean section, a baby is delivered by surgically opening the mother's womb, usually via the abdomen. This procedure may be performed for a variety of reasons—because a baby is too large, or a woman's pelvis is too small, or a combination of both. It also is often done to prevent a baby from becoming infected with a disease the mother has, such as herpes or **AIDS**. About one in five births in the United States is by cesarean section.

Contrary to popular belief, the cesarean section is not named after Julius Caesar (100–444 B.C.), and the Roman emperor was not delivered by this method. The operation was certainly performed in ancient times and in the Middle Ages, but usually only when the mother was dying or dead.

The first documented cesarean section on a living woman was performed in Germany in 1610. The mother lived for 25 days. In Virginia, the country doctor Jesse Bennett (1769–1842) performed the first cesarean section in the United States in 1794, on his wife.

The operation remained rare in the next century; by 1878 only about 80 cesarean sections had been performed in the United States, and the mortality rate for mothers was more than half. It was only until antiseptic and aseptic technique became widespread, and physicians began suturing the incision in the uterus after performing the operation (previously, it had been left open), that the operation became safe. (*See also* antisepsis; asepsis.)

Additional reading: Speert, *Obstetrics and Gynecology,* pp. 297–316.

Chagas' disease

Chagas' disease is a parasitic infection, common in South America, that the Brazilian physician Carlos Chagas (1879–1934) discovered in 1909. He began investigating the disease after hearing about a blood-sucking bug called the "barbiero," or barber bug, while heading an antimalaria campaign in a small Brazilian town where railroad workers lived.

The disease kills about 10 percent of people in their first bout with it, and can leave survivors with lasting symptoms including heart arrythmias. It plagues mainly poor people and children and is the second most common insect- or animal-borne disease in Latin America, after **malaria**. The disease is carried by a tiny organism called a trypanosome that is transmitted through bug bites. There is no cure for the chronic stage of Chagas' disease when organ damage has occurred.

Additional reading: Kiple, *The Cambridge World History of Human Disease,* pp. 636–38.

chemotherapy

Chemotherapy is the use of chemicals to fight disease. Today, the word is most often used to describe drugs used to fight **cancer**. Chemotherapy drugs for cancer are toxic and can have serious side effects, since most of them work by destroying rapidly growing cancer cells and thus they destroy some healthy cells in the process. Also, tumor cells can develop resistance to cancer drugs.

Pharmacologist and immunologist Paul Ehrlich (1854–1915) pioneered the chemical treatment of disease. He launched his study by looking for chemical agents that

would attack the disease microbe but not its animal host, like a "magic bullet." He began his investigation with dyes, which were easy to observe under a microscope. The 606th compound he looked at, **Salvarsan,** proved to be the first effective treatment for **syphilis**. Ehrlich announced his discovery of the first chemotherapeutic agent in 1910.

The era of cancer chemotherapy began in the 1940s, when the first effective drugs for treating cancer were introduced. The first modern cancer chemotherapy was an alkylating agent called **nitrogen mustard,** first used in patients in the 1940s.

Today there are dozens of chemotherapy drugs for cancer that fall into several classes based on their source and mode of action: **alkylating agents**; **antimetabolites**; natural products such as the **vinca alkaloids**, **taxol**, **podophyllotoxin** derivatives, and **anti-tumor antibiotics**; and **hormones** and hormone-antagonists such as forms of **estrogen, tamoxifen,** and corticosteroids.

In 1955, a Cancer Chemotherapy National Service Center was established at the National Cancer Institute to develop and evaluate drugs for cancer chemotherapy and coordinate clinical trials.

In the 1960s, a new era of cancer chemotherapy began when Howard E. Skipper (1915–) and Frank M. Schabel (1918–) set forth a series of principles of chemotherapy and cancer growth, based on research in mice, that remain in use today. A central point of their principles was that a single cancerous cell can multiply and eventually kill its host. They also observed that tumors grew exponentially at first; that cancer drugs killed a consistent proportion of tumor cells, no matter how many were present; and that the number of cancer cells was inversely related to the curability of a cancer with chemotherapy. Basically, they showed that certain types of cancers could indeed be cured if chemotherapy was delivered in the right doses at the right time.

Today a person receiving chemotherapy treatment for cancer will generally receive several different drugs, which are chosen to maximize tumor-killing action while minimizing the destruction of normal tissue.

Additional reading: Hellman and Vokes, "Advancing Current Treatments for Cancer."

chicken pox

Chicken pox is a highly contagious infection with the varicella-zoster **virus**. Once people have caught chicken pox, they are immune to it, although the virus can remain dormant in the body. Shingles, a painful infection of the nerves in the torso, occurs when the virus is reactivated, usually when the immune system is weak. In children, chicken pox is a mild disease, but the infection can be serious and even fatal in adults and in people with weak immune systems.

The Italian physician Giovanni Filippo Ingrassia (1510–1580) is thought to have first distinguished between chicken pox and **scarlet fever** in 1553. The British doctor William Heberden (1710–1801) provided a clinical description of chicken pox in 1785.

The name "chicken pox" first appeared in medical literature in 1694 in the writings of English physician Richard Morton (1637–1698).

Thomas Milton Rivers (1888–1962) and William Smith Tillet (1892–1974) isolated the varicella-zoster virus in 1924.

In 1995, a **vaccine** for chicken pox became available for the first time. People who are infected with chicken pox and are at a high risk of developing complications may be given **antibodies** to help fight the virus.

Additional reading: Kiple, *The Cambridge World History of Human Disease*, pp. 1092–94.

Chinese medicine

Chinese medicine is an ancient system of remedies and diagnostic techniques.

Medical historians divide Chinese medicine into three stages: Chinese Folk Medicine, which probably dates back to prehistoric times and held sway until about 1000 B.C.; Traditional Chinese Medicine, dating from that time until the beginning of the twentieth century; and the New Chinese Medicine of the twentieth century, which attempts to meld Eastern and Western medicine.

Chinese medicine in all its stages focuses on treating illness by maintaining and restoring the proper flow of *qi*, the life force. **Acupuncture** and moxibustion are intended to reroute *qi*.

Major figures in the history of Chinese medicine include Fu Hsi, a mythical person credited with inventing the fundamentals of civilization such as the calendar and family structure, in 4000 B.C.; Shen Nung, of roughly 3000 B.C., who is considered the inventor of **herbal medicine** and the author of a work called *Great Herbal*; and the Yellow Emperor, the author of Chinese civilization's first major medical work, dated around 2700 B.C. This book, the *Yellow Emperor's Canon of Internal Medicine,* describes acupuncture extensively and could be considered analogous to the **Hippocratic Corpus** in terms of its subsequent influence on medical theory and practice.

The concept of *qi* comes from the philosopher Chuang Tze (369–286 B.C.). Another ancient concept of Chinese medicine, intriguingly similar to early medical ideas of the West and of **Ayurveda**, is the idea that health is based on the balance of five elements. Chinese medicine also calls for a balance of the male and female principles, yin and yang. An important diagnostic technique in early Chinese medicine was the reading of the pulse.

In the beginning of the first millennium, pioneering Chinese medical theorists included Chun Yu I who developed a system of medical records; Chang Chung Ching, who wrote a book of disease classifications and drug formulations; and Hua T'o (141–208), considered the father of Chinese surgery.

With the revolution of 1911, Chinese leaders attempted to modernize the nation's health with public health efforts, medical schools, and doctors' groups and medical journals. Pharmaceutical research in the 1920s established the effectiveness of some long-used Chinese herbs, such as ephedra, the source of **ephedrine**.

In 1929, the Chinese government attempted to ban old-style Chinese medicine. Despite restrictions on the training and practice of traditional medicine, the techniques and treatments did not disappear, but were sustained by the large rural population as well as the effectiveness of these therapies and the relative cheapness and wide availability of medicinal plants.

Tan Zonghai was one of the first scholars to recommend, in the mid-nineteenth century, that traditional Chinese medicine and Western medicine be reconciled into a single system. This was also a goal sought by public health leaders in Communist China, spelled out at the 1950 National Conference on Health. In 1965, Chairman Mao Tse-Tung (1893–1976) called for medicine to concentrate on the rural population, and "barefoot doctors" who treated this population made their first appearance in the following year.

Today the benefits of many traditional Chinese medical techniques, such as acupuncture and t'ai chi, are increasingly recognized and being incorporated into Western medicine. (*See also* alternative medicine)

Additional reading: Hoizey, *A History of Chinese Medicine;* Porter, *Medicine*, pp. 102–05.

chiropractic

Chiropractic is a school of medical thought based on the idea that many neurological and musculoskeletal problems are caused by misalignments of the spine, and that realigning or "adjusting" the spine will cure these problems.

Daniel David Palmer (1845–1913) was the originator of chiropractic. He founded the Palmer School in Davenport, Iowa, in 1898. Five of his first 15 students were medical doctors.

Chiropractic, like other alternative medical systems such as **osteopathy**, struggled for acceptance throughout the twentieth century. Early on, many osteopaths and chiropractors were granted licenses through correspondence courses. For this reason, and others, the American Medical Association (AMA) has been one of chiropractic's chief enemies; the *Journal of the American Medical Association's* (JAMA) editor in 1925 called osteopathy a means of entering medicine by the back door, and chiropractic an entry through the cellar.

Because so many patients felt that chiropractic had helped them, the medical establishment eventually began to accept the treatment. The **U.S. Public Health Service** conducted a study of chiropractic, holding a conference in 1974, and that same year the Council on Chiropractic Education was designated by the government to be the official accrediting body for chiropractic colleges.

Now, students who want to become chiropractors in the United States must have two years of college training in the basic medical sciences and four years of chiropractic college. Congress voted to cover chiropractic under **Medicare/Medicaid** in 1972, and today, many health plans cover chiropractic adjustments. After being sued, the AMA in 1980 changed its code of ethics to allow members to refer their patients to chiropractors. (*See also* alternative medicine)

Additional reading: Wardwell, *Chiropractic*.

chloral hydrate

Chloral hydrate came into use as a sedative and sleeping draught in 1869.

This bad-tasting liquid loses its effectiveness if used frequently, and can be addictive. Criminals used chloral hydrate in "Mickey Finns," sedating drinks given to put prospective victims to sleep.

Chloral hydrate, which was the first safe hypnotic drug to be discovered, is still used today as a sedative for children.

Additional reading: Breimer, *Pharmacokinetics of Hypnotic Drugs*.

chloroform

Chloroform was one of the first effective drugs used for **anesthesia**.

Samuel Guthrie (1782–1848), an American chemist, invented chloroform in 1831.

The Scottish physician James Young Simpson (1811–1870) first tried chloroform as an anesthetic. He used it to ease a patient's childbirth pains for the first time in 1848.

Queen Victoria (1819–1901) promoted acceptance of chloroform among the people (and the medical establishment) when she used it during labor for the birth of two of her children in 1853 and 1857. Of the first birth, the queen wrote in her journal, chloroform's effect was "soothing, quieting, and delightful beyond measure."

The use of chloroform was discontinued after it became clear that the gas would damage the liver and also caused many more patient deaths than **ether.**

Additional reading: Friedman and Friedland, *Medicine's 10 Greatest Discoveries*, pp. 110–11.

chlorothiazide

Chlorothiazide, or Diuril, a drug used to treat high **blood pressure**, was the first **diuretic** drug not based on mercury.

Chemists at Merck, a pharmaceutical company, synthesized chlorothiazide in 1955 while looking for a drug that would share the diuretic properties of the sulfa drugs without causing the body to excrete bicarbonate. The drug reduces blood pressure by increasing the release of salt and water from the kidneys.

The first patient to receive the drug, in 1956, was a 60-year-old man suffering from heart failure. He lost 20 pounds of water weight, and his blood pressure fell. The **Food and Drug Administration (FDA)** approved chlorothiazide in 1958. Millions of people with high blood pressure or heart failure have taken Diuril, which is safe and effective, although it can cause **cholesterol** levels to rise and potassium to be depleted.

Additional reading: Sneader, *Drug Discovery*, p. 158.

cholera

Cholera is a diarrheal disease caused by infection with the *Vibrio cholerae* bacterium. The bug secretes a toxin that prevents the small intestine from absorbing salts and water, resulting in a massive loss of fluids and electrolytes that can be fatal. Cholera is spread by water contaminated with human stool containing the bacteria.

Cholera erupts in epidemics in some areas and then disappears for years; the trigger is unknown. Many scientists believe that weather plays a role.

Cholera is endemic to the Ganges River delta of India and Bangladesh, and has spread to the rest of the world in a series of seven pandemics that began in 1817. Cholera first struck Europe in 1831, and appeared in North America the following year. The seventh pandemic began in 1961, and continues today. The first descriptions of cholera in Western literature were from sixteenth century Portuguese explorers, who had seen the disease in their travels to India.

Cholera has a mortality rate of up to 70 percent if it is left untreated, but **oral rehydration therapy** can bring mortality down to 1 percent. Treatment generally consists of replacing lost fluids and electrolytes orally or intravenously. There is currently no vaccination against cholera.

Early treatment for cholera—as for many diseases of the time—consisted of purging and bleeding. A popular treatment in India was to apply a red-hot iron to the heel.

Scottish doctor Thomas Latta administered injections of saline solution to treat cholera for the first time in 1832. About a third of the patients who received the therapy recovered. Although Latta was ahead of his time, he was treating very ill patients, which was probably the reason for his poor success rate. His contemporaries condemned his approach. Intravenous rehydration for cholera was perfected by Leonard Rogers (1868–1962), working in Calcutta in the early twentieth century.

British physician John Snow (1813–1858), who believed correctly that cholera was an intestinal disease transmitted by an organism found in drinking water, proved his theory with the famous analyses of water and cholera in London neighborhoods in his 1855 book, *On the Mode of Communication of Cholera*. He found that neighborhoods getting their water from the Thames downstream from sewage outflows had high cholera mortality rates, while those that got their water from the river above the outflows had no cholera deaths. At the time, however, Snow's claims were doubted. His experiment did not become an epidemiological classic until the 1930s. The prevailing view was that "miasma" (fog or vapors) transmitted cholera, or that the disease had something to do with elevation above sea level.

Robert Koch (1843–1910) discovered the bacillus that spreads the disease in Egypt in 1884. However, Filippo Pacini (1812–1883) of Florence had reported in 1854 that *miriadi di vibrioni*—"many vibrios"—were seen in cholera, and he also had described the disease correctly as a massive loss of fluid and electrolytes due to the action of the vibrio in the small intestine. In recognition of Pacini's discovery, the vibrio was renamed *Vibrio cholerae Pacini 1854* in 1965.

The Indian physician Sambu Nath De showed in 1958 that a toxin produced by the cholera vibrio is responsible for fluid and electrolyte loss.

Additional reading: Kiple, *The Cambridge World History of Human Disease*, pp. 642–49.

cholesterol

Cholesterol is a nutrient found in eggs and animal foods that the body uses to make steroid hormones. High levels of cholesterol can lead to heart disease.

After a series of experiments in which they fed eggs to animals, Nikolai Anichkov (1885–1964) and his colleagues reported in 1913 that cholesterol was the main substance responsible for inducing **atherosclerosis.**

In 1924, Anichkov adjusted his theory, suggesting that since some animals that are fed cholesterol did not develop atherosclerosis, it was necessary for the animals also to develop high levels of blood cholesterol—hypercholesterolemia—in order for plaques to form in the blood vessels. He also posited that inflammation of the artery lining and high **blood pressure** might play a role in atherosclerosis development in humans.

In 1950, John Goffman (1918–) of the University of California at Berkeley and his colleagues first distinguished between high-density lipoprotein (HDL) and low-density lipoprotein (LDL), now popularly known as "good" and "bad" cholesterol, respectively. They also observed that high levels of LDL appeared to be associated with heart attack and heart disease. The role of LDL as "bad" cholesterol was confirmed by epidemiological studies in the 1960s and 1970s.

Researchers showed in 1952 that humans could lower their blood cholesterol by staying away from animal fats and eating plant foods. Edward H. Ahrens (1915–) of Rockefeller University and his colleagues demonstrated that this was because vegetable fats were less saturated than animal fats.

The medical community's interest in the issue was minimal until William Dock (1898–1990) wrote a powerful editorial in the journal *Circulation*, in 1958, chastising his colleagues for ignoring the role of dietary cholesterol in heart disease.

Understanding of how cholesterol is synthesized, absorbed, and destroyed in the body became more clear in the 1960s and 1970s. Researchers also learned that cholesterol consumption is not solely responsible for high cholesterol, but that emotional and genetic factors also play a role.

Today cholesterol levels can be controlled with a new generation of **cholesterol-lowering drugs**, although diet and exercise remain crucial in cholesterol control and heart-disease prevention. (*See also* hypertension)

Additional reading: Friedman and Friedland, *Medicine's 10 Greatest Discoveries*, pp. 153–67.

cholesterol-lowering drugs

Cholesterol-lowering drugs reduce the level of fats in the blood, thus protecting a person against heart disease and heart attack.

The newest of these drugs, which are also known as antilipemic drugs, work by inhibiting the action of HMG-CoA reductase, an enzyme involved in the synthesis of **cholesterol**.

Several drugs were introduced to lower cholesterol in the 1950s and 1960s, including nicotinic acid, D-thyroxine, cholesteryamine, clofibrate, neomycin, and **estrogen**. Of these drugs, clofibrate had been the most commonly used; it accelerates the breakdown of fat particles, but it lowers cholesterol only slightly for most people. The other drugs all had troublesome side effects.

Japanese scientists began searching in 1971 for HMG-CoA reductase inhibitors that could be used as cholesterol-lowering drugs, looking for them among compounds produced by microorganisms. The team had determined the structure of the first, mevastatin, by 1973. This substance was produced by a strain of **penicillin** mold.

Clinical trials of mevastatin in patients with a genetic condition that causes them to have very high cholesterol began in 1976; the drug lowered total cholesterol and LDL cholesterol in most. But the drug was found toxic in animal trials, so clinical trials in humans were suspended in 1980. Merck, a pharmaceutical company, isolated a drug similar to mevastatin, lovastatin, in 1979. After clinical trials found lovastatin was safe and more effective than mevastatin in reducing cholesterol levels, the **Food and Drug Administration (FDA)** approved the drug in 1987. Pravastatin, a drug derived from mevastatin, was released in 1989. Other similar drugs include simvastatin and fluvastatin.

These drugs have been found to be effective in slowing the progression of heart disease and in some cases reversing it.

Additional reading: "Cholesterol Drugs," *Consumer Reports.*

chorionic villus sampling (CVS)

Chorionic villus sampling is a technique for prenatal genetic testing. Between the ninth and twelfth week of pregnancy, cells are obtained from the villi, which are hairlike projections from the chorion, the outer tissue of the sac surrounding the embryo.

From 1968 to 1975, Danish and Swedish researchers were performing the procedure by inserting instruments through the pregnant woman's cervix. Their efforts were experimental, as the women were volunteers who planned to have **abortions**. The researchers experienced several problems and didn't obtain useful samples.

Scientists in Moscow performed the first sampling of the chorion while using **ultrasound** to visualize their instruments and the structures within the body. They tested 110 patients without serious complications, reporting their results in 1982. Two years later it became possible to test the sampled tissue without culturing it first, which led to results in hours rather than weeks.

Dr. Laird Jackson (1930–) in Philadelphia opened the first CVS program in the United States.

CVS carries a slightly higher risk of miscarriage and fetal damage than **amniocentesis**, and may result in false positives because placental cells can carry abnormalities that the fetus doesn't. CVS had originally been introduced as an earlier alternative to amniocentesis, but the time in which the two procedures can be offered is getting closer.

Additional reading: Galton, *Med Tech,* pp. 122–25.

chromosome

Chromosomes are structures found in cell nuclei that carry the genetic material known as **DNA**. The name chromosome, which means "colored bodies," comes from the fact that chromosomes take up dye more readily than other cell structures. During a special type of cell division called meiosis, the normal number of chromosomes is halved and germ cells—eggs or sperm in humans—are created. In sexual reproduction, each germ cell carries half the number of chromosomes of the parent animal, and the two germ cells unite to form a new individual.

Ernst Haeckel (1834–1919) proposed in the 1860s that the cell nucleus played a role in passing along inherited traits. Working with egg and sperm cells from seahorses in 1875, Oskar Hertwig (1849–1922) observed that when the two cells united their nuclei joined to form a single structure. Walther Flemming (1843–1905), a German chemist, first observed chromosomes four years later, noting that they looked like minuscule bunches of thread. He called the material "chromatin," and they were later dubbed chromosomes. Belgian researcher Pierre Joseph van Beneden (1809–1894) observed in 1883, while studying the germ cells of worms, that sperm and egg chromosomes mixed during fertilization.

In 1903, two scientists working independently—Walter Sutton (1877–1916) in the United States and Theodor Boveri (1862–1915) in Germany—observed that chromosomes were retained in normal cell division but halved in sperm and egg cells, which united to form a new full set of chromosomes in fertilized eggs.

In 1910, the American geneticist Thomas Hunt Morgan (1866–1945) noticed that a mutant trait among fruit flies followed the inheritance of the male chromosome. He also observed that sex is determined by the pairing of two X chromosomes, for a female, or an X and a Y, for a male. Morgan won the Nobel Prize in 1933 for his work with genetics.

Once **chromosome banding** was invented in 1970, it was possible for scientists to identify each of the 24 human chromosomes based on the unique pattern in which each of them absorb dye. Scientists are now able to analyze chromosomes at the molecular level using a number of different techniques.

Additional reading: Therman, *Human Chromosomes.*

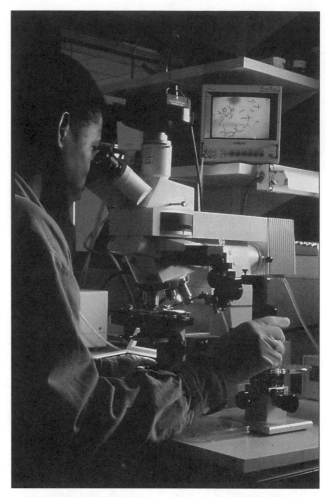

A scientist at the NIHGR performs a chromosomal microdissection using a compound microscope. Similar techniques have been used to identify genes linked to certain types of cancer, such as BRCA1 and 2 (breast cancer). (Courtesy of National Institute for Human Genome Research.)

chromosome banding

Chromosome banding is a technique for identifying **chromosome** pairs and analyzing regions within chromosomes. Dye is added to the chromosomes, which absorb the coloring in patterns that reveal the composition of nucleic acids within. Each of the 24 human chromosomes has a distinctive banding pattern.

Before chromosome banding, it was impossible to visualize the composition of chromosomes, or even to identify which chromosome was which. Torbjorn O. Caspersson (1910–) of the Karolinska Institute in Sweden was the first to perform this procedure, in 1970. Caspersson and his colleagues treated chromosomes with quinacrine mustard and then exposed them to fluorescent light. After analyzing 5,000 chromosomes, they established that each of the 24 human chromosome pairs had a unique fluorescence pattern. He and his colleagues also devised a system for numbering the chromosomes, which was officially accepted at the Paris Conference on Standardization in Human Cytogenetics in 1971.

Banding, now a routine procedure, paved the way for **DNA fingerprinting,** detection of genetic defects, **gene mapping**, and other technologies.

Additional reading: Aldridge, *The Thread of Life,* pp. 58–65.

cimetidine

Cimetidine is a drug released in 1977 that revolutionized ulcer treatment.

Ulcers are places where the stomach lining has been eroded. Stomach acid secretions can worsen ulcers and slow healing. Cimetidine works by repressing the secretion of stomach acids, which allows ulcers to heal.

James W. Black (1924–) began a search for an ulcer drug in the early 1960s based on the idea that it would be possible to block the stomach's secretion of acid. In 1972, he and his colleagues discovered a group of drugs that did this and named them H2 blockers. These drugs, including cimetidine, are called H2 **antihistamines** because they block receptors in the stomach that release acid when exposed to **histamine**. (Allergies are treated with H1 antihistamines.) Cimetidine helps ulcers heal, and low doses can prevent new ulcers from forming.

Researchers have since discovered that ulcers are almost always caused by infection with the **H. pylori (Helicobacter pylori)** bacterium, so treatment with antibiotics can eradicate them, but patients may also require treatment with cimetidine to help the ulcers heal.

Additional reading: Bindra and Lednicer, eds., *Chronicles of Drug Discovery, Vol. 1,* pp. 1–38.

cingulotomy

Cingulotomy is a surgical procedure in which the cingulate gyrus, a structure within the brain, is partially removed.

This structure is part of the limbic system, which controls emotions, and altering connections within it can affect the perception and expression of emotions. This operation is performed today to ease intractable pain and to treat mood and anxiety disorders that do not respond to other types of treatment.

John Fulton (1899–1960) first suggested the surgery in the 1940s. Eldon Foltz (1919–) of the University of California and his colleagues performed the first cingulotomy to treat chronic pain in 1962.

Cingulotomy can relieve pain immediately, but when the operation is performed to treat anxiety, these symptoms don't abate until months after surgery. However, cingulotomy produces relatively few side effects on personality and does not permanently impair cognition.

H. Thomas Ballantine (1912–) began popularizing the surgery in the late 1960s, and developed guidelines for which patients should have cingulotomy.

Additional reading: Herbert, "Psychosurgery Redux."

circulation

Circulation is the continuous path blood follows from the heart to arteries, **capillaries**, and veins, and back to the heart again, first described by William Harvey (1578–1657) in 1628.

In 1603, Harvey's teacher Fabrici (1537–1619) published the results of an experiment proving that veins in the

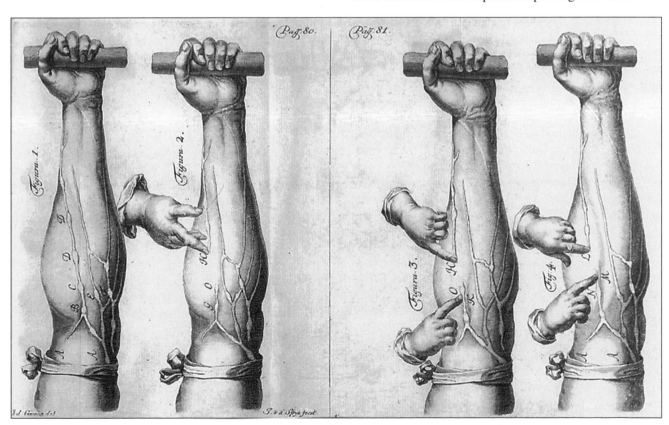

Woodcut from William Harvey's 1628 book, *De Motu Cordis,* illustrating the principle of circulation. (Courtesy of New York Academy of Medicine.)

arms contain valves that allow blood to flow in only one direction, toward the heart. He tied a tourniquet around a person's arm above the elbow tightly enough to block blood flow. The veins swelled below the tourniquet, proving that the blood couldn't flow "backward." Harvey went further, using the same experiment setup, by manually pushing all of the blood out of the veins toward the upper arms so the veins were flat. The veins refilled beginning at the fingers. Harvey proposed, correctly, that the heart pumps the blood through the body, back to the right heart, out through the lungs, and back to the left heart where the cycle begins again.

The discovery that blood circulates through the body was a major milestone in medicine because it paved the way for the understanding that blood distributes oxygen and nutrients throughout the body and collects wastes for excretion. Also, understanding of the mechanism of circulation was central to the ultimate understanding of the heart's function and structure.

Additional reading: Callahan, et. al, *Classics of Cardiology, Volume III,* pp. 13–79; Friedman and Friedland, *Medicine's 10 Greatest Discoveries,* pp.18–36.

circumcision

Circumcision is an operation, usually performed shortly after a boy's birth, in which the foreskin of the penis is removed. The surgery is part of Jewish and Islamic tradition. Many parents also have their sons circumcised for reasons of hygiene and personal preference.

The surgery is one of the oldest in human history. In the ancient Egyptian Book of the Dead, the hieroglyph for "penis" shows a circumcised organ. In his writings, the tenth-century Arab physician Albucasis recommends using shears to perform circumcision, but suggests that the surgeon hide them in his sleeve or under his foot until the last possible moment.

Circumcision can prevent urinary tract infections and sexually transmitted disease, and penile **cancer** occurs half as often in circumcised men as in uncircumcised men. Both the Jewish physician Moses Maimonides (1135–1204) and the father of psychoanalysis, Sigmund Freud (1856–1939) suggested that circumcision also reduces sexual pleasure for the male, although there have been no studies proving or disproving this theory.

In 1999, the American Academy of Pediatrics issued a statement on circumcision that declared there is no strong medical reason for boys to be circumcised, and that if circumcision is performed, the child should be given a local anesthetic to dull the pain.

Additional reading: Speert, *Obstetrics and Gynecology,* pp. 324–30.

Clean Air Act

The Clean Air Act of 1970 marks the beginning of efforts to put air pollution control in the hands of the federal government.

Air pollution control is important to health because air contaminated with certain chemicals can cause **cancer**, respiratory problems, reproductive problems, and other ailments.

The first local attempts to control air pollution in the United States were laws passed in 1881 in Chicago and Cincinnati, to curb smoke and soot emissions from factories in which were soon emulated by other cities. The first state to pass air pollution control legislation was Oregon in 1952, and the first federal law addressing air pollution was the Air Pollution Control Act of 1955, which provided grants to states.

The broader Clean Air Act of 1963 funded federal research, provided additional support for states, and directed the U.S. government to become involved in air pollution cases that crossed state boundaries. Two years later, an amendment ordered the Department of Health, Education, and Welfare to establish emission standards for automobiles, trucks, and other motor vehicles. The Air Quality Act, passed in 1967, provided more support to states and required them to establish Air Quality Control Regions.

The Clean Air Act of 1970 marked a major change in air pollution control policy, because it redirected responsibility for this issue to the federal government. President Richard Nixon (1913–1994) and Maine Senator Edmund Muskie (1914–1996) were the leaders in this effort. For the first time, limits were set on emissions of specific substances: lead, carbon monoxide, ozone, nitrogen dioxide, particulate matter (fine particles of soot, heavy metals, and other substances), and sulfur dioxide. The **Environmental Protection Agency (EPA)**, also created in 1970, was required to establish emissions standards for these chemicals. Separate requirements were set for automobile emissions to dramatically cut production of carbon monoxide, hydrocarbons, and nitrogen oxide by 1975. An amendment to the law passed in 1977, which had been supported by environmentalists, protected air that was of better quality than Clean Air Act standards, such as the air in national parks and wilderness areas.

Amendments to the act stalled during the administration of Ronald Reagan (1911–), but his successor George H. Bush (1924–) and another Maine senator, George Mitchell (1933–), led efforts to pass new amendments to the act in 1990. The main components of the law were requirements for major reduction in sulfur dioxide and nitrogen oxide emissions to prevent acid rain; new regulations for 189 toxic chemical air pollutants; tougher requirements on automobile emissions; and eventual banning of three types of chemicals implicated in the depletion of the ozone layer: chloroflourocarbons, hydrochlorofluorocarbons, and methyl chloroform. The law also allowed factories and power plants to "trade" pollution credits among themselves. Cities with the most pollution, such as Los Angeles and New York, were required to adhere to stricter emissions standards. The 1990 act also regulated emissions from small businesses, such as dry cleaners, for the first time.

Clean air legislation has been most successful in controlling lead, carbon monoxide, and sulfur dioxide levels. Lead has been dramatically reduced because of the gradual phase-out of leaded gasoline.

Additional reading: Bryner, *Blue Skies, Green Politics.*

Clean Water Act

The Clean Water Act, first passed in 1972, shifted efforts to control water pollution in the United States into the hands of the federal government.

Water contaminated with sewage and agricultural and industrial runoff poses many dangers to human health. Dirty water can spread disease and it may also be implicated in the development of certain **cancers**.

Congress passed the Water Pollution Control Act in 1948, which provided states with funding for water pollution control, and federal funding for these efforts grew through the 1950s and 1960s. In 1965, the Water Quality Act created the Federal Water Pollution Control Administration to set and enforce water quality standards.

Amendments passed in 1972, after some dispute between President Richard Nixon (1913–1994) and Congress over how to respond to public concerns over water pollution, which set forth the goal of improving water quality to the point where fish, wildlife, and shellfish would be protected. The amendments also required that all pollution discharge into navigable waters be ended by 1985. To achieve these goals, the government provided funding for research into pollution control technology, waste treatment plants, and local pollution control. Funding for sewage treatment facility construction was boosted from $1.25 billion in 1971 to $7 billion in 1975.

Industries that polluted water were given two deadlines: "Best Practicable Technology" for effluent control had to be in place by 1977, and "Best Available Technology" was to be installed by 1985.

These requirements were scaled back with 1977 amendments to the federal law, because most major municipalities had not met scheduled requirements. The Water Quality Act of 1987 substituted loans for grants for establishing wastewater treatment plants, which would be completely phased out by 1994. It also included grants to clean up water in specific areas, such as Boston Harbor and the Chesapeake Bay.

Some critics say the Clean Water Act has been stalled during the 1990s. In 1998, President Bill Clinton proposed a $2.3 billion Clean Water Action Plan to control agricultural runoff and initiate other water pollution prevention measures.

Additional reading: Loeb, "Very Troubled Waters."

cleft lip/cleft palate repair

Cleft palate is a congenital condition in which the upper part of the palate fails to close. Cleft lip, also known as harelip, usually accompanies cleft palate, although a person may have a cleft lip alone.

The first surgical repair of a cleft lip was reported in China in about 390 A.D. The 18-year-old boy who received the surgery went on to become governor general of six provinces. By 1000 A.D., Arab surgeons had refined their technique for repairing cleft lip, and British surgeons wrote about using silk to close cleft lips in about 950 A.D. But it was centuries later before the first successful surgical closure of the palate was reported, by Karl Ferdinand von Graefe (1787–1840) in Berlin in 1816.

In the eighteenth century, European surgeons—Ambrose Pare (c.1510–1590) was the first—developed a number of different obdurators, used to close off the palate and separate the mouth from the nasal cavity, making eating and breathing easier for people with cleft palate.

From von Graefe's time to the present, surgeons have tried dozens of techniques to repair cleft palate and lip in children without impairing facial growth. Today, **plastic surgery** can do a great deal to give people with cleft palate a more normal appearance and better oral function, although the surgery is still not perfect.

Additional reading: LeVay, *The History of Orthopaedics.*

clinical trials

Clinical trials are scientific experiments designed to evaluate the effectiveness of medical treatment. James Lind (1716–1794) is credited with conducting the first clinical trial, in 1747. His subjects were 12 patients with **scurvy**, and Lind found those given oranges and lemons improved the quickest.

Throughout the nineteenth century, similar studies were done on treatments for **smallpox**, **diphtheria**, and **cholera**.

Today, the prospective, randomized, controlled trial is considered the gold standard for clinical trials. Patients are chosen for the study and assigned to either a control group or a group receiving the treatment being evaluated. The control group may receive a **placebo**, or they may be given a different treatment. These trials are often double-blind, meaning neither the patients nor the investigators know which treatment is being used. The first placebo-controlled trial was performed in 1948; it was an evaluation of **streptomycin** treatment for **tuberculosis (TB)** performed by the British Medical Research Council.

Today, clinical trials in humans in the United States follow three stages. In Phase I, the treatment is first evaluated in humans and given to people with advanced disease. These trials determine the best dosage and evaluate the drug's safety. In Phase II trials, patients with less-advanced disease receive the treatment. Phase III trials are larger, and are used to find specific effects of a treatment in terms of an individual's survival and quality of life. After these trials are complete, the **Food and Drug Administration (FDA)** decides whether to approve a treatment.

Additional reading: "Trial and Error," *The Economist*; Brody, "A Study Guide to Scientific Studies."

club foot treatment

Club foot is a deformation of the foot, also known as equinovarus, in which the foot is abnormally curved, making walking difficult.

Hippocrates (c.460–c.377 B.C.) wrote about treating club foot by moving the foot into proper alignment and then fixing it in place with stiff bandages and a foot-plate made of lead or leather. He suggested that treatment begin as early as possible.

Italian anatomist Gabriele Falloppio (1523–1562) recommended correcting the malformation gradually, so "nothing is to be done with violence." Other experts of the time suggested delaying treatment until early childhood. During the Middle Ages, correction of club foot was not strictly a medical matter, but was often performed by roving barber-surgeons and other semi-professionals.

Splints used to brace club feet gradually lengthened to cover the shin and then the knee by the 1700s. Jean-Andre Venel (1740–1791) developed his *sabot de Venel* for club foot, which used a rod attached to the outer side of the leg. He also recommended warm baths and manipulation of the foot.

Johann F. Dieffenbach (1792–1847) recommended casts similar to those used for fractures for treating club foot. Antonio Scarpa (1752–1832) added a spring to Venel's device.

Tenotomy, the cutting of the Achilles tendon to correct club foot, was first performed by Moritz Gerhard Thilenius (1745–1809) in 1784. This and other early operations were performed by surgically exposing the tendon. Jean-Mathieu Delpech (1777–1832) recommended performing tenotomy through a tiny incision without opening the skin further. The operation was popular in Europe and the United States in the first half of the nineteenth century.

Today, measures much like those recommended by Hippocrates are used to correct club foot, and surgery may be used in more severe cases.

Additional reading: LeVay, *The History of Orthopaedics.*

cocaine

Cocaine is an anesthetic substance found in leaves of the coca plant. The people of South America's mountainous regions, where this plant grows wild, have known about its numbing, hunger-easing, energizing, and hallucinogenic powers for thousands of years, but the substance responsible for these effects—cocaine—was not isolated until 1860.

Europeans discovered coca when the Spanish arrived in Peru, where people had been cultivating the plant for at least a thousand years. The Spanish conquerors were the first to create a market for the plant as a cash crop. They also supplied workers in Bolivian silver mines with coca leaves to chew to make the work more tolerable. Because demand became so high for the plant in South America, little was exported for centuries.

In 1860, a German doctoral student, Albert Niemann (1834–1861), developed a method for isolating cocaine from coca. He also observed that the pure cocaine numbed the tongue. The drug company Merck began producing cocaine on a small scale shortly afterwards. During the 1870s, European researchers began studying the effects of coca leaves, and the small amounts of cocaine that were available, on athletic performance.

Angelo Mariani (1838–1914) developed a coca-based wine, Vin Mariani, that he began selling in 1870 and marketed using the first-ever celebrity endorsements. Imitators in Europe and the United States developed their own coca wines.

Commercial production of pure cocaine on a large scale began in the 1880s, after German chemists learned how to extract the material from coca leaves economically.

German researchers soon observed that cocaine solutions had a locally anesthetizing effect. Sigmund Freud (1856–1939), an advocate and user of cocaine, published a monograph on the drug in 1884. Freud believed it might be possible to use cocaine to cure **morphine** addicts, although cocaine was later found to be addictive itself. Freud's friend Carl Koller (1857–1944) hit upon the idea of using cocaine to numb the eye before surgery, and his animal experiments showed this would indeed work. He published his findings in 1884, and news of cocaine's usefulness as a local anesthetic, especially for **dentistry**, sped around the world. The surgeon William Steward Halsted (1852–1922) and his colleagues discovered that injections of cocaine could be used to block the nerves.

Doctors began prescribing cocaine for a wide variety of maladies, such as colds and hay fever. As production of the drug grew, it got cheaper, and cocaine became the main ingredient of many patent medicines. Abuse soon became widespread.

In 1913, Congress passed the Harrison Act to regulate cocaine distribution, and President William Howard Taft (1857–1930) called the drug "Public Enemy No. 1." Cocaine abuse eventually dropped off, but came back in the 1970s. Users of powdered cocaine inhale the substance through the nostrils, and many became addicted to the drug, which produces nervous system stimulation and euphoria. Continued use can lead to erosion of the nasal passages and heart damage, and overdoses can produce fatal heart arrythmias and respiratory arrest. "Crack," a cheap and powerful form of cocaine that is smoked rather than "snorted," became widely available in the 1980s and has resulted in a new epidemic of cocaine **addiction**.

Cocaine is now used legitimately as a local anesthetic, particularly in dentistry; it is applied to the mucous membranes and numbs the area. (*See also* anesthesia)

Additional reading: Karch, *A Brief History of Cocaine.*

cochlear implants

Cochlear implants are devices that stimulate the auditory nerves of profoundly deaf people to provide them with some semblance of hearing, basically by partially replacing the function of an inner-ear structure called the cochlea. These devices are surgically implanted in the skull for permanent use and cost upwards of $14,000.

In the 1930s, researchers made several attempts to stimulate the auditory nerves of deaf people using electrodes. The first cochlear implant was performed in France in 1957. It consisted of a copper wire placed inside the cochlea of a profoundly deaf 50-year-old man, which allowed him to hear speech rhythms. During the 1960s and 1970s, U.S. scientists developed increasingly complex devices that were actually implanted in a handful of patients.

The **Food and Drug Administration (FDA)** approved multichannel cochlear implants for adults in 1984 and for children in 1990. Multichannel cochlear implants have been found to be more effective than single-channel implants, helping some patients to understand speech better.

Although cochlear implants are helpful for totally deaf people who lose their hearing after learning to speak, it remains unclear if they truly help deaf children who haven't yet learned to communicate. Some experts argue that since these children will have rudimentary hearing at best, they should instead be taught to communicate with sign language and lip reading.

Additional reading: Carpenter, "Learning to Hear Takes More than Hardware."

colchicine

Colchicine is a drug derived from the autumn crocus, *Colchicum autumnale*, that has long been used to treat **gout** and other disorders. In 1763, Anton Storck (1731–1803) of Vienna recommended using a vinegar extract of the root of the crocus with honey as a **diuretic.**

An officer in the French army developed a secret remedy, *Eau Medicinale*, that he said would cure just about every disease but was especially good for **gout.** In 1814, the secret was revealed when a chemist demonstrated that the active ingredient in the panacea was colchicum and showed that the plant treated gout effectively.

Colchicine eventually replaced *Eau Medicinale* for treating gout and was also used frequently to treat rheumatism and various types of inflammation.

Although the mechanism by which colchicine treats gout remains unknown, the drug is still used for this purpose.

Additional reading: Sneader, *Drug Discovery,* p. 95.

colorectal cancer

In the United States, colorectal cancer is the second leading cause of **cancer** death in both men and women. About 131,000 new cases of colorectal cancer were reported in the United States in 1998, and about 55,000 people die of the disease each year.

People older than 40, as well as those with inflammatory bowel disease, are at greater risk of developing this type of cancer. Two types of inherited colon cancer discovered in the 1990s, familial adenomatous polyposis and hereditary nonpolyposis colorectal cancer, account for about a quarter of cases of colon cancer.

In 1925, Cuthbert Esquire Dukes (1890–1977) first suggested that colorectal cancer followed an orderly progress and originated in the mucous membrane lining the colon. He observed that the lining first formed benign polyps, which could progress into cancers.

To date, the best chemotherapeutic drug for colorectal cancer that has metastasized is 5–fluorouracil, an **antimetabolite**. However, a combination of 5-FU with leucovorin (folinic acid) may hold promise in selected cases.

Colonoscopies, a type of **endoscopy** in which the colon is examined by a scope inserted through the rectum, as well as tests for blood in the stool, are now recommended to screen for colorectal cancer in people who are at risk, so that polyps can be removed before the cancer grows and spreads. A person whose colorectal cancer is detected and removed early has a 90 percent chance of surviving for five years, but once the cancer has spread to the lymph nodes that chance drops to 50 percent.

Mutated **tumor-suppressor genes** have recently been implicated in some types of colorectal cancer. (*See also* chemotherapy)

Additional reading: Weinberg, *One Renegade Cell,* pp. 79–85.

colposcopy

Colposcopy is the technique of viewing the cervix of the uterus through a microscope to detect and examine abnormal tissue.

Hans Hinselmann (1884–1959) invented the colposcope in 1925. Shortly afterwards, physicians began sampling and studying cervical cells to detect **cancer**. The **Pap smear**, in which cell samples are taken from the cervix and analyzed for abnormalities, was invented later that decade. Medical students in the United States began learning the technique in the 1950s.

Thanks largely to this instrument, scientists have learned that mild changes in the cells of the cervix are not a separate condition from invasive cancer of the cervix, but are in fact an early—and much more treatable—stage of the disease.

Treating **cervical cancer** also is easier because of the colposcope. Using the instrument, gynecologists can see where to sample for abnormal cells and can also excise abnormal cells with a variety of techniques. An early technique for treating cervical cancer, conization, which can weaken the cervix, is now much less common thanks to the precision the colposcope affords.

Additional reading: O'Dowd and Philipp, *The History of Obstetrics and Gynaecology,* pp. 550–52.

computerized axial tomography. *See* CAT scanning

condom

A condom is a sheath for the penis that acts as a contraceptive by retaining semen after ejaculation, and is also used to prevent the spread of sexually transmitted disease. Condoms are fairly reliable when used properly but not foolproof, as they may burst while in use or may contain holes through which sperm or disease-transmitting **viruses** or bacteria may escape. The first mention of a condom-like device appeared in the writings of Gabriele Falloppio (1523–1562), who described testing a linen cloth shaped to fit the penis on 1,100 men to prevent **syphilis**.

Condoms made of animal intestine became popular in the eighteenth century. Two London condom-makers, Mrs. Philips and Mrs. Perkins, advertised their wares through handbills. The discovery of vulcanization in 1839 made rubber condoms possible, with seamless versions produced by the end of the century. Poured latex, invented in the 1930s, further advanced condom technology, as did **Food and Drug Administration (FDA)** rules on quality control issued during that decade. U.S. soldiers fighting abroad in World War II were supplied with condoms. Lubricated condoms became available in the 1950s.

With the scourge of **AIDS** and **public health** efforts promoting "safe sex," condoms are enjoying renewed popularity; they protect against transmission of the herpes virus and HIV, as well as pregnancy. A condom for women, called "Reality," was introduced in the late 1980s. This "female condom" is a latex sac that is placed within the vagina, with a ring at the opening of the vagina that anchors it in place. (*See also* birth control pills; contraception)

Additional reading: Murphy, *The Condom Industry in the United States*.

contact lenses

A contact lens is a device used to correct vision. Placed directly on the eyeball, contact lenses fix the abnormalities in the curvature of the cornea that cause vision problems.

In about 1508, Leonardo da Vinci (1452–1519), suggested a design for a contact lens made of glass and filled with water. Several scientists subsequently suggested strategies for contact lens design.

Adolf Eugen Fick (1852–1937), who coined the term "contact lens," made the first contact lens for vision correction out of glass in 1887. He fit lenses made of glass to rabbit eyes, and then made lenses molded to the eyes of cadavers. He switched to lenses made by Ernst Abbe (1840–1905) of the Zeiss Optical Laboratories.

Before instruments were developed that would measure the curvature of the cornea, contact lenses were fitted by taking a mold of the eyeball.

Attempts were made to produce plastic contact lenses in the late 1930s, but these lenses were difficult to use because they did not allow tears to circulate beneath them. A plastic contact lens that floated above the tears covering the cornea was introduced in 1948. As fitting improved and the lenses became smaller, it became possible to wear the plastic lenses throughout the day.

Larger "soft" contact lenses made of a water-absorbing plastic gel, which were more comfortable and could be worn for longer periods of time, were developed in the 1970s. In the 1980s, long-wear soft lenses were introduced that could be worn for weeks at a time. The first disposable soft contact lenses, called "Acuvue," were introduced by

Johnson and Johnson in 1987. These are safe if used as recommended and replaced every two weeks.

Additional reading: Albert and Edwards, *The History of Ophthalmology*, pp. 119–22.

contagion theory

Contagion is the transmission of disease from one person to another, and also refers to the virus, bacteria, or other organism that causes the disease.

The first contagion theory was put forth by the Italian physician Girolamo Fracastoro (1483–1553), who proposed in 1530 that human contact spread "seeds" that carried **syphilis**. He outlined three types of contagion: diseases spread by person-to-person contact, diseases spread by infected objects as well as by contact, and diseases spread by contact, infected objects, and at a distance.

Fracastoro's work was basically ignored until 1840, when Friedrich Gustav Jacob Henle (1809–1885) published an examination of contagious disease. This work was carried on famously by Louis Pasteur (1822–1895) and Robert Koch (1843–1910) in their research on **germ theory.**

Contagion theory represents a milestone in the history of medicine because it was the first accurate articulation of how disease is spread. The successor of contagion theory, germ theory, defined how infection occurs and made it possible to prevent the spread of disease.

Additional reading: McGrew, *Encyclopedia of Medical History*, pp. 77–79.

contraception

Contraceptives are devices, medications, or techniques for preventing pregnancy.

The Greeks and ancient Egyptians recommended covering the vagina and cervix with cedar oil to prevent conception, while the **Hippocratic Corpus** suggests shaking out semen with bodily movement after intercourse.

The Arab physicians Rhazes (c.850–c.923) and Avicenna (980–1037) recommended coitus interruptus, or withdrawal of the penis before ejaculation, as well as cedar oil, pessaries made of pomegranate pulp, several potions, and an early version of the rhythm method (which would not have worked, because it was based on incorrect assumptions about when women were most fertile during their menstrual cycle). Women also have used a variety of herbs since antiquity to "bring on menstruation," but this is more of an **abortion** technique than a contraceptive method.

The **condom** first appeared in the sixteenth century. Two important female contraceptive methods were introduced in the nineteenth century: the cervical cap and the diaphragm, both of which block sperm from entering the cervix. The invention of the vulcanization process for rubber in 1839 allowed these devices to be mass-produced inexpensively, and also improved condom technology.

The modern birth control movement began in Britain and the United States in the early 1800s, with writers such as Robert Owen (1801–1877) and Francis Place (1771–1854) advocating contraception rather than abstinence.

Owen's 1831 book, *Moral Physiology,* described condoms, the sponge, and coitus interruptus, while Charles Knowlton's (1810–1850) *Fruits of Philosophy,* published one year later, recommended douching with a number of different solutions including red rose leaves, green tea, vinegar, and sodium bicarbonate.

The birth control movement brought on a backlash. In 1873, Congress passed the Comstock Law, which made dissemination of birth control information by mail illegal. Abortions became more common. Margaret Sanger's (1883–1966) *Family Limitation,* published after World War I, and the establishment of the National Birth Control League brought contraception closer to the mainstream, but vestiges of the Comstock Law remained in place until 1966.

More advanced methods of contraception, including the **intrauterine device (IUD)** and the **birth control pill**, became available in the 1950s and 1960s, respectively. **Clinical trials** of long-term contraceptive methods consisting of an injection of **progesterone** or implantation of materials containing the **hormone** beneath the skin began in the 1960s. With these methods, fertility is restored when the hormone implant is removed, or when the effectiveness of the injection runs out. One of these methods, the Norplant, consists of six matchstick-sized rubber capsules filled with levonorgestrol that are implanted in a woman's arm. The implant can prevent conception for up to five years, and can be implanted in a doctor's office. It is made by the drug company Wyeth-Ayerst and was approved by the **Food and Drug Administration (FDA)** in 1990. Depo-Provera an intramuscular injection of medroxyprogesterone acetate, is effective for 90 days. Made by Upjohn, Depo-Provera was approved in 1992. For both methods, irregular menstrual bleeding is the most common side effect.

A method for preventing pregnancy known as the "morning-after pill" can be used within 72 hours of unprotected intercourse, and works by preventing ovulation, fertilization, or implantation of a fertilized ovum, depending on when in the cycle the unprotected intercourse took place. It will not dislodge an implanted fertilized egg from the uterine wall, so it is considered a contraceptive method, not an abortifacient.

The method is known as the Yuzpe method, after Albert Yuzpe, the Canadian physician who developed it. He began research on this method in 1972. It consists of a high dose of estrogen and progestin, followed by a second dose 12 hours later. In 1997, the FDA ruled that the morning-after pill is safe and effective.

Today, there is a continuing battle over whether making contraceptives available to young people encourages them to have sex.

Additional reading: Riddle, *Contraception and Abortion from the Ancient World to the Renaissance; A History of Abortion and Contraception in the West.*

convulsive therapy

Convulsive therapy was an early technique for treating **mental illness**, usually psychosis, by inducing convulsions.

Ladislas J. Meduna (1896–1964), a psychiatrist in Budapest, Hungary, tried this technique for the first time, injecting schizophrenic patients with camphor in 1934. He had observed that patients with **schizophrenia** and **epilepsy** seemed to become less psychotic after a seizure, so he thought that artificially inducing seizures might have the same effect. He replaced camphor with pentylenetetrazol (Metrazol) because it induced seizures in a shorter time and was more comfortable for the patient. Manfred Sakel (1900–1957), who had invented the technique of coma therapy the year before, later claimed to have invented convulsive therapy.

Ugo Cerletti (1877–1963) and Lucio Bini (1908–) developed **electroconvulsive therapy** (also called "electroshock" treatment) after learning of Meduna's work and theorizing that electric shock would be a more effective means of inducing convulsions. They ran animal tests for years and gave the treatment to a human patient for the first time in 1938.

Another chemical method for inducing convulsions, the drug Indoklon, was given to patients by inhalation along with muscle relaxants to prevent fractures during seizures. This was introduced in 1957, and had the advantage of not being associated with electric shock and the disadvantage of producing nausea, but the makers stopped manufacturing it.

Electroconvulsive therapy is still used today to treat depressed patients who do not respond to other therapies. The treatment remains controversial because of its perceived cruelty and its relatively high cost, but it has been shown to be effective. (*See also* depression)

Additional reading: Shorter, *A History of Psychiatry,* pp. 207–24.

corneal transplant

In a corneal transplant, the clear outer covering of the eye is taken from a deceased donor and grafted onto the eye of a person whose cornea has been damaged by disease or injury.

European interest in the possibility of corneal transplantation arose in the late 1700s after an infectious disease known as Egyptian ophthalmia (infection of the eye with *Chlamydia trachomatis*, which causes conjunctivitis) was brought back to the continent from Africa. Charles Darwin's grandfather Erasmus (1731–1802) first suggested the possibility of corneal transplant to treat the disease in 1797.

While visiting Egypt in 1835, Samuel Bigger performed the first corneal transplant, in a pet gazelle that had lost its vision. The donor cornea was removed from another gazelle that was wounded but not yet dead. Bigger found that the graft healed and the animal's vision wasn't obstructed by scarring. When he returned to his home country of Ireland, he performed further experiments with corneal transplantation in animals. Henry Power (1829–1911), a London surgeon, also carried out a series of experiments in animals and humans, reporting on them in 1872.

The first successful corneal transplant, from a boy whose eye was removed to a man whose corneas were scarred from chemical burns, was performed in 1905 by the Czech surgeon Edward Zirm.

The New York Eye Bank was founded in 1959 to store donated corneas for transplantation, and a national group, the Eye Bank Association of America, was established two years later.

Additional reading: Schmeck, "Sight Restored for Thousands Yearly."

coronary care unit (CCU)

A coronary care unit is a specialized hospital division equipped to care for patients who have just had heart attacks, who are in danger of having them, or who suffer from life-threatening heart arryhthmias. The first CCUs opened in the early 1960s, in the United States, Australia, and Canada, after the introduction of **CPR** and **cardioversion** in 1960. These advances meant that heart attacks and ventricular fibrillation, a type of heart arrhythmia that is fatal if not treated, were no longer a death sentence.

The United States' first CCU was established at the Bethany Medical Center in Kansas City, with 11 beds and a nursing staff trained to handle cardiac emergencies. Bethany doctors described the CCU to colleagues at a meeting of the American College of Chest Physicians in 1962, and the college helped establish a training program for coronary care nurses. Manufacturers of monitoring equipment encouraged the founding of the first CCUs with generous donations.

As CCUs developed, diagnosis and treatment of heart attacks and arrythmias advanced further. During the 1960s, new techniques including **cardiac catheterization** at the patient's bedside, drugs to limit damage from heart attacks, and mechanical devices to assist the heart were introduced.

Additional reading: Acierno, *The History of Cardiology,* pp. 368–69.

cortisone

Cortisone is a **hormone** manufactured by the **adrenal gland** which is also produced synthetically as a drug to treat inflammation. This hormone is largely inactive in the body until it is converted to the closely related hormone cortisol. Both hormones are important in regulating the metabolism of fats, proteins, carbohydrates, potassium, and sodium. Cortisone and cortisol are steroid hormones, meaning they share a basic molecular building block known as perhydrocyclopentanophenanthrene.

Julius Rogoff (1884–1966) of Case Western Reserve University in Ohio showed, in 1927, that extracts of the adrenal gland could be used to keep dogs alive after their adrenal glands were removed. He was working with the cortex of the gland. An extract was developed and sold by Parke-Davis for treating **Addison's disease.**

During the 1930s, several different steroid hormones were isolated from the adrenal cortex by a number of researchers working independently, including Edward C. Kendall (1886–1972) of the Mayo Clinic in Rochester, Minnesota, and Tadeus Reichstein (1897–1996) of the University of Basel in Switzerland. Reichstein also developed an artificial adrenal steroid from plants, which was the first adrenal steroid hormone to be used clinically and went on the market in 1937.

In 1940, Hans Selye (1907–1982) of McGill University in Montreal reported that corticosterone, one of these hormones, was an effective treatment for **shock.** As World War II was approaching, various governments became interested in the hormone for treating soldiers and pilots. At the behest of the U.S. Office of Scientific Research and Development (on behalf of the Air Force), Kendall worked at the drug company Merck to develop a system for making the hormone, which he had previously isolated and called "Compound A." Lewis Sarrett (1917–), also at Merck, synthesized the related hormone "Compound E."

Compound E was renamed cortisone and used in 1949 by Philip Hench (1896–1965) of the Mayo Clinic to treat patients with **rheumatoid arthritis**. Hench had been investigating treatments for rheumatoid arthritis since 1929.

Hench and Kendall shared the 1950 Nobel Prize for their discovery of cortisone.

Cortisone is an excellent treatment for rheumatoid arthritis and other inflammatory, autoimmune conditions. However, the hormone is usually used as a last resort and only on a short-term basis, if possible, because it has severe side effects that include bone thinning, psychological changes, and Cushing's syndrome.

Cushing's syndrome is caused by excessive secretion of cortisol hormones from the adrenal gland. Other causes include medications such as oral corticosteroids or ACTH treatment. Some symptoms include florid complexion, high blood pressure, osteoporosis, facial swelling, purple eruptions on the abdomen and forearm, or, in some cases, **diabetes mellitus.** If overproduction of ACTH is caused by a tumor of the pituitary gland, the disease is called Cushing's disease.

A number of synthetic forms of cortisone and other adrenocortical steroids were developed in the 1950s and remain in use today. The first, fluodrocortisone, was synthesized by Josef Fried (1914–) at the drug company Squibb in 1954. Others include prednisone and prednisolone.

Additional reading: Shorter, *The Health Century,* pp. 32–37.

COX-2 inhibitors

COX-2 inhibitors are **nonsteroidal anti-inflammatory drugs** (**NSAIDs**) that reduce inflammation without being toxic to the stomach lining. They are useful for treating **rheumatoid arthritis**, and may also help prevent **colon cancer** and **Alzheimer's disease**.

Cyclooxygenase (COX) is the main enzyme involved in the synthesis of **prostaglandins** in the body. Sir John Vane (1927–) and his colleagues reported in 1971 that **aspirin** and related drugs worked by inhibiting the action of COX, thus halting the production of prostaglandins. COX was purified in 1976 and cloned in 1988. A second form of COX, now known as COX-2, was discovered in 1996.

The drug celecoxib, sold under the name Celebrex, was approved by the **Food and Drug Administration (FDA)** in 1998. This medication, made by the pharmaceutical company G.D. Searle, was the first COX-2 inhibitor to go on the market.

COX-1 is believed to help protect the gastrointestinal tract and also to maintain normal blood flow in kidneys damaged by disease. COX-2 is rarely found in normal tissues, but appears in association with inflammation and also in the central nervous system, where it may play a role in nerve transmission. The stomach and intestinal problems produced by NSAIDs are thus thought to be related to inhibition of COX-1, while their effects in reducing inflammation have to do with COX-2 inhibition. Once this was determined, scientists began looking for drugs that would inhibit COX-2 without affecting COX-1.

Animal research has shown that COX-2 inhibitors prevent colorectal tumor formation. Aspirin appears to have similar properties, but long-term aspirin use isn't practical for many people because of the effects of the drug on the stomach. Clinical trials of COX-2 inhibitors for preventing colon cancer in humans and for slowing the progress of Alzheimer's disease are now underway.

Additional reading: Kolata, "Drug Makers Say New Painkillers Work Without Side Effects."

CPR (cardiopulmonary resuscitation)

Cardiopulmonary resuscitation is a technique for keeping a person alive whose heart has stopped, using mouth-to-mouth resuscitation and rhythmic compression of the chest. This ensures that oxygenated blood continues to flow to the brain.

In 1958, William Bennett Kouwenhoven (1886–1975) and Charles H. Knickerbocker (1922–) discovered that chest compression could maintain blood flow in patients whose hearts had stopped, and began using the technique in patients with cardiac arrest immediately.

A Norwegian dollmaker had produced the Resusci-Anne doll in 1959 to train people in mouth-to-mouth resuscitation. When Kouwenhoven and his colleagues published their findings on closed-chest compression in 1960, the dollmaker modified Resusci-Anne so the doll could be used to teach CPR.

The American Heart Association (AHA) and the American **Red Cross** developed the first CPR training program, directed at medical and paramedical professionals, in 1966, and subsequently decided to begin teaching the lay public the technique as well. Now, CPR training is available in nearly every town and city in the United States, usually through the Red Cross, and has saved thousands of lives.

Additional reading: Khan and Marriott, *The Heart Trouble Encyclopedia*, pp. 51–56.

cryosurgery

Cryosurgery is the use of extremely cold temperatures to remove abnormal growths from the skin, such as warts and **cancers**, as well as to destroy abnormal **tissue** within the body.

This technique was pioneered in the nineteenth century, when refrigeration became available, although the anti-inflammatory and pain-killing effects of cold have been known for centuries.

The first cryosurgeon was James Arnott (1797–1883), who developed an apparatus for removing tumors and published several works on cryosurgery from 1851 and 1854. In 1850, he suggested using cryosurgery to destroy breast tumors. Cryosurgery for skin cancers was introduced around the beginning of the twentieth century.

The neurosurgeon Irving Cooper (1922–) developed an apparatus for performing cryosurgery that was first used on humans in 1962 to treat **Parkinson's disease** and to destroy **brain tumors**. The device consisted of a hollow metal tube through which liquid nitrogen circulated. It was insulated everywhere except at the tip, which was the operating instrument.

Today cryosurgery is used in neurosurgery; gynecology; urology; dermatology; gastroenterology; ear, nose, and throat surgery; and operations on the mouth and teeth. Cryosurgery not only destroys tumors, it also may encourage the body to fight the tumor on its own by inducing resistance to **antigens** produced by the abnormal cells. It can also be performed with local or no **anesthesia**. In the late 1980s, guidance of cryosurgery with **ultrasound** was introduced.

Additional reading: Galton, *Med Tech*, pp. 136–39.

cryptosporidium

Cryptosporidium is a parasite spread by water or food contaminated with fecal matter.

Healthy people infected with cryptosporidium usually suffer from diarrhea and other gastrointestinal symptoms for a week and then recover on their own. But the parasite can be deadly to people with weak immune systems, such as people with **AIDS,** causing dehydration and eventual death in some cases. There is no treatment for cryptosporidium infection, aside from rehydration and other supportive therapy.

Cryptosporidium was first observed in 1907, but it was only discovered to infect humans in the 1980s. The largest outbreak of water-borne illness in United States history was caused by cryptosporidium. In 1993, more than 400,000 people were sickened in Milwaukee, Wisconsin, and about 100 people died after a defective pump allowed sewage containing cryptosporidium to enter the water supply and contaminate it with the parasite. *Cryptosporidium* cannot be destroyed with chlorine, but boiling water for about a minute usually will kill the parasite.

There were six major outbreaks of water-borne cryptosporidium infection in the 1990s, and several outbreaks caused by eating contaminated food.

Additional reading: Fox. *Spoiled*, pp. 272–73, 386–91.

c-section. *See cesarean section.*

CSF. *See cerebrospinal fluid.*

CT scanning. See CAT scanning

cupping

Cupping is an ancient technique employed to remove un-healthful substances from the body, or to draw them closer to the surface of the body where they will do less harm.

Cups were applied to the skin and the air inside the cup was drawn out by various methods, producing a vacuum. In "wet" cupping, the skin was slashed or punctured so the suction would draw out blood. "Dry" cupping of uncut skin was intended to produce blisters.

Herodotus (c.484–c.430 B.C.) wrote that the Egyptians used both methods for headache, digestive problems, men-strual regulation, and to either promote restful sleep (when applied behind the ears) or do away with a tendency to sleep too much. The ancient Greeks used gourds for cupping. Hippocrates (c.460–c.377 B.C.) recommended dry cupping, and suggested using shallow, wide cups to treat sickness close to the surface of the skin and small, cone-shaped cups for deep-seated illnesses.

Cupping was popular in Rome and throughout the Middle Ages for treating **gout** and arthritis.

Methods for creating a vacuum changed as technol-ogy advanced. In ancient times, the cupper may have sucked out the air through a tube with his or her mouth, but more advanced methods included creating a vacuum with **syringe** pumps or by heating the air with a blow torch.

In the mid-seventeenth century, a device called a "spring scarificator," a box holding about a dozen spring-loaded lances that could make several cuts relatively pain-lessly at once, was introduced. The eighteenth and nine-teenth centuries saw the use of glass cups, which were called "glass leeches."

Although wet cupping fell out of favor, along with **bloodletting**, in the mid-nineteenth century, dry cupping continued to be used in the early twentieth century for pneu-monia and swellings of the joints. Barbers in New York City in the 1920s, hailing back to their long-ago days as barber surgeons, would offer "cups for colds."

A technique related to cupping, moxibustion, in which herbs are burned near the surface of the skin to "draw out" sickness-causing materials, is still used today by some **acu-puncture** practitioners.

Additional reading: Root-Bernstein, *Honey, Mud, Maggots and Other Medical Miracles*, pp. 180–83.

curare

Curare is a nerve poison made from the bark of Amazon-basin plants that people indigenous to the region use for hunting. They tip arrows with the poison, which paralyzes prey. Curare has also proved extremely useful in medicine.

The German explorer Alexander von Humboldt (1769–1859) was the first westerner to describe how hunters col-lected and prepared the poison. But because there are so many varieties of curare, made from several different plants, it was difficult to research.

In 1851, Claude Bernard (1813–1878) identified the motor end plate where nerves connect with muscle as the site of curare's paralyzing action. After Bernard's discov-ery, a handful of doctors used curare to treat muscle spasms from **tetanus** and **rabies**.

Welsh pharmacologist Harold King (1887–1956) pu-rified d-tubocurarine in 1935. King used samples of the nerve poison brought to Britain by explorers.

Meanwhile, the American researcher and explorer Ri-chard Gill (1901–1958) had been diagnosed in 1934 with multiple sclerosis, and his physician suggested that the ar-row poison of South America might help to ease his spasms. Gill went to the jungle and collected 25 pounds of curare, which he sold to the pharmaceutical company E.R. Squibb and Sons in 1938.

E.R. Squibb and Sons made the first commercial curare preparation out of the sample, calling it Intocostrin. The initial use of the drug was for patients undergoing **convul-sive therapy**, to relax their muscles so they would be less likely to injure themselves.

Anesthetized patients' muscle activity was a problem for surgeons of the time. Although patients were uncon-scious, their muscles still reacted, interfering with opera-tions. In 1942, Harold Griffith (1894–unknown) used the drug to paralyze a man who was having his appendix re-moved, with excellent results. Because Griffith and his con-temporaries had extensive experience in mechanically ven-tilating patients, the paralyzation of the lungs wasn't a prob-lem. This is considered one of the greatest advances in **an-esthesia**, because muscle relaxation has made it possible to anesthetize patients more lightly and to perform surgeries that had not been possible before.

A synthetic version of curare, gallamine (Flaxedil) became available in 1947. Since then a number of synthetic muscle relaxants have been manufactured with increasingly specific action.

Additional reading: Altman, *Who Goes First?,* pp. 74–85.

CVS. See chorionic villus sampling.

Cushing's syndrome. *See cortisone.*

cyclosporine

Cyclosporine is a drug that suppresses the immune system. It has revolutionized organ transplantation, because people treated with the drug are much less likely to "reject" for-eign organs. Rejection occurs because the organ recipient's immune system, recognizing cells that are not "self," at-tacks and kills the transplanted **tissue**.

For years, organ transplants from donors not closely related to recipients were impossible, because rejection would destroy the new organ shortly after it was implanted. Attempts to suppress the immune system by irradiating the bone marrow or by treatment with early immunosuppressant drugs weren't dependable, and few people survived long after such operations.

Researchers at Sandoz pharmaceuticals in Basel, Switzerland, discovered Cyclosporine A while investigating the properties of a number of different substances produced by fungi. The group had begun looking at these chemicals in 1957, originally as part of a search for potential antifungal drugs. Cyclosporine A, later called cyclosporine, is produced by fungus of the species *Beauveria nivea*. Sandoz chemists published a paper on the substance's powerful immunosuppressive powers in 1972. The first article on using Cyclosporine A to treat organ transplant patients appeared four years later.

Cyclosporine's action isn't completely understood, but the drug is thought to block the action of the immune system's "killer" **T cells**, which hunt down and destroy foreign invaders.

Cyclosporine has greatly improved survival after transplantation. Because of its side effects, such as kidney damage, cyclosporine is usually now used in low doses as part of triple immunotherapy along with the older drug azathioprine and the artificial **cortisone** prednisone. (*See also* bone marrow transplant; immunosuppression; heart transplant; kidney transplant; lung transplant)

Additional reading: Galton, *Med Tech,* pp. 142–46.

cystic fibrosis

Cystic fibrosis is a hereditary disease in which abnormal secretions from certain glands block the lungs and the digestive tract. The gene for cystic fibrosis, which is recessive, appears in about 5 percent of white people of European heritage.

The "cystic fibrosis gene" in normal form produces a protein that regulates the transfer of chloride and sodium across cell membranes. When the gene is mutated, the protein doesn't function properly. This interrupts the transfer of these ions, resulting in dehydration and extremely sticky secretions. This sticky mucus fills the lungs, making breathing difficult. Babies with cystic fibrosis are often born with meconium ileus, in which the intestine is blocked with a similar sticky substance.

Some European folktales hold that a child whose sweat is salty will die soon; these tales probably referred to children with cystic fibrosis.

Karl Landsteiner (1868–1943) first described meconium ileus in 1905, and Swiss researcher Guido Fanconi (1892–1979) first described cystic fibrosis in 1936. Two years later, Dorothy Anderson (1901–1963) of the Columbia University Babies Hospital provided an extensive description of the disease. After analyzing family histories of 103 children with cystic fibrosis, Anderson suggested that the disease was inherited by a recessive trait.

After first noting that a disproportionate number of children who came to his hospital with heat prostration had cystic fibrosis, in 1952 Paul Di Sant-Agnese (1914–) found that the disease produced a high concentration of sodium

and chloride in sweat. Testing the levels of these ions in sweat was soon used to diagnose cystic fibrosis.

The Cystic Fibrosis Foundation was established in 1955. At this time, children with cystic fibrosis rarely lived past childhood. In the 1960s, the technique of pounding cystic fibrosis patients' chests to dislodge mucus from their lungs began to extend their lives. The **antibiotics** flucloxacillin and tobramycin, introduced in the early 1970s, helped clear up the severe lung infections that often strike people with cystic fibrosis.

The first **lung transplant** in a cystic fibrosis patient, who received a new heart as well, was performed in 1984. To date more than 500 cystic fibrosis patients have received lung transplants.

In 1985 a marker was identified that made it possible to diagnose cystic fibrosis in a fetus as early as the seventh or eighth week of pregnancy, and the first successful prenatal diagnosis of cystic fibrosis was made two years later. The cystic fibrosis gene was identified in 1989.

In 1991, the cystic fibrosis gene was discovered to be a chloride channel. The defective gene that leads to cystic fibrosis prevents the chloride channel from opening. Attempts to correct the defect in cells in the laboratory have met with some success, raising the possibility that the disease could one day be treated with **gene therapy.**

Additional reading: Hopkins, *Understanding Cystic Fibrosis.*

cytokine

Cytokine is a collective name for a number of peptides that cells produce to communicate with one another. Cytokines are intercellular messengers, like **hormones**, but they act locally rather than being carried to remote locations by the bloodstream. Cells make cytokines in response to emergencies.

Cytokines shore up the ability of the immune system to identify self and nonself. They regulate immunological and inflammatory processes, and also help to repair cells and regulate normal cell growth and differentiation.

Stanley Cohen (1922–) and colleagues suggested the name "cytokine" in 1977; these substances had originally been called lymphokines, for the lymphocytes that produced them, but it became clear that other types of cells made these substances as well.

The first cytokine discovered was **interferon**, which was identified in 1957. A series of cytokines that stimulate **T cell** function, known as interleukins, were discovered in the 1970s. Trials of interleukin-2 for treating **cancer** that began in the 1980s have so far not found significant therapeutic benefit.

About 80 cytokines have been identified to date. Researchers are investigating their potential for treating **AIDS, autoimmune disease**, and cancer. The potential of cytokine therapy is huge, since nearly every disease involves some type of imbalance in the cytokine communication system.

Additional reading: Lowenstein, *The Touchstone of Life,* pp. 165–321.

D

decompression

Decompression is a technique for preventing "the bends" in deep-sea divers and people who work far underground where pressure is much higher than at sea level. Instead of rising to sea-level pressure immediately, which can cause nitrogen bubbles to form in the blood (the bends), the person stays in a decompression chamber where the pressure is slowly lowered. People are at risk of the bends if they have been under water or under the earth's surface 30 feet or more for enough time for the **tissues** to become saturated with nitrogen.

Robert Hooke (1635–1703) performed the first human experiments under lowered atmospheric pressure, on himself, in about 1670. He sat inside a giant barrel with a tube that passed through the barrel wall to a vacuum pump. By opening the tube he could release air, lowering the pressure inside the chamber. He felt "some pain in his ears at the breaking out of the aire included within him," but didn't notice much else.

Paul Bert (1833–1886) led the study of decompression in the nineteenth century, conducting his experiments in a large steel chamber and publishing his landmark book *Barometric Pressure* in 1878. Among his findings: altitude sickness occurs because of a lack of oxygen; decreasing and increasing the concentration of oxygen in the air counteracts some of the effects of high and low pressure on the body; rapid decompression can cause bubbles to form in nitrogen that has been dissolved at high pressure in the tissues and the blood; and gradual decompression prevents the bends.

Additional reading: Altman, *Who Goes First?,* pp. 221–24.

defibrillator

Fibrillation occurs when the electrical system that controls the heartbeat is not functioning properly. In defibrillation, the heart receives a jolt of electricity timed to make all of the heart's chambers contract at once. When the heart relaxes, it can begin responding to its own pacemaker again and can resume a steady beat.

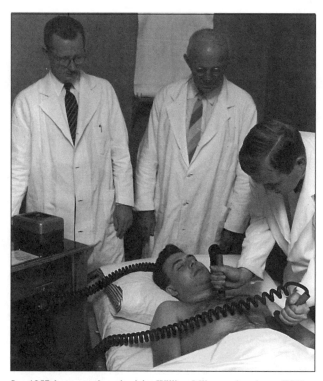

In a 1957 demonstration, physician William Milnor and engineers William Kouwenhoven and Guy G. Knickerbocker show the proper use of closed-chest cardiac defibrillator that they developed at Johns Hopkins. (Courtesy of The Alan Mason Chesney Medical Archives of the Johns Hopkins Medical Institutions.)

Ventricular fibrillation is the most dangerous type of fibrillation, leading to death if left untreated. A cardiac surgeon from Cleveland, Claude Beck (1894–1971), was the first person to successfully defibrillate a patient's heart during surgery, in 1947. He delivered the shock directly to the exposed heart.

In 1956, Paul Zoll (1911–1999) and his colleagues reported using external electric shocks to successfully treat 11 episodes of ventricular fibrillation in 4 patients. Along with external cardiac massage or **CPR** (developed shortly afterward), and a growing understanding of the heart's electrical system, these techniques provided the foundations for the cardiac resuscitation techniques used in emergency rooms today.

Additional reading: Jordaens, *The Implantable Defibrillator.*

dengue

Dengue fever is caused by a **virus** carried by mosquitoes. There is no effective treatment for the disease itself.

Symptoms include a sudden, high fever; pain in the bones and muscles; rash; and swelling. Dengue fever usually is not fatal, and infection with one strain of the virus confers immunity to that strain. However, people who have had a single infection are much more prone to develop a more deadly disease, known as dengue hemorrhagic fever or dengue shock syndrome, if they are infected with a second strain. Children, particularly malnourished youngsters, are at particularly high risk of developing dengue hemorrhagic fever or shock syndrome.

Dengue has been known for hundreds of years. Philadelphia physician Benjamin Rush (1745–1813) provided the first description of the disease in a 1780 account of an epidemic of "breakbone fever" in that city. The name "dengue" is believed to come from the Swahili phrase *Ki denga pepo,* meaning a sudden seizure caused by an evil spirit.

Thomas L. Bancroft (1860–1933) demonstrated in the early twentieth century that mosquitoes transmit dengue. The first of the four different types of dengue virus was identified in 1940. Dengue hemorrhagic fever appeared for the first time in Asia in the 1950s, in Thailand.

The Pan American Health Organization launched an effort to eliminate the strain of mosquitoes that carries dengue and malaria in 1942, and by 1962, 18 countries had done so, but subsequently the insects recolonized most of these countries. Today, the only Western Hemisphere countries free of the mosquito are Canada, Chile, and Bermuda.

Additional reading: Kiple, *The Cambridge World History of Human Disease,* pp. 660–64.

dentistry

Dentistry is the care of the teeth and gums.

Many ancient peoples practiced decorative dentistry; the Mayas of Mexico, for example, placed jade and turquoise inlays in their teeth. Filing the teeth into points for aesthetic purposes was a common practice in many cultures. Early dentists also made attempts at restorative dentistry. Bridges made of human and animal teeth bound with gold wire have been found in Phoenician tombs dating back to 400 B.C.

The world's first dentist may have been the Egyptian Hesi Re, whose skills are extolled in a papyrus of 3000 B.C. Among other operations, Egyptian dentists drilled holes in the jawbone to relieve pressure from abscesses.

The ancient Romans used gold crowns to restore rotted teeth. They employed a variety of abrasive substances as dentifrices, including talc, pumice, coral powder, and iron rust. The Romans, as well as the Greeks, also performed tooth extractions. The Greeks used a tool called an

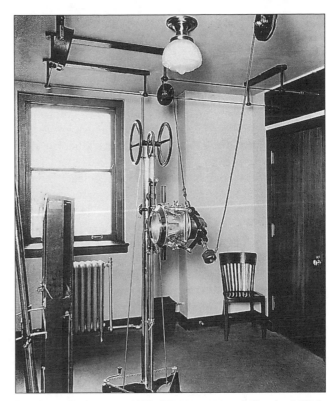

Dental examination room, 1921. (Photo courtesy of Cleveland Clinic Archives.)

odontagogon that was made of lead and looked like a giant pair of forceps. They may have believed that teeth that couldn't be removed with an instrument made of such soft metal should be left alone. The Romans had a similar instrument that they called the dentiducem, and professional tooth-pullers performed the procedure.

The job of extracting teeth remained a specialty, and doctors did not become involved in dentistry until well after the Middle Ages were over. Some English barber-surgeons began specializing in dentistry in the mid-1600s.

Historians of dentistry believe Aulus Cornelius Celsus (25 B.C.–50 A.D.) made the first cavity fillings. He used a mixture of lint and lead, but these fillings were used only to prevent a tooth from collapsing as it was being pulled.

Despite the sophistication of some ancient dentistry, since the time of Hippocrates (c.460–c.377 B.C.) and possibly before, westerners thought a creature known as the toothworm caused cavities and toothaches. Up until the eighteenth century, many remedies recommended burning noxious substances near the teeth to drive out the toothworm.

However, the ancient Greeks also suggested that sweet foods could cause tooth decay, a hypothesis that wasn't proven until the twentieth century.

The Spanish Arab physician Albucasis (c.976–1013), writing in the tenth century, had a more advanced understanding of dental health. He knew that plaque on the teeth led to periodontal disease and he developed instruments for removing it. The Chinese also were ahead of their time;

a 659 A.D. medical manuscript from that nation recommends silver fillings.

Claudius Galen (129–c.199), the influential Greek doctor and writer, thought that teeth were bones. The Italian anatomist Gabriele Falloppio (1523–1562) disproved this, and described the difference between primary ("baby") and permanent teeth. In 1563, the Italian anatomist Bartolommeo Eustachio (1520–1574) published the first book on the anatomy of the teeth. The first textbook of dentistry was published in Leipzig in 1530.

France was the first government to regulate dentistry, enacting a law in 1699 that required dental practitioners to pass an exam before practicing in Paris. The founder of modern dentistry, Pierre Fauchard (1678–1761), was a leading dentist of this time. In his 1728 book, *The Surgeon Dentist, or Treatise on the Teeth,* he rejected the toothworm theory. Fauchard filled cavities with lead or tin, and recommended scaling teeth. He also afforded patients some dignity by having them sit in an armchair during examinations and procedures; previously, people had sat on the floor. One of his less progressive beliefs was that rinsing the mouth each morning with fresh urine promoted dental health.

Fauchard's method for tooth extraction was typical of the time. He used a series of tools including a lancet to cut the gums if necessary; a punch to push the tooth aside and loosen it in its socket; a pincers; a lever to lift the tooth from the socket; and the pelican, a type of pincers with hooks facing inward toward the tooth.

A major advance in extraction was the dental key, first described in 1725. It had a head similar to a pelican and a handle set at a right angle. The key allowed teeth to be extracted with a quick twist. However, tooth extraction would not become a painless procedure until the introduction of **anesthesia** in the next century.

The first professional dentist in the United States began advertising his services in 1776. The American Josiah Flagg invented the first dental chair in 1790. It had an adjustable headrest and an extension of the arm to hold instruments. The first reclining chair was built in 1832.

The first mixed materials, or amalgams, used to fill cavities were introduced in the late eighteenth century and included mercury and other metals. These were not ideal because mercury is toxic. Early materials also had to be poured into the cavity while molten, which required them to be at a very high temperature. American dentist Greene Vardiman Black (1836–1915) developed an easy-to-use, safe amalgam in 1895.

Horace Hayden (1769–1844) and Chapin Harris (1806–1860) are considered to be the fathers of professional dentistry in the United States. They helped found the world's first dental college, the Baltimore College of Dental Surgery, in 1840. Four years later, laughing gas (**nitrous oxide**) began to make dentistry truly painless.

The first electric dentist's drill was invented in 1868. Earlier drills had been powered by clockwork mechanisms or pedals. Carl Koller (1857–1944) also contributed greatly to painless dentistry when he introduced **cocaine** for local anesthesia in 1884.

Willoughby D. Miller (1853–1907), an American dentist working in Berlin, discovered the cause of dental decay or caries. In his 1890 book, *Micro-organisms of the Human Mouth*, he explained that acid in fermented foods softens teeth, and then bacteria invades these tissues. In 1954, Frank J. Orland, at the University of Notre Dame, proved that decay couldn't take place without bacteria. In the 1960s, plaque was confirmed to be the cause of gum disease.

Charles Henry Land (1847–1919), the grandfather of pioneering aviator Charles Lindbergh (1902–1974), invented the porcelain jacket crown, introducing it in 1903.

Dentists got a helping hand from Dr. Alfred Civilion Fones (1869–1938), the originator of the dental hygiene movement. He started the first school for dental hygienists in his garage in Bridgeport, Connecticut, in 1913.

The faster and less-painful air-turbine dental drill was introduced in the 1950s.

Several short-acting drugs for intravenous sedation during dental procedures (usually wisdom-tooth removal) have been introduced since the 1960s, although many dentists still use nitrous oxide to anesthetize patients before such procedures. The first official guidelines for anesthesia and sedation in dentistry were introduced by the American Academy of Pediatric Dentistry and the American Academy of Pediatrics in 1985. The American Dental Association adopted separate guidelines in 1996.

The introduction of **fluoridation** in the United States in the mid-twentieth century has contributed greatly to the dental health of Americans.

In the 1980s, advances in treating periodontal disease, the inflammation of the gums that is the leading cause of tooth loss, include the development of tooth implants to restore lost teeth and techniques for directing gum regrowth.

Additional reading: Ring, *Dentistry;* Wynbrandt, *The Excruciating History of Dentistry.*

dentures

Dentures, or false teeth, are used to restore teeth lost to disease or injury.

The Japanese had developed what were probably relatively comfortable dentures made entirely of wood by the 1500s. They took an impression of the mouth using beeswax, from which a model was made. The dentures were then carved, based on this model, from a single piece of wood. Early, more primitive dentures have been found in Japanese tombs dating back to the 700s. Later dentures were decorated with bone, real teeth, and minerals. Women's dentures were dyed black, in keeping with the fashion of the time for married women to darken their teeth.

A set of dentures made of bone found in Switzerland and dating back to the 1500s appears to have been made for aesthetics alone, and would have been difficult to chew with. This set and the pair roughly from the same era from Japan are the oldest full sets of dentures that have been found.

In the eighteenth century, some dentists worked from plaster impressions to make false teeth. This was a painful and cumbersome process; the plaster was molded around the teeth and then chipped away once it was dry. The physician then pieced the mold back together again. In 1756, Prussian dentist Philip Pfaff (1715–1767) published a step-by-step description of how to make wax impressions and casts of missing teeth, which made the uncomfortable plaster method obsolete.

Early materials for dentures included wood, ivory, and tortoiseshell for the gum, and ivory and porcelain for the teeth. These dentures were attached to the jaw with hooks and clamps. Some French denture wearers even had their upper jaws pierced so dentures could be attached to them with hooks.

Pierre Fauchard (1678–1761) invented dentures in which the upper set was attached to the lower with springs, holding them in place. The French chemist Alexis Duchateau invented a formula for making porcelain that was suitable for use in dentures and published a book on his method in 1788.

Great advances in the comfort of dentures came with the invention of vulcanized rubber and plastic in the mid-nineteenth century. Thomas W. Evans (1823–1897) began using vulcanite, a hard rubber, after the material was invented and patented the material in 1851. John A. Cummings won a patent in 1864 for making dentures out of rubber, which the Goodyear Dental Vulcanite Company bought and controlled until the patent expired in 1881.

Today's dentures are held to the jaw by the capillary action of water, and employ a base made of acrylic resin. During the second half of the twentieth century, dentists began giving patients permanent dental implants to replace lost teeth.

Additional reading: Wynbrandt, *The Excruciating History of Dentistry,* pp. 148–72.

deoxyribonucleic acid. *See DNA.*

depression

Depression is a form of **mental illness** that is estimated to affect nearly 10 percent of adult Americans in any given year. It is characterized by loss of interest in usually pleasurable activities, changes in sleep patterns, feelings of hopelessness and worthlessness, difficulty concentrating, and persistent thoughts of suicide. While some people suffer severe or major depression, others may experience less severe depression over a longer period of time, which is called dysthymia. Both types of depression tend to recur.

Perhaps the first description of depression appears in the Bible in the story of Saul in the Book of Samuel, written in the eighth century B.C. Melancholia and mania were both described in the **Hippocratic Corpus.**

There are several theories about the causes of depression, including imbalances in brain chemistry, genetic or hereditary factors, and hormonal causes. Treatment can in-clude psychotherapy, cognitive therapy, and medication with **antidepressants.**

Dr. Aaron Beck (1921–) of the University of Pennsylvania, who developed the theory of cognitive behavior, suggested that depression is caused by negative thinking patterns and could be treated by teaching a person to change these patterns. Some people do respond to this type of therapy.

The first effective antidepressant drugs, the MAO inhibitors and the tricyclic antidepressants, became available in the late 1950s. These drugs, though effective, may have severe side effects. The selective **serotonin** reuptake inhibitors (SSRIs), which include the popular drug Prozac and have less severe side effects than older drugs, were introduced in the late 1980s. St. John's wort, an herbal antidepressant, has also become increasingly popular and has fewer side effects than any prescription antidepressant drugs. The effectiveness of medications in treating depression—about 70 percent of depressed people experience at least a 50 percent improvement in their symptoms upon taking an antidepressant drug—has added weight to the theory that depression is related to imbalances in brain chemicals called neurotransmitters. (*See also* herbal medicine)

Additional reading: Klein, *Understanding Depression.*

diabetes mellitus

Diabetes mellitus occurs when the body cannot make or react to **insulin,** a **hormone** the pancreas produces to maintain proper blood sugar levels and metabolize sugar efficiently.

People with Type 1 or insulin-dependent diabetes, who generally are born with this condition, don't secrete the hormone at all and require insulin injections to stay alive. In Type 2 diabetes, which tends to strike later in life, people secrete some insulin but not enough, and may also be less sensitive to the effects of the hormone. Because the blood vessels and nerves of people with diabetes tend to deteriorate, they may develop heart disease and problems such as blindness, impotence, and numbness of the feet and hands.

In the second century A.D., the Greek writer Aretaeus (120–200) described the symptoms of diabetes including excessive urination, thirst, and emaciation, and hypothesized that the disease was caused by bladder or kidney problems. Indian writings of the sixth century describe the "honey urine" disease, so-called because the urine of diabetics contains abnormally high amounts of sugar, and note that patients with this disease are very susceptible to infections. The Arab doctor Avicenna (960–1037) wrote that people with diabetes often had abnormally large appetites and experienced loss of sexual function.

The Yorkshire doctor Matthew Dobson (unknown–1784) was the first person to suggest that the urine and blood of people with diabetes was sweet because it contained sugar.

In 1788, Thomas Cawley suggested that diabetes was caused by injury to or deterioration of the pancreas, having noted that patients with the disease often had atrophy in this organ. A number of other researchers confirmed this suggestion with autopsies. The understanding of the disease was advanced further by Claude Bernard (1813–1878), who discovered and described how the body uses and stores sugar, but he believed that diabetes was caused by a disorder of the liver.

Meanwhile, Paul Langerhans (1849–1888) observed distinct cell formations within the pancreas that were subsequently called the islets of Langerhans, which were later discovered to play a key role in diabetes.

Oscar Minkowsky (1858–1931) and Josef von Mering (1849–1908), working in Strasbourg in about 1889, showed that removing a dog's pancreas would produce diabetes in the animal. In 1902, in a series of **autopsies** on people with diabetes, Eugene Lindsay Opie observed that they all had atrophied islets of Langerhans. Edward Sharpey-Schafer (1850–1935) suggested that the islets secreted a substance that controlled carbohydrate metabolism, which he named "insulin."

Effective treatment for diabetes was impossible until researchers isolated and identified insulin and determined how to collect it in sufficient quantities. Early treatments for diabetes included various diets and exercise. Frederic Madisson Allen introduced starvation diets in 1912 that were up to that point the most effective treatment for the disease.

Today, newer **antidiabetes drugs,** longer-acting forms of injected insulin, and the development of home **glucose tests** have helped people with diabetes to manage and control their disease. **Public health** campaigns are underway to identify people who may be at risk of diabetes, so they can receive treatment before the illness has a chance to inflict permanent damage. By controlling their blood sugar levels carefully, people with diabetes can stave off deterioration of their health.

The incidence of Type 2 diabetes, which is linked to obesity and genetic factors, is on the rise in the United States, and the disease is appearing in young children.

Additional reading: Papaspyros, *The History of Diabetes Mellitus.*

Diagnostic and Statistical Manual of Mental Disorders (DSM)

U.S. psychiatrists and psychologists have used the Diagnostic and Statistical Manual of Mental Disorders to diagnose **mental illness** since 1952, when the first version was published by the American Psychiatric Association.

DSM-I was 130 pages long, and divided mental disorders into two categories: those caused by impairment of brain function ("psychotic") and those that resulted from a person's difficulty in adjusting to society ("psychoneurotic"). Psychotic disorders included **schizophrenia**, manic **depression**, and paranoia, while psychoneurotic disorders included depression, phobia, anxiety, and other disorders. Following the prevailing thought of the time, DSM-1 was largely based on psychoanalytic and psychodynamic concepts, and referred to various disorders as "reactions."

DSM-1 was developed because psychologists working during World War II found existing classification manuals from public mental hospitals weren't suited to the patients they were seeing. Military doctors frequently saw neurotic disorders, personality disturbances, and psychosomatic disorders in the servicemen they treated, but the manuals only briefly described these conditions.

The second edition of the DSM was published in 1967. The third, published in 1980, was three times longer. DSM-III attempted to make the diagnosis of mental illness less subjective by introducing specific criteria. A revised version that omitted homosexuality as a mental disorder, DSM-III-R, was published in 1987.

As ideas about mental illness have become more complex and nuanced, the DSM has become more complex and nuanced as well. The DSM-IV, published in 1994, is 886 pages long. Also, the uses of the manual extend beyond diagnosis of individual patients.

Today, the DSM is used for health-care reimbursement, mental health care budget allocations, and to help make legal decisions.

Additional reading: Friedman, *Encyclopedia of Mental Health,* pp. 29–42.

dialysis

Dialysis is the process of filtering liquid by passing it through a membrane that traps larger molecules while letting smaller ones pass.

In kidney dialysis, a machine replaces the action of the kidneys, maintaining the balance of fluids and electrolytes in the body by regulating their excretion in urine and also clearing wastes from the blood. Peritoneal dialysis is performed by infusing the abdominal cavity with a balanced electrolyte solution through a permanent plastic entry site.

John Jacob Abel (1857–1938) performed the first successful kidney dialysis on a dog in 1914, using colloidon as a membrane and **hirudin** (a substance extracted from leeches) as an **anticoagulant**. The machine consisted of a membrane formed into tubes, held in a glass cylinder containing dialysis fluid. Blood was passed through the tubes and waste products diffused into the surrounding fluid.

The first dialysis on a human patient was performed in 1924. Dr. Willem Kolff (1911–) created a new dialysis machine using cellophane sausage casing as a dialyzing membrane and had his first real success using the machine to treat a comatose patient in 1945.

Through these and several other advances in machine design, long-term kidney dialysis for patients in renal failure began to become practical in the 1960s. Part of the Medicare Act of 1972 included a provision to pay for dialysis for patients who needed it. Now, people with end stage kidney problems routinely have periodic dialysis.

Additional reading: Weisse, *Medical Odysseys,* pp. 89–96.

digestion

Digestion is the process by which the body breaks down food so it can be used as fuel. Enzymes secreted in the saliva and released by the stomach, pancreas, and small intestine all play a role in digestion. Peristalsis, in which the muscles of the digestive tract move rhythmically to pass food along, is also an important part of digestion.

In Hippocrates' (c.460–c.377 B.C.) time, digestion—like the incubation of a child—was seen as a process analogous to cooking, while Claudius Galen (129–c.199) thought the stomach, intestine, and liver cooked food in a series of steps and then converted it into blood. Paracelsus (1493–1541), a Swiss alchemist-physician, proposed correctly that the stomach contained acid, which was necessary for digestion, but he incorrectly suggested that this acid came from drinking spa water. Jean Baptiste van Helmont (1574–1644) described digestion as fermentation.

Two schools of thought on digestion subsequently developed: it was seen as either a chemical breakdown process, or a mechanical process in which the stomach physically milled the food into smaller pieces.

In 1777, Edward Stevens (1755–1834), proved that the stomach juices themselves contained acid. William Prout (1785–1850) suggested correctly that this was hydrochloric acid in an 1823 paper.

The unfortunate case of Alexis St. Martin (1803–1886) advanced the scientific understanding of digestion a great deal. St. Martin sustained a gunshot wound in his upper abdomen that left an open passage from his stomach to the outside of his body. The physician William Beaumont (1785–1853) took advantage of the man's injury and performed a series of experiments in which he suspended food in St. Martin's stomach by a silk string. In an 1833 book, Beaumont made many novel observations about digestion, including how long the process took, what environmental factors stimulated the flow of gastric juice, which foods are difficult to digest, and the motions of the stomach walls during digestion.

Beaumont reported in his book that it was not the acid contained in stomach juice that digested meat; he suggested that some other "principle inappreciable to the senses" was responsible. Theodor Schwann (1810–1882) isolated the responsible substance from the stomach lining, calling it "pepsin" in the 1836 report of his discovery.

During the 1890s, Ivan Petrovich Pavlov (1849–1936) showed in experiments with dogs that gastric secretion was a reflex response, controlled by the vagus nerve.

In 1901, William Bayliss (1860–1924) and Ernest Henry Starling (1866–1927) discovered that a substance they called secretin stimulated the pancreas to release digestive enzymes. Another substance that stimulated gastric secretion, called "gastrin," was discovered four years later and isolated in the 1960s. **Histamine** was, in the late twentieth century, also confirmed to stimulate acid secretion. A drug that blocks the action of histamine, **cimetidine**, was discovered in the 1970s and proved to be the first effective treatment for ulcers. Ulcers were later confirmed to be associated with a bacterium called **H. pylori**.

Researchers have subsequently found that cells in the stomach lining have receptors for gastrin, histamine, and cholinergic **hormones**, meaning all three types of substances can influence the secretion of stomach acid.

Additional reading: Davenport, *A History of Gastric Secretion and Digestion.*

digitalis

Digitalis is a drug for congestive heart failure made from the dried leaves of the foxglove plant. William Withering (1741–1799), a prominent British physician and botanist, published the first account of digitalis's effects in 1785, and the medication is still used today. The foxglove had been known and used in folk medicine for centuries before Withering's report. The natural product is no longer used. Instead, synthetic digitalis is used for better dosage control. The most common product is digoxin, a tablet.

Withering's *An Account of the Foxglove* warned that the medication should be used carefully, which remains true today. Digitalis strengthens the heart's contractions and helps the body excrete excess fluid. It is useful for treating some types of heart arrhythmia, but dangerous for patients with others.

Additional reading: Sneader, *Drug Discovery,* pp. 136–40.

dilantin

Dilantin, also called phenytoin, is a drug for controlling epileptic seizures that was discovered in 1936 and remains a mainstay of treatment.

Harvard neurologists H. Houston Merritt (1902–1979) and Tracy J. Putnam (1894–unknown) theorized that they could find an anticonvulsive drug by producing convulsions in animals with electric shock, and then determining whether certain chemicals protected the animals from suffering seizures. At this point, the only treatments for **epilepsy**—a condition affecting 1 percent of the U.S. population—were **barbiturates** and bromides, which had a sedating effect; a special diet; or restricted fluid consumption. In 1936, Merritt and Putnam and their colleagues began testing compounds from the Detroit drug company Parke-Davis for their ability to prevent convulsions.

After they found that compound sodium diphenyl hydantoinate protected against electric shock, and did more animal tests to check safety and dosage, Merritt and Putnam began conducting clinical tests on humans in 1937. The drug protected most patients against seizures without producing sedation. Parke-Davis began selling dilantin in 1938. Some patients taking the medication can develop serious hematopoietic complications and also dermatologic and lymphatic problems can occur.

Additional reading: Scott, *The History of Epileptic Therapy,* pp. 87–96.

diphtheria

Diphtheria is an inflammation of the throat caused by the *Corynebacterium diphtheriae* bacillus.

Some people with diphtheria develop a pseudomembrane that narrows the airway and may even close it off completely. The membrane resembles a shield, and the name diphtheria comes from the Greek word for rough leather. Thanks to vaccination, diphtheria is rare in developed countries, although a large outbreak occurred in the former Soviet Union in the early 1990s.

When the diphtheria bacterium itself is infected with a virus, it produces a toxin that causes the disease to be much more virulent. This toxin can damage the heart and nervous system.

Pierre Bretonneau (1778–1862) first described and named diphtheria in the 1820s. Diphtheria was a leading cause of death in children in the nineteenth century, killing half of those infected. In 1883, Edwin Klebs (1833–1913) at the Pasteur Institute identified the bacterium by culturing the bleeding surface beneath the membrane covering a patient's throat. Frederich Loeffler (1852–1915) developed an improved medium for growing the bacteria the following year, and both Klebs and Loeffler demonstrated that the bacterium was responsible for causing the disease. Loeffler also suggested that a toxin was involved.

In 1888, Pierre-Paul-Emile Roux (1853–1933) and Alexandre-Emile-John Yersin (1863–1943) at the Pasteur Institute provided more evidence for Loeffler's theory by showing that filtered material from the bacteria that did not contain the organism itself could cause diphtheria.

For children who developed the disease in the nineteenth century, a **tracheotomy** had often been the only effective treatment; this procedure allowed them to breathe through a hole cut in the trachea. Otherwise the obstruction caused by the infection would have suffocated them. **Endotracheal intubation,** developed around in the 1880s in the United States, involved inserting a tube down the throat to allow a child to breathe and prevent the trachea from closing off; this technique allowed many children to survive diphtheria infection without surgery.

Emil von Behring (1854–1917) and Shibasaburo Kitasato (1852–1931) found in 1890 that animals injected with toxins from diphtheria and tetanus would produce antitoxins that protected them; they also found that this immunity could be passed along with injections of serum. The following year, diphtheria antitoxin was given to a human for the first time, and soon many children were receiving injections of the antitoxin. The serum wasn't totally effective; about a quarter of the children who received it still died. However, it remained the only treatment for diphtheria for years.

In 1913, von Behring introduced active immunization, in which children were given some toxin along with the antitoxin. This treatment resulted in a few children getting infected. Treating the diphtheria toxin with formalin was found to inactivate the toxin, while still allowing it to confer immunity, resulting in a safer **vaccine.** The diphtheria toxin was licensed in 1926, while a combination called DPT that contained **pertussis** and **tetanus** vaccine along with diphtheria was licensed in 1948. The United States provided free diphtheria **immunization** to all children for the first half of the twentieth century. By 1935, diphtheria was no longer the leading killer of U.S. children.

The **virus** responsible for infecting the diphtheria bacillus and producing the toxin was identified and isolated in the early 1950s.

Today, children in the United States routinely receive diphtheria vaccines, often in the DPT form.

Additional reading: Hammonds, *Childhood's Deadly Scourge.*

diuretics

Diuretics are drugs that increase excretion of water in the urine and are used to treat swelling and also to reduce **blood pressure**.

Several herbs were known in ancient times to have diuretic effects. The diuretic properties of caffeine were known in the late nineteenth century, and this led to the investigation of theophylline, an extract from tea, as a diuretic. Theophylline was found to be three times more effective than caffeine.

The diuretic properties of a mercurial drug for **syphilis**, merbaphen, were dicovered in the early 1900s. The drug was found by Viennese researchers to reduce swelling and relieve pressure on the heart, allowing it to function normally. Unfortunately merbaphen could be toxic to the intestines and kidneys.

Scientists from the drug company Merck, Sharp, and Dohme discovered the thiazide diuretics in 1957. The first of these drugs was **chlorothiazide**. These drugs also increase salt excretion, and are still used today as first-line treatment for **hypertension.**

Drugs known as "loop diuretics," because their effect is on the kidney's loop of Henle, were introduced beginning in 1962 with furosemide, or Lasix, by the German drug company Hoechst. These drugs have the disadvantage of increasing **calcium** excretion, which can lead to **osteoporosis** with long-term use. Potassium loss can also occur with long-term use of chlorothiazide and furosemide.

Additional reading: Comroe, *Exploring the Heart,* pp. 289–308.

DHEA. *See* **androgens**.

DNA

DNA, or deoxyribonucleic acid, is the substance that makes up our **chromosomes** and carries genetic information. Technology that has allowed us to "read" the genetic code carried in DNA has made it possible to screen embryos for genetic disease and understand how the nucleus of the cell directs metabolic processes.

While analyzing pus-cell nuclei in 1869, Swiss chemist Friedrich Miescher (1811–1887) extracted a material containing phosphate that he called "nuclein." Miescher presciently suggested that this large, complex molecule might somehow carry encoded hereditary information.

One of Miescher's colleagues, Richard Altmann (1852–1900), removed the protein from nuclein in 1889 and called the remaining substance nucleic acid. The German biochemist Albrecht Kossel (1853–1927) found that nuclein contained purines and pyrimidines.

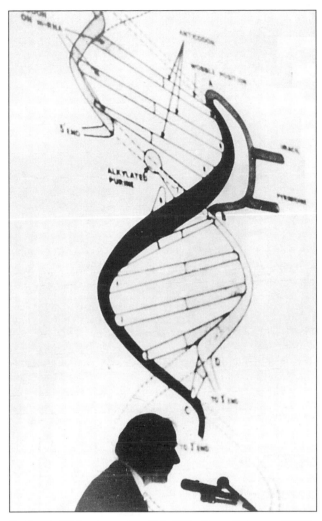

Dr. Francis Crick, winner of the Nobel Prize for co-discovery of DNA's double-helix structure, speaks at Columbia University with a diagram of the DNA molecule as a backdrop. (Photo by Elizabeth Wilcox, Archives and Special Collections, Columbia University Health Sciences Division.)

In 1927, British doctor Fred Griffith (1877–1941) observed that when he injected mice with dead, virulent bacteria along with a live, harmless strain, the mice died within days. He proposed that some substance carried the virulence trait from the dead bacteria to the live bacteria, making it virulent as well.

Rockefeller Institute scientist Oswald Avery (1877–1955) began looking for this substance, which he called the "transforming principle," in 1931. Colin MacLeod (1909–1972) joined Avery four years later, and Maclyn McCarty (1911–) followed in 1941. Both were physicians. The researchers eventually concluded that DNA was indeed the transforming principle, announcing their results to their Rockefeller colleagues in 1943 and publishing them early the following year.

Maurice Wilkins (1916–), a biophysicist at Kings College in London, began investigating the structure of DNA in 1950. He employed **X-ray** crystallography, in which the shadow of a crystal on an X-ray image is used to reveal a molecule's atomic structure. Rosalind Franklin (1920–1958), a young crystallography expert, joined the

lab at the suggestion of its chief John Randall (1905–) a year later.

The researchers secured a miniature X-ray machine called a microfocus generating tube that projected a narrow beam of light, making it possible to examine a single strand of DNA. Franklin made a series of images of DNA, which included an image taken in 1951 that clearly showed DNA's double helix structure. Franklin kept the image a secret from Wilkins, with whom she had an acrimonious relationship, but turned it over to him in 1952 after Randall asked her to leave the lab.

Around the same time, James Watson (1928–) and Francis Crick (1916–) at Cambridge University began working with a giant model of wire and brass to puzzle out the structure of DNA. With the help of information from Franklin and Wilkins, Watson and Crick determined the proper structure of DNA in 1953. The three teams—Watson and Crick; Franklin and Raymond Gosling; and Wilkins, Alex Stokes, and H.R. Wilson—each published papers on their DNA discoveries in the same issue of the journal *Nature*.

In the Watson-Crick model, sugar and phosphate molecules act as the rails of the double spiral, while the base pairs—cytosine and guanine or adenine and thymine—are the steps. Watson and Crick reported that the steps followed a pattern: cytosine bonded to guanine, adenine to thymine, and vice versa, so that one side of the molecule could act as a template for the construction of a whole molecule. They also proposed that the order of the nucleotide bases made up the **genetic code**. Watson, Crick, and Wilkins shared the 1962 Nobel Prize for their discovery of DNA's structure.

Additional reading: Friedman and Friedland, *Medicine's 10 Greatest Discoveries,* pp. 192–227.

DNA fingerprinting

DNA fingerprinting is a test for identifying and matching genetic material, usually for forensic purposes. It also has applications related to medicine and health. For example, DNA fingerprinting can be used to identify infectious microbes, to characterize cancerous tumors, and to match donors and recipients for organ transplants. Also, it is one of the main technologies being used to map the **human genome**.

DNA fingerprinting takes advantage of a phenomenon known as restriction fragment length polymorphism. **Restriction enzymes** cut **DNA** at a point where a certain sequence is found. This point on the DNA molecule varies from person to person. When restriction enzymes are added to genetic material, a series of fragments of varying lengths results. These fragments are then placed in an electrophoretic gel, through which they will travel for a certain distance based on their length. The fragments are then transferred to a sheet of nitrocellulose material and exposed to a radioactive probe that will bind to genes of a particular sequence. A piece of **X-ray** film is placed against this sheet and developed. The resulting "fingerprint" looks like a bar code, and describes the proportion of fragments of various lengths found in a sample. No two people will have the same DNA fingerprint.

The technique was developed in the 1970s by the English scientist Alec Jeffries. DNA fingerprints were first used in criminal study in 1986.

Additional reading: Begley, "Blood, Hair and Heredity."

Down syndrome

Down syndrome is a genetic condition resulting in delayed mental and physical development. People with Down syndrome have small heads, slanting eyes, a large tongue, and short hands with a single crease across the palm. They also often have heart defects. One in 1,000 children has Down syndrome.

Edouard Seguin (1812–1880) described this condition as a mental retardation syndrome accompanied by multiple genetic abnormalities in 1846. In an 1866 paper, J. Langdon H. Down (1828–1896) called the syndrome that would come to bear his name "mongoloid idiocy." He was attempting to classify the "feeble-minded" by their resemblance to various ethnic groups, a scientifically invalid as well as a racist pursuit.

Jerome Lejeune (1926–) discovered the chromosomal defect responsible for 95 percent of cases of Down syndrome in 1959. In this defect, called trisomy 21, the 21st **chromosome** pair contains three chromosomes instead of the normal two. Older women are at greater risk of giving birth to a Down syndrome child.

People with Down syndrome develop **Alzheimer's disease**-like lesions in their brain at a very young age; nearly 90 percent of people with Down syndrome who are older than 30 have these lesions, which lead to dementia. People with Down syndrome are also at higher risk of **leukemia**, and tend to have heart defects. They generally live until their 30s or 40s.

Additional reading: Kiple, *The Cambridge World History of Human Disease,* pp. 683–86.

Drinker respirator (iron lung)

This device, known popularly as the iron lung, provides breathing assistance to a person whose lungs are paralyzed.

The American industrial hygienist Philip Drinker (1894–1972) began developing the iron lung with his colleague Louis Shaw (1886–1940) in the 1930s, and built the first device in 1937.

The entire body, except for the head and neck, is placed inside the device. Raising and lowering the pressure within the capsule causes the lungs to contract and expand, expelling and then drawing in air to make breathing possible. These devices were widely used during the American **poliomyelitis** epidemic that began in the late 1940s.

The iron lung fell out of use in the late 1950s, after the polio **vaccine** had vanquished the disease. Today, the Drinker respirator has been replaced by other **artificial respiration** techniques, usually positive pressure ventilation apparatuses that push air rhythmically into the lungs. The

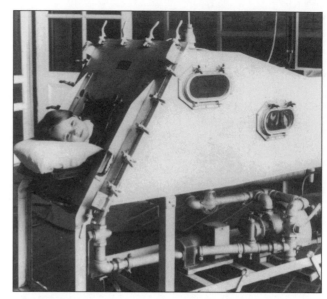

Child in a Drinker respirator, also known as an iron lung, at Johns Hopkins. (Courtesy of The Alan Mason Chesney Medical Archives of the Johns Hopkins Medical Institutions.)

air is passed into the lungs either by **endotracheal intubation** or through a **tracheotomy.**

The newer systems, though less cumbersome, actually tend to produce more complications than the older device. A patient in an iron lung can speak and they also face less risk of infection. A handful of research published in the late 1990s demonstrated that the less-invasive iron lung may be helpful in treating patients with certain types of injury to the chest. In some parts of the world, in fact, iron lungs are making a comeback for treating patients who require long-term breathing assistance.

Additional reading: Shorter, *The Health Century,* pp. 61–63.

DSM. *See Diagnostic and Statistical Manual of Mental disorders.*

dysentery

Dysentery is a collective term for several diseases characterized by inflammation of the colon; bloody, loose stools; and painful defecation. Known as the "bloody flux," dysentery has plagued the poor, armies, and sailors since ancient times.

One form of the disease, amebic dysentery, is caused by the organism *Entamoeba histolytica* and spread by fecal contamination of food and water. The Russian doctor Frederic A. Losch (1840s–1875) described this microorganism in 1875.

Bacillary dysentery may be caused by several types of bacteria, including *Campylobacter, Salmonelle, Yersinia,* certain strains of E. coli, and *Shigella,* which is the main culprit. Like amoebic dysentery, bacillary dysentery is spread by contaminated food or water. In 1898, Kiyoshi Shiga (1870–1957) discovered the first dysentery-causing bacteria, *Shigella dysenteriae,* and others were found in the early twentieth century. Campylobacter was not known to cause dysentery until the 1970s.

Dysentery remains a serious health problem in communities without good sanitation. It also is frequently spread by poor hygiene. Food poisoning with bacteria and other organisms, such as **E. coli 0157:H7** and **cryptosporidium,** has become an increasingly large **public health** problem. Dysentery can also be fatal to people with vulnerable immune systems, such as older people, infants, and people with **AIDS**.

E

E. coli 0157:H7

E. coli 0157:H7 is a strain of the *Escherichia* bacterium that can cause bloody diarrhea. Infection in 5 percent to 10 percent of cases can lead to hemolytic uremic syndrome, a potentially fatal disease. This usually occurs in children younger than five. The bacterium causes 250 deaths and 20,000 illnesses in the United States annually.

E. coli 0157:H7 is the most common of a group of related bacteria known as Shiga toxin-producing E. coli, so called because they produce a toxin similar to that released by the bacterium *Shigella dysenteraie*. Very low concentrations of the bacterium can cause illness; some researchers believe as few as five organisms are necessary.

The bacterium is believed to infect cattle, and usually is spread to humans by consumption of contaminated food, particularly undercooked ground beef and unpasteurized fruit juices. The bacterium can survive in extremely acidic foods and at low temperatures.

Public health experts believe these bacteria typify a type of food contamination that will become more and more common in the developed world, as food production becomes increasingly centralized and distribution more far-reaching.

First recognized in 1975 in a single case by researchers from the **Centers for Disease Control and Prevention**, the bacterium has been implicated in a growing number of food-poisoning outbreaks in the United States since 1982. In the 1990s, cases were reported in Europe and Japan.

The largest outbreak of E. coli 0157:H7 to date occurred in 1993 in the western United States after hundreds of people ate contaminated hamburgers from a restaurant chain. There were 500 confirmed cases and four deaths.

Public health experts believe one reason for the increase in E. coli 0157:H7 is the change in how meat is produced. Dairy and cattle farms are becoming much larger, increasing opportunities for spread of infection among animals. Ground beef producers may also buy meat from several sources and process it in lots as large as 30 tons, meaning a hamburger or package of ground beef typically contains meat from several animals—perhaps even hundreds. Researchers also suggest that the disease is becoming more common because more and more Americans are eating beef from fast-food restaurants, rather than cooking it at home where they can be sure the meat is well-done.

The U.S. Department of Agriculture and the Department of Health and Human Services launched a multiagency effort in 1997 to improve the safety of the food supply. A major focus of this effort, which continues today, is on hazard analysis and critical control point (HACCP) systems for food production. As of January 25, 2000, all meat and poultry producers were required to have HAACP systems in place. Companies that do not have these systems will not be inspected by the **Food Safety and Inspection Service** and thus will not be able to sell their product in the United States.

Additional reading: Fox, *Spoiled*, pp. 211–63.

ECG. *See electrocardiogram (ECG, EKG)*

echocardiography

Echocardiography is the use of **ultrasound** to provide a "picture" of the structures within the heart, namely the valves and muscular components. Also it shows disorders of the membrane covering the heart, the pericardium. A transducer delivers sound waves into the area around the heart, and a computer reads the returning echoes. Echocardiograms are the second most commonly used diagnostic test for the heart, after **electrocardiograms (EKG).**

The technology used for echocardiography is an adaptation of sonar, which had been developed during World War II for military applications such as detecting enemy subs underwater.

Wolf Dieter Keidel (1917–) was the first physician to use ultrasound to image the heart, in 1950, but he used it more as an **X-ray** to portray a shadow of the organ. Cardiologist Inge Edler (1911–)and physicist Carl Hellmuth Hertz (1920–), both Swedish, were the first to use the technique to examine structures within the heart, publishing their results in 1954. Japanese investigators focused on

Doppler ultrasound technology, which measures the velocity of blood flow, and began publishing their results in the 1950s as well.

Throughout the 1960s and 1970s, researchers developed echocardiographic instruments and refined the diagnosis of heart ailments with ultrasound. The first academic course on echocardiography in the United States was taught in 1968, and the first book on the subject was published in 1972.

Today, researchers are working on developing three-dimensional ultrasound techniques and digital recording of echocardiographic images, rather than video recording.

Additional reading: Comroe, *Exploring the Heart,* pp. 128–36.

eclampsia

Eclampsia is a deadly condition that strikes women late in pregnancy and is marked by coma and convulsive seizures. Although the cause of eclampsia is unknown, high **blood pressure** and certain types of kidney disease can predispose a woman to developing it.

Eclampsia is signaled by preeclampsia, a collection of symptoms that include high blood pressure, swelling of the legs, and headache. About 1 in 200 women with preeclampsia will go on to develop eclampsia.

Eclampsia was thought to be identical to **epilepsy** until 1739, when Francois Boissier deSauvages (1706–1767) wrote that epilepsy was chronic and occurred throughout life; he dubbed acute convulsions "eclampsia." He later described convulsions related to labor, which he called "eclampsia parturientium." Francois Mauriceau (1637–1709) had noted in his 1668 book that women pregnant for the first time were more likely to suffer convulsions, an observation that several subsequent studies over the centuries have confirmed. Less accurately, he said convulsions were caused by hot blood flowing from the uterus and stimulating the nerves, or possibly by vapors arising from a dead fetus.

From the seventeenth to the nineteenth century, doctors relied on purging and bleeding to treat eclampsia. Their rationale was that a woman suffering from eclampsia was "replete," or too full of blood. In the later 1800s, anesthetic and narcotic drugs also were used. Around this time two different courses of treatment for eclampsia emerged: **cesarean section** and the conservative method, in which the child was usually delivered with **forceps** as soon as the cervix dilated sufficiently. A study published in 1922 found that conservative management with vaginal delivery had the lowest rate of mortality.

The major advance in treatment of eclampsia came with the use of magnesium sulfate to treat eclampsia in the 1920s. The mineral had been shown in the early twentieth century to control convulsions in tetanus. This remains the best treatment for eclampsia.

Preeclampsia cannot be prevented, but one of the main benefits of regular **prenatal care** is to monitor pregnant women for it and treat them so that it will not get worse.

In 1960, Leon Chesley (1909–) and his colleagues suggested that the tendency for preeclampsia may be inherited, and subsequent studies have borne this out; women with a sister or mother who had preeclampsia are much more likely to develop it themselves.

Antiseizure drugs such as diazepam and phenytoin also have been used to treat eclampsia, but studies completed in the 1990s showed that magnesium sulfate was safer and more effective. Today, the death rate for eclampsia is about 5 percent.

Additional reading: Kiple, *The Cambridge World History of Human Disease,* pp. 704–07.

ECT. *See electroconvulsive therapy.*

EEG. *See electroencephalography.*

egg donation

In egg donation, a woman who cannot produce healthy eggs on her own uses an egg donated by another woman to become pregnant. For the donation to be successful, the menstrual cycles of the donor and the recipient must be synchronized with drugs.

The first cases of successful pregnancies with donated eggs were reported in 1984, and the technique became available in the United States in 1987. The American pioneers were Maria Bustillo (1951–) and her colleagues at the UCLA Medical Center in Torrance, California. The group used a donated embryo from a woman who had been artificially fertilized with the future father's sperm. A group at the Queen Victoria Medical Center in Victoria, Australia, used a donor egg inseminated in vitro.

Donors receive gonadotropin to stimulate egg maturation, and women who receive the donated eggs must undergo hormone therapy in order to maintain the pregnancy.

When egg donation first became available, the Ethics Committee of the American Fertility Society had discouraged payment for donors, but now advertisements regularly appear in magazines offering women $5,000 or more for their eggs.

Additional reading: Angier, *Woman,* pp. 1–16.

electrocardiogram (ECG, EKG)

An electrocardiogram is a recording of the electrical impulses that govern the heartbeat. Cardiologists read this record to diagnose heartbeat irregularities, heart muscle damage from a coronary occlusion, and insufficiency of blood flow through heart muscle (ischemia).

In the nineteenth century, researchers noted that the muscles and the heart—which is a muscle itself—produced electrical activity. Augustus Waller (1856–1922) was the first to publish a recording of the heart's electrical activity as measured on the surface of the body, in 1887. Waller used a device called a capillary electrometer, a thick glass tube containing mercury and sulfuric acid. When the tube was placed in the proper place on the chest, the mercury column moved as electrical current from the body changed.

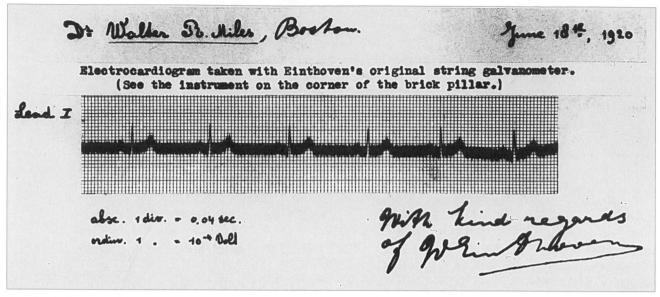

A reading from the string galvanometer echocardiograph invented by William Einthoven to record the electrical activity of the heart, dated 1920. (Courtesy of National Library of Medicine.)

The mercury's movement was observed through a microscope, enlarged, and projected on photographic paper. This device wasn't sensitive or precise enough to provide a truly accurate picture of the heart's electrical activity.

In 1901, Dutch physiologist and pathologist William Einthoven (1858–1930) used a new device—based largely on the work of French engineer Clement Ader (1841–1923)—to produce a more accurate recording. Einthoven suspended a silver-plated quartz string between two poles of an electromagnet. The string changed position depending on the strength of the current passing through it. Einthoven used a **microscope**-and-photographic-paper system similar to Waller's to record the activity. He published a paper on using his device to record a patient's heart activity in 1906, and won the 1924 Nobel Prize for his work.

Einthoven's **echocardiograph** weighed 800 pounds and required five people to operate it. The patient undergoing the test had to immerse each hand and each foot in a separate bucket of water.

By the 1930s, ECGs were available to general practitioners in the United States. About half of all U.S. general practitioners had an ECG in their office by the 1950s.

The Holter monitor, which a patient can wear around his or her waist, is capable of recording up to 24 hours of heart activity and weighs less than 2 pounds. It uses the same calibration system for recording that Einthoven developed.

Additional reading: Bynum, et al., *The Emergence of Modern Cardiology,* pp. 53–76.

electrocautery

Electrocautery is the use of high-energy electricity to stop bleeding or destroy abnormal **tissue**.

Albrecht Theodor von Middeldorpff (1824–1868) of Breslau, Poland, designed several galvanocautery instruments, publishing a treatise on electrocautery in 1854.

An instrument with a current strong enough to cut tissue only became available in 1907, after Lee De Forest (1873–1961) invented the triode tube. Johns Hopkins neurosurgeon Harvey Cushing (1869–1939) worked with a Harvard physicist, William Bovie (1882–1958), to develop a tool that would produce currents suitable for both cutting tissue and coagulating blood. The machine was completed in 1926 and is similar to those used today.

Additional reading: Ellis, *Famous Operations,* pp. 71–76.

electroconvulsive therapy (ECT, electroshock therapy)

Electroconvulsive therapy is the act of passing an electric current through the brain to induce a seizure in hopes of treating various types of mental illness. ECT is also often referred to as electroshock therapy.

Ugo Cerletti (1877–1963) and Lucio Bini (1908–) performed the first ECT in 1938, on a Roman man with schizophrenia. They reported that the treatment worked. The two Italian researchers studied the use of electricity to induce seizures in dogs for several years before applying the technique to a human.

ECT descends from **convulsive therapy**, introduced by Ladislas J. Meduna (1896–1964) in 1934. Doctors had observed that schizophrenics stopped being psychotic for a time after having seizures, which usually had been caused by **epilepsy** or induced by drug withdrawal. Meduna theorized that intentionally giving schizophrenics seizures would be an effective treatment for their psychoses.

ECT was performed on a patient in the United States for the first time in 1940, in New York City. Lothar Kalinowsky (1922–), who also established an ECT unit in New York, helped popularize the therapy in the United States, building his own machine.

A serious drawback of ECT was that it caused patients to make violent thrashing movements, which could result in fractured limbs and vertebrae. Abram Bennett (1898–unknown), an Omaha psychiatrist, used the muscle relaxant drug **curare** in patients receiving ECT at the suggestion of Walter Freeman (1895–1972) beginning in 1940. The safer drug succinylcholine, which worked similarly to curare, was introduced into ECT therapy in 1952, along with a short-acting anesthetic called Brevital (methohexital sodium).

By 1959, ECT was considered in the United States to be the best treatment for manic-depressive illness and major **depression.**

Although ECT was controversial because of its perceived cruelty, and the fact that it was used in public **mental hospitals** sometimes against patients' will, ECT remains a respected treatment today. The mechanism by which ECT improves mental health, however, remains a mystery. (*See also* schizophrenia)

Additional reading: Shorter, *A History of Psychiatry,* pp. 218–24.

electroencephalography (EEG)

Electroencephalography is the recording of the brain's electrical activity.

In 1870, two German researchers, Edouard Hitzig (1838–1907) and Gustav Fritsch (1838–1927), observed that dogs under **anesthesia** would move in response to electrical stimulation of their brains. This work was based on an earlier experience of Fritsch's. He was dressing a patient's open head wound, and noticed that when he touched the brain the limbs on the opposite side of the patient's body moved. Sir David Ferrier (1843–1928) did similar work in England on animals.

Richard Caton (1842–1926) was the first to record the electronic activity of the brain, using a mirror galvanometer to track activity from electrodes placed on the exposed brains of rabbits and monkeys, reporting his work in 1875.

Several different researchers subsequently tried to develop more sensitive instruments and better methods for recording electrical activity, always using animal subjects. Hans Berger (1873–1941) recorded the electrical activity of a human brain in 1924, the first time that this had been done. After he had made 1,133 recordings of brain activity in 76 people, he published his findings in 1929. Berger identified the alpha wave and the beta wave, two types of normal brain waves people exhibit when awake and relaxed.

Both Caton and Berger had to demonstrate their work "live" to colleagues by projecting recordings of electrical activity, as it occurred, onto a wall in a dark room, since they had no method for making permanent recordings of this activity.

Herbert H. Jasper (1906–) of the University of Montreal was the first American to confirm Berger's work, and his EEG research paved the way to monitoring epileptic seizures and localizing the foci of these seizures, which made surgical treatment possible.

Researchers built their own EEG equipment until the mid-1930s, when commercial manufacture of EEG systems began. Dr. Reginald Bickford (1913–) made a portable EEG unit in the 1940s that he used to monitor the brains of injured World War II pilots. By the mid-1950s most teaching hospitals had EEG departments, and by 1960 most hospitals and private practices had them.

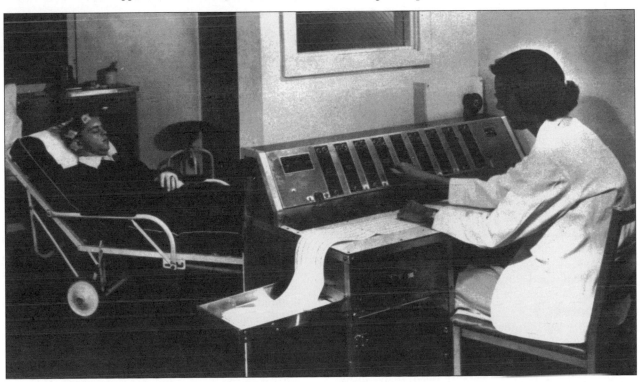

A patient undergoing an electroencephalogram at George Washington University Hospital in Washington, DC. (Courtesy of National Library of Medicine.)

In the late 1930s researchers began using cameras to record a patient's physical activity simultaneously with the brain's electrical activity, which was especially useful for observing epileptic seizures. Dr. Eli Samuel Goldensohn (1915–) of New York developed the first split-screen video/ EEG recording in 1963, reporting on it in 1966.

Most recently digital EEGs have come into use, although computerized recording of brain activity actually has some disadvantages compared with the old paper-based system. For example, producing images requires massive amounts of computer memory. However, digital EEGs can record more sensitively and store information more cheaply.

Although brain imaging techniques such as **magnetic resonance imaging**, **CAT scanning**, and **PET scanning** now provide ways to "look at" structural defects and metabolic activity within the brain, EEG remains a vital diagnostic tool, especially for patients with **epilepsy**.

Additional reading: O'Leary and Goldring, *Science and Epilepsy,* pp. 119–52.

electron microscope

Electron microscopes use streams of electrons, rather than light, to magnify objects for viewing, and can magnify by up to 25,000 times.

Louis de Broglie (1892–1987) paved the way for the development of electron microscopes when he suggested in 1924 that electron beams could be seen as wave motion, with a wavelength much smaller than that of light, meaning an electron microscope could be produced with resolution much better than that of a light **microscope**. Ernst Ruska (1906–1988) built the first electron microscope in Berlin in 1931. He shared the 1986 Nobel Prize in Physics for this achievement.

Early electron microscopes were difficult to use because they heated up the specimens to be magnified; this problem was not solved for several years.

Commercial construction of electron microscopes began in England in 1935 and soon followed in Germany, by the electrical engineering and electronics company Siemens, and in the United States by the electronics company RCA. Electron microscopes revolutionized biology, because they made it possible for scientists to see minuscule structures within cells as well as **viruses.**

Subsequent advances in microscopy include acoustic microscopy in 1940, which made it possible to visualize the interior of structures; and scanning tunneling microscopy, which measures changes in electric current between the specimen and the microscope probe. With this device it is possible to "see" individual atoms.

Additional reading: Rasmussen, *Picture Control.*

electrophoresis

In electrophoresis, the movement of charged particles suspended in a solution is observed to determine the composition of the solution.

Arne Tiselius (1902–1971), a Swedish chemist, wrote his 1930 thesis on electrophoresis and went on to build an electrophoretic machine in 1936. In his thesis, he had observed that globulin in the blood displayed great heterogeneity, which was surprising because globulin was thought to be a single type of protein. Working with his new machine, he found four classes of materials in a serum sample, and he named three of them alpha-, beta-, and gamma-globulin, which are now known to be different classes of **antibodies**. He won the 1948 Nobel Prize in Chemistry for this and other work with electrophoresis.

Many researchers used Tiselius's electrophoresis machines, which became commercially available soon after the first machine was built, to study proteins. The method could be used to gauge protein purity and detect abnormal proteins, but it is cumbersome because a single run of the machine takes an entire day. A less complex method called zone electrophoresis was developed, which is now in common use in clinical laboratories.

Starch gel electrophoresis, introduced in 1955 by Oliver Smithies (1925–), broke down the different globulins on the basis of molecular size as well as ionic charge. It also required much less sample material, and was less cumbersome to perform.

Additional reading: Andrews, *Electrophoresis.*

electroshock therapy. *See* electroconvulsive therapy.

endorphins

The brain produces endorphins—natural opiates—to dull pain, to elevate mood, and for many other purposes. Endorphins are a type of neurotransmitter.

Researchers in the 1940s noted that the action of opiate drugs in the brain was extremely specific. In 1973, two teams of scientists discovered independently that the brain contained sites for the binding of these drugs, which suggested that chemicals similar to opiates occurred in the body naturally. John Hughes (1942–) and Hans Kosterlitz (1903–1996) at the University of Aberdeen and Avram Goldstein (1919–), Eric Simon (1924–), Lars Terenius (1940–), and Solomon Snyder (1938–) discovered these binding sites.

Once the receptors were discovered, researchers began searching for the natural chemicals, reporting their existence in 1974. In 1975, Hughes isolated and characterized the first of these chemicals, which he named methionine and leucine enkephalin. Simon coined the term "endorphin" as a contraction of "endogenous morphine."

There are now known to be 15 opiate-like peptides that naturally occur in the brain. All are believed to come from three precursors: proenkephalin, proopiomelanocortin, and prodynorphin. Endorphins can be found in tissues beyond the brain, and fall into two families: the enkephalin system and the endorphin system.

The discovery of these chemicals has helped scientists begin to understand how the body fights pain. Pharmaceutical researchers are also searching for new pain-killing drugs based on the structure of these endorphins.

Additional reading: Davis, *Endorphins.*

endoscopy

Endoscopy is the observation of the interior of the body through an instrument that may be inserted via a natural opening or through an incision.

German Rudolf Schindler (1888–1968) built the first useful gastroscope, an instrument for examining the inside of the stomach. Flexible at the end inserted into the esophagus and stiff at the viewing end, the gastroscope employed lenses and prisms to transmit the view to the clinician. Schindler published instructions for using the new instrument in 1923.

Further advances in endoscopy required the development of fiberoptics, which uses a bundle of glass fibers to transmit an image. With fiberoptics, an image could be transmitted along a curved, flexible tube, meaning endoscopic instruments could be passed into the body further, and also more comfortably for the patient. In 1954, Narinder Singh Kapany (1927–) and his colleagues announced that they had built an endoscope using fibroscopic technology.

Refining this instrument, Basil Hirschowitz (1925–) built a prototype of a flexible gastroscope, and showed the instrument to a gathering of the American Gastroenterological Association in 1957. Bergein Overhold built a flexible sigmoidoscope for viewing the lower intestine in 1963.

Today, endoscopic instruments use photographic and video technology to record the appearance of the interior organs, and can also be used to take tissue samples for biopsies. These instruments are extremely useful as screening and diagnostic tools.

Additional reading: Galton, *Med Tech*, pp. 184–90.

endotracheal intubation

Endotracheal intubation is the insertion of a tube into the trachea to allow breathing, either when a person cannot breathe on his or her own due to disease or injury or during **anesthesia**.

The Flemish anatomist Andreas Vesalius (1514–1564) performed the first endotracheal intubation of an animal, but humans were not intubated successfully until the nineteenth century.

Joseph O'Dwyer (1841–1898) of New York developed a tube that he used to open the windpipes of children with **diphtheria**, who otherwise would have had to have **tracheotomies**. He reported the first recovery of a child in whom the tube was used in 1884. By the end of the 1880s, many physicians were using the O'Dwyer tube. He wrote a textbook of instructions on its use that was published in 1889.

Endotracheal intubation during surgery began with Sir William Macewen in 1878. He practiced his method for inserting the tube on cadavers. His method was adapted from that of the German surgeon Friedrich Trendelenburg (1814–1924), who had inserted the tube through a tracheotomy.

Additional reading: Dao, "Paramedics Can Practice Life-Saving Process on Cats."

Environmental Protection Agency (EPA)

The Environmental Protection Agency was established in 1970 by an executive order of President Richard Nixon (1913–1994) to oversee environmental protection efforts, which had been previously been handled by more than a dozen different government programs. The EPA thus assumed responsibility for waste management, air and water pollution control, radiation standards, and regulation of pesticide levels in the environment and in food.

Headquartered in Washington, D.C., the EPA has 10 regional offices and field laboratories. The central office issues pollution permits to companies, and regional employees ensure that businesses adhere to the limits set in these permits.

In 1974, the Safe Drinking Water Act required the EPA to set standards for safe levels of pollutant in drinking water. The Superfund act, formally known as the Comprehensive Environmental Response, Compensation, and Liability Act of 1980, provided funds for cleanup of areas contaminated with toxic waste. Taxes on chemical companies paid for the cleanup.

Improving the environmental health of the United States' coastal areas became a major focus of EPA policy during President William Clinton's second term. In December 1999, the United States joined 26 other nations in signing the first-ever international agreement on controlling emissions in order to reduce smog, acid rain, and other types of environmental damage caused by air pollution. In early 2000, the Clinton administration announced the largest-ever increase in the EPA's operating budget.

Additional reading: Marwick, "New Focus on Children's Environmental Health"; Landy, et al., The *Environmental Protection Agency*; Andrews, *Managing the Environment, Managing Ourselves*.

ephedrine

Ephedrine is a drug with effects similar to those of the neurotransmitter **epinephrine**. Also called Ma Huang, the drug has been used in China since 3100 B.C. to promote sweating, ease fever, and halt coughing.

Ephedrine comes from a type of desert shrub from the genus Ephedra. Nagajosi Nagai of Tokyo University first isolated ephedrine from the plant in 1887.

Ku Kuei Chen (1898–unknown) at the Peking Union Medical College, with Carl Schmidt (1893–1988), developed and tested extracts of Ma Huang and observed that it increased **blood pressure** and heart rate and caused the blood vessels to constrict. They also found out that, unlike epinephrine, ephedrine could be given orally. They sent a supply to physicians at the University of Pennsylvania and the Mayo Clinic for tests, and the drug was approved for use in the United States in 1926.

Ephedrine is now used in medications for hay fever, **asthma**, and nasal congestion. It is, however, addictive and can lead to drug abuse.

Additional reading: Tyler, "The Two Faces of Ma Huang"; Leary, "A Federal Panel Suggests Restriction of an Herbal Stimulant."

epidural anesthesia

Epidural **anesthesia** is a technique for pain relief during childbirth in which local anesthetics such as lidocaine are injected into the space outside the dura, the membrane covering the spine.

This is currently the preferred method for pain relief during labor, but it also may slow the labor process and can cause certain side effects.

The Romanian obstetrician Eugen Bogdan Aburel (1899–1975) pioneered epidural anesthesia for women in labor, reporting on it in a paper at a professional meeting in Paris in 1931. The development of lidocaine, chloroprocaine, and mepivacaine in the 1940s and 1950s allowed for continuous administration of the anesthesia during labor, and in the 1960s bupivacaine was introduced.

When opioid receptors on the spine were discovered in the 1970s, opioid drugs such as fentanyl were used for epidural anesthesia, allowing for better pain relief and less motor blockage. Today, about one-third of women in the United States opt for epidural anesthesia during childbirth.

Additional reading: Shute, "No More Hard Labor."

epilepsy

Epilepsy is a condition in which abnormalities within the brain give rise to seizures, in which the body's muscles contract and a person loses consciousness. The name comes from "epilepsia," the Greek word for seizure. About 1 percent of the U.S. population suffers from epilepsy. Medication can control most cases of epilepsy, while severe forms of the condition may require surgery in which the part of the brain from which seizures arise is removed or destroyed.

Epilepsy has most likely affected humans since prehistoric times; some medical historians believe **trepanation,** an ancient operation in which a hole was cut in the skull, was performed to treat epilepsy. Up until the nineteenth century, epilepsy was considered by many to have a supernatural cause; some saw it as evidence of demonic possession, while others believed the gods caused it. However, Hippocrates (c.460–c.377 B.C.)wrote that epilepsy originated in the brain and made many correct observations about the disease, including that it most often appears in early life and rarely first strikes a person after age 20. Ancient Greek physicians also described the aura that can precede a seizure, and knew what steps to take to prevent a person from being injured during convulsions.

The Greek doctor Claudius Galen (129–c.199) believed that epilepsy originated in the ventricles, the hollow areas within the brain. His incorrect view was held to be correct for centuries afterwards.

In the Middle Ages, epilepsy was referred to as the "falling sickness." Remedies prescribed for epilepsy included peony and mistletoe. **Cauterization** of the brain and trepanning were also performed, the latter operation well into the seventeenth century.

The prominent London doctor Thomas Willis (1621–1675) proposed in 1667 that the epileptic attack, as well as the aura preceding it, originated from the cerebellum.

The first drugs capable of reducing the frequency of epileptic seizures, bromides, were introduced by London doctor Charles Locock (1797–1875) in 1857.

In the 1860s, John Hughlings Jackson (1835–1911), proposed that epilepsy was due to excessive discharge from the gray matter of the brain and that certain seizures arose from abnormal electric discharge in the cortex. Seizures would manifest themselves differently depending on where they arose and how they spread through the brain, Jackson concluded.

Jackson's colleague, Victor Horsely (1857–1916), performed the first modern surgery for epilepsy in 1886, on a patient whose seizures issued from a scar on the cortex. Horsely and his followers over the next four decades used **X-rays** and pneumoencephalography to locate the site of the lesion, and would test the electric field of the brain after the skull had been opened.

The first modern medication used to treat epilepsy was phenobarbitol, a **barbiturate** drug. Alfred Hauptmann (1881–unknown), a German physician, first reported using the drug in patients with epilepsy in 1912. He found that it reduced the number of seizures patients suffered as well as the severity of the attacks.

The ancient Greeks had observed that fasting could control epileptic seizures. Interest in carefully controlled "ketogenic" diets, so called because they contained a great deal of fat but little protein and carbohydrates and thus caused the body to produce ketone bodies, grew in the 1920s. Such diets, when administered with care, could indeed prevent seizures in some patients and allowed them to take fewer antiseizure drugs. A drug that produces a similar effect as the ketogenic diet, acetazolamide, continues to be used as an adjunct to therapy today.

Hans Berger (1873–1941) was able to show in his work with the **electroencephalogram** in the 1920s that people with epilepsy had abnormal electrical activity within the brain.

The next antiseizure drug to be discovered, **dilantin**, was first tested in humans in 1937 and represented a major advance in epilepsy treatment. Unfortunately the drug, which is still used today as a first-line epilepsy treatment, has many side effects including nausea, vomiting, headache, dizziness, and sometimes abnormalities in the blood.

Carbamazepine was discovered at the Swiss drug company Geigy and introduced as an anti-epilepsy drug in 1954. The drug was found not only to control seizures but to lift patients' moods as well. This was beneficial, because people with epilepsy commonly suffer from **depression**. The **Food and Drug Administration (FDA)** did not approve the drug until 1974.

Valproate, a drug that was first synthesized in 1881, was found in 1962 to be useful for treating every type of epileptic seizure. **Clinical trials** began two years later, and the drug was introduced in France in 1967.

Several new drugs are being studied for epilepsy that affect the brain's use of the neurotransmitter GABA, which is believed to play a role in epilepsy.

Since **magnetic resonance imaging (MRI)** was introduced in the 1980s, imaging of epileptogenic lesions has become much more precise, and has clarified which patients can benefit from this surgery. The great majority of epilepsy surgeries—90 percent to 99 percent—involve the cortex. Most of these are temporal lobectomies.

Very rarely, more radical operations such as hemispherectomy—in which a large section of the brain is removed—or surgery on the corpus callosum to disrupt the spread of seizures are performed. These surgeries are usually only performed on children who suffer from severe, disabling seizures.

Additional reading: Temkin, *The Falling Sickness.*

epinephrine

Epinephrine, or adrenaline, is a **hormone** associated with fear and anxiety.

The sympathetic nervous system triggers the **adrenal gland** to release adrenaline, and the hormone causes blood vessels to constrict.

Epinephrine is available in artificial form as a medication, and is used to treat **asthma** attacks, hemorrhage, and heart arrythmias. It also improves the action of local anesthetics by constricting blood vessels so the numbing drug is absorbed more slowly.

The British researchers George Oliver (1841–1915) and Edward A. Schafer showed, in 1894, that extracts from the adrenal gland had strong effects on the skeletal muscles, heart, and blood vessels, and also caused **blood pressure** to rise. John Jacob Abel (1857–1938), a pharmacology professor at Johns Hopkins University in Baltimore, isolated the hormone responsible for this effect, which he called epinephrine, reporting on his method in 1897. Epinephrine was the first hormone to be isolated.

Jokichi Takamine (1854–1922), a Japanese scientist working in the United States, developed a more effective process for isolating this substance, which he called "adrenaline," and published his findings in 1901. He won five U.S. patents on the substance, name, and method in 1903. The pharmaceutical company Parke-Davis licensed the name.

Hoechst Dyeworks chemists developed a process for synthesizing and producing epinephrine, and the company began producing the hormone in 1906. It was sold to increase the effectiveness of another Hoechst product, the local anesthetic Novocaine, as well as to treat **shock** and control bleeding.

Synthetic epinephrine is widely used today, especially as an emergency treatment for anaphylactic shock. (*See also* anaphylaxis)

Additional reading: Sneader, *Drug Discovery,* pp. 96–105.

epo. *See* erythropoietin

ergot

Ergot is produced by *Claviceps purpurea*, a fungus that grows on rye, corn, and wheat and has neurotoxic effects. Ergot poisoning produces convulsions and partial paralysis. Several derivatives of this natural substance have been developed as medications.

Epidemics of ergot poisoning were common in the Middle Ages, when they were called "St. Anthony's fire" because poisoned people suffered burning sensations in the limbs as well as blackening of the skin from gangrene.

Before ergot became known as the substance responsible for St. Anthony's fire, midwives had used it to speed labor. The German author Adam Lonicer (1528–1586) provided the first description of using ergot for this purpose in 1582. After the cause of St. Anthony's fire became known in the 1600s, the use of ergot in established medicine ended, although midwives may have continued to use it.

In the United States, where ergot poisoning was basically unknown, John Stearns (1770–1848) of New York popularized the use of ergot to speed labor in an 1808 letter. He had heard of the substance from a German woman who had emigrated to the United States. Stearns warned that the drug shouldn't be used in cases where labor was slowed by an obstruction, but his admonition was ignored. Overly enthusiastic use of ergot led to many maternal deaths and stillbirths. Its use was soon limited to treating postpartum hemorrhage.

Ergotamine, a derivative of ergot, was isolated by the Swiss chemist Arthur Stoll (1887–unknown) in 1918 while he was working at the Sandoz Company. He described its chemical structure 33 years later. His successor as director of research at Sandoz, Albert Hofmann (1906–), synthesized ergotamine in 1961. The drug, which constricts the blood vessels and counteracts the effects of **epinephrine**, is still used to treat **migraine** headache.

John Chassar Moir at University College Hospital in London reported using ergot extract to strengthen labor contractions in 1932. Working with Harold Dudley (1887–1935) of the National Institute for Medical Research, Moir isolated the responsible substance in 1935, naming it ergometrine. Stoll and Hofman synthesized ergometrine two years later.

Because ergometrine is unstable and can have side effects including **hypertension,** nausea, and vomiting, oxytocin is the preferred drug for stimulating uterine contractions. (*See also* LSD)

Additional reading: Sneader, *Drug Discovery,* pp. 105–09.

erythropoietin (epo)

Erythropoietin is a **hormone** the kidney produces to stimulate **red blood cell** formation in response to low oxygen.

The existence of epo was first hypothesized in 1906 by French scientists, who suggested that there was something in the blood that instructed the bone marrow to form more red blood cells when little oxygen was available. Work with animals in the 1940s and 1950s added evidence for their theory. In 1953, the factor was identified as an alpha globulin by Allan Erslev (1919–) of Thomas Jefferson University and his colleagues, and in 1957 Leon Jacobson and his colleagues learned that epo came from the kidneys. Eugene Goldwasser (1922–) of the University of Chicago and his coworkers described the amino acid sequence of epo in the late 1970s, which made it possible to begin mass-producing recombinant epo in 1985. Studies confirmed two years later that kidney **dialysis** patients treated with epo produced enough red blood cells; previously they had needed transfusions.

In the 1990s, athletes illicitly used epo for "blood doping," sometimes with fatal results.

Additional reading: Longman, "Lifesaving Drug Can Be Deadly When Misused."

estrogen

Estrogen is a general term for **hormones** that exert effects on the uterus, specifically estradiol and estrone, which are produced by the ovaries. The word "estrogen" comes from "estrus," a state of sexual receptiveness to the male, or "heat," that appears in many female animals—although not in humans. With **progesterone**, estrogen regulates a woman's menstrual cycle.

Estrogen, along with progesterone, is given to menopausal women in **hormone replacement therapy**, and is the main ingredient of **birth control pills.**

Led by Charles-Edouard Brown Sequard (1817–1894), a number of researchers in the late nineteenth century began investigating extracts of various glands for their use in medicine. This and other research soon led to the discovery of hormones. Around this time, Viennese gynecologist Emil Knauer (1867–unknown) proved that there was some sort of female hormone in the ovary. He found that transplanting ovaries from older female animals into younger ones sped up the recipients' sexual development.

Researchers developed ovarian extracts, of which one was marketed by the Swiss chemicals manufacturer Ciba in 1913, but these extracts varied widely in their effectiveness, mainly because there was no way to determine how much of the hormone they actually contained.

In 1917, Georges Papanicolaou (1883–1962) had shown that guinea pigs' vaginal cells changed with the estrus cycle, in work that provided the foundation for the **Pap smear** screening test. This also provided the foundation for a test to identify the presence of the ovarian hormone in extracts, which was developed and reported in 1923 by endocrinologist Edgar Allen (1892–1943) and biochemist Edward Doisy (1893–1986), both of whom worked at the Washington University School of Medicine in St. Louis.

Selman Ascheim (1878–1965) and Bernhard Zondek (1891–1966) developed the first **pregnancy test** in 1927, which was based largely on Allen and Doisy's work. They also discovered that the urine of pregnant animals contained large amounts of the ovarian hormone. Once Aschiem and Zondek announced their discovery, researchers around the world began competing to be the first to isolate the hormone from urine.

Doisy was the first to do so, reporting his results in 1929. German researcher Adolf Butenandt (1903–1995) isolated the hormone shortly afterwards, and in Amsterdam Ernst Laqueur (1901–1947) did so the following year. In 1935, The League of Nations agreed to call this hormone oestrone. Other related hormones, including oestriol and oestradiol, were soon isolated.

In 1930, Charles Dodds (1898–1973) at London's Courtauld Institute of Biochemistry began searching for an artificial, more powerful estrogenic hormone. With chemist James Cook (1900–unknown), he began synthesizing compounds, eventually finding one that was three times as powerful as oestrone, and reported his discovery in 1938. This chemical was called stilboestrol in Britain, and diethylstilbestrol in the United States.

Research into other similar chemicals yielded the fertility drug Clomid, which was found in 1962 by Robert B. Greenblatt (1906–1987) to stimulate ovulation, and the cancer drug **tamoxifen**.

Additional reading: Speert, *Obstetric & Gynecologic Milestones Illustrated,* pp. 640–41.

ether

Ether is a volatile gas that was one of the first agents used in **anesthesia**, but is rarely used now because of its side effects, which can include nausea.

Ethers are made by distilling alcohol with an acid, and had been known for hundreds of years before first being used for anesthesia in the 1840s. Early in the 1800s some people would inhale ether recreationally, for the giddiness and euphoria it produced.

Crawford Long (1815–1878) first used ether as an anesthetic in 1842, after noticing that friends who inhaled ether at parties felt no pain after falling down or being struck. Long didn't write about the surgery he performed to remove a tumor from a young man's neck until 1849.

William Morton's (1819–1868) use of ether in a similar operation performed at Massachusetts General Hospital in 1846 got more attention because an account of the surgery was published in the *Boston Journal* newspaper the following day.

When the effectiveness of **chloroform** as an anesthetic was discovered in the early 1850s, this less-toxic chemical became the anesthetic of choice.

Additional reading: Friedman and Friedland, *Medicine's 10 Greatest Discoveries,* pp. 98–101, 104–06.

eyeglasses

Eyeglasses are used to improve vision and have been with us in gradually improving forms for more than 700 years.

The name of the inventor of eyeglasses is not known, but spectacles probably originated in Italy in the thirteenth century. These early spectacles were hinged in the middle and propped on the nose, and made of glass or a clear mineral such as beryl. The oldest pair in existence, which probably belonged to a nun, were found under the floorboards of a cloister in Germany.

The work of Francesco Maurolyco (1494–1575) and Johannes Kepler (1571–1630) provided the foundation for the understanding of optics, which was necessary to make glasses that truly corrected near- and far-sightedness.

Maurolyco suggested in his work *Photismi*, published in 1521, that the lenses of farsighted people were not curved enough, while nearsighted people's lenses were overly curved. This is fairly close to our current knowledge of the cause of these problems.

In 1623, Benito Daca de Valdes (c.1591–1634) published what is believed to be the first book on vision testing and eyeglass-fitting.

Eyeglasses were custom-made until a London spectacle maker developed a method for grinding good-quality lenses in batches. The Royal Society endorsed his method in the 1690s, and soon all of the nation's opticians were using it.

Temple pieces to hold the lens in place, like those used today, were introduced in the early eighteenth century.

Famous American Renaissance man Benjamin Franklin (1706–1790) invented bifocals in 1784, two-piece glasses that allowed him to see distances clearly from the top half, and use the bottom for close-up perusal. He probably had two sets of lenses—one for distance-viewing and one for close vision—cut in half and stuck together to make the set. Trifocals were first described in 1826 by the civil engineer J.I. Hawkins. Lenses for correcting astigmatism became available in the middle of this century. In the 1800s, several German companies were founded that were devoted to making lenses based on scientific principles and the best knowledge of optics of the time. During this century, several advances were also made in understanding the dioptrics of the eye. Swedish ophthalmologist Alvar Gullstrand (1862–1930) invented the photokeratoscope and the slit lamp, and spelled out the basic understanding of the optics of the eye in 1896. He won the 1911 Nobel Prize for his work.

Plastic lenses made of hard resin were developed by the Pittsburgh Plate Glass Company in the 1930s. The company manufactured the first eyeglasses using the new material, called CR-39, in 1937. The next advance in plastic eyeglass technology, in the 1970s, was the introduction of polycarbonate as a lens material. Polycarbonate had originally been developed for Air Force flight helmets and visors. (*See also* contact lenses)

Additional reading: Albert, *The History of Ophthalmology,* pp.107–23.

F

FDA. *See Food and Drug Administration*

fetal monitoring

Fetal monitoring is the use of various techniques to check the health of a fetus.

Two physicians were independently the first to report hearing fetal heart tones: Matthias Mayor (1795–1847) in Geneva in 1818, and Jacques Alexandre Lejumeau, Viscount de Kergaradec (1787–1877), in 1821. The Irish physician Evory Kennedy (c.1806–1886) wrote an 1833 book on fetal heart tones. He described several heartbeat patterns and their significance, and made a number of observations that hold true today.

Throughout the mid- and late-nineteenth century, physicians made a series of successive recommendations on when a heart rate signified fetal distress and required intervention.

In the early twentieth century an obstetric head stethoscope, or "fetoscope," was designed to make monitoring the heartbeat easier. Around this time obstetricians began recording fetal heart sounds.

Fetal monitoring techniques have improved with technology in this century, as physicians have used **electrocardiograms (ECGs), ultrasound,** and other techniques to measure the strength and regularity of the heartbeat.

Additional reading: Acierno, *The History of Cardiology,* pp. 512–13.

fetal surgery

Fetal surgery is an operation performed to correct defects before an infant is born. The fetus is taken from the womb, operated on, and returned to the uterus to finish its development.

The earliest attempts at fetal surgery were made in the 1960s, to treat babies in danger of death from erythroblastosis fetalis, which can occur when a woman who is negative for **Rh factor** is pregnant with an Rh positive child. A. William Liley (unknown–1983) attempted to transfuse a fetus with blood in 1963. A subsequent patient, before his birth and christening as Grant Liley MacLeod, was the first fetus to undergo successful fetal surgery. The transfusion was performed through the mother's skin, without cutting her body open.

Vincent Freda (1927–) and Karliss Adamsons (1926–), Columbia University doctors working in Puerto Rico, attempted to perform a similar procedure in which they surgically opened the woman's uterus. Their first patient, operated on in 1963, survived the operation, as did her fetus, but she delivered the baby prematurely two days later and the child died. Although there were several attempts at an open version of the surgery by this team, none of the babies survived. The single early success at an open fetal operation was by Stanley Asensio (1925–) in 1965, also in Puerto Rico.

Because the closed operation was sufficient to treat Rh disease, open fetal surgery was abandoned until the 1980s.

In the mid-1980s, Michael Harrison (1943–) of the University of California at San Francisco and his colleagues attempted to correct a defect of the urethra in two fetuses. The first child died shortly after birth, but the second child lived. At about this time attempts began to be made to correct **hydrocephalus** in the womb, with mixed results.

In the 1990s fetal surgery for lung malformations, urinary tract obstructions, and certain **cancers** became more common. The infant death rate for all of these procedures has been about 50 percent.

In 1998, a team at the Center for Fetal Diagnosis and Treatment at the Children's Hospital of Philadelphia repaired a 23-week-old fetus' open spinal cord, a defect known as spina bifida. The child did not experience the neurological damage that normally accompanies spina bifida, and at six months of age had met all appropriate developmental milestones.

Fetal surgery today remains a risky endeavor. Although to date no woman has died from fetal surgery, many woman suffer serious complications, often from the drugs used to prevent premature labor after the surgery has been performed.

Additional reading: Casper, *The Making of the Unborn Patient.*

Flexner report

The Flexner Report, published in 1910, was a survey of medical education in the United States written by Abraham Flexner (1866–1958). His conclusion that American medical training was in a shambles resulted in the most extensive series of reforms of the establishment ever undertaken.

Although the release of the report is considered a milestone, reform was already underway in 1910, as Flexner himself noted. More medical students were pursuing premedical training, as well as training in the clinic after they received their medical degrees. Many American doctors had pursued their education in the great schools of Germany and Vienna. The Johns Hopkins School of Medicine, modeled on these schools and others, opened in Baltimore in 1893, and was the first medical school that required students to have a bachelor's degree and to study for four years.

Physicians in the United States were not regulated or licensed by the government between 1830 and 1875. The American Medical Association (AMA) established a council to regulate and inspect medical schools in 1904, and along with the Carnegie Foundation, funded Flexner's research.

In his report, Flexner recommended that the existing 155 medical schools be trimmed to 31. The number was never brought down that low, but was reduced to 76 by 1930. He also said medical schools should require at least two years of college for admission, mostly science courses. He called for doctors to take a more scientific approach to their patients, and for medical school faculty to conduct scientific research. He also said medical schools should have hospital beds at their disposal for clinical training of students.

Flexner's report brought public attention to the problem of poor medical education and the need for reform.

Additional reading: Barazansky and Gevitz, *Beyond Flexner*, pp. 1–18.

flu. See influenza.

fluoridation

Fluoridation is the use of the mineral sodium fluoride to protect teeth against decay, either by adding fluoride to drinking water or by using it in toothpaste and mouthwash. Fluoride can also be consumed in pills.

Dr. Frederick S. McKay made the observations that led to the discovery of fluoride's tooth-protective properties. After moving to Colorado Springs in 1901, he noticed that many of his patients had brown stains on their teeth. He also noticed that people with stained teeth tended to have fewer cavities. By 1915 he determined that the stains were probably caused by something in the water supply. The responsible substance was identified as fluoride in 1933.

Dr. H. Trendley Dean (1893–1962) of the **U.S. Public Health Service** began investigating whether it would be possible to give people fluoride safely to protect their teeth, without causing stains. Dean helped initiate the first ex-

perimental water fluoridation program, in Grand Rapids, Michigan, in 1945. The experiment was halted early because it was so successful. Fluoridated water can bring down the incidence of dental caries (tooth decay) by 17 to 40 percent.

Today, more than 144 million people in the United States drink fluoridated water, while many also get fluoride through treatments at their dentists and from toothpaste and mouthwashes. Fluoride is believed to be completely safe, although anti-fluoridation movements have existed since the first fluoridation experiments, when detractors called fluoridation a Communist plot to poison Americans. The **Centers for Disease Control and Prevention** lists fluoridation of drinking water as one of the 10 great public health achievements of the twentieth century.

Since people today consume fluoride from so many sources, efforts are now underway to determine if water should be fluoridated at a lower level.

Additional reading: Wynbrandt, *The Excruciating History of Dentistry*, pp. 194–98.

fluoroscope

A fluoroscope is a fluorescent screen used to view **X-ray** images of the body in real time. Because fluoroscopes require exposing the patient to more radiation than other types of imaging, they are rarely used today.

Princeton professor and physicist William F. Magic (1858–1943) invented a similar machine that he called a "skiascope," reporting on his discovery in early 1896.

Thomas Edison (1847–1931) invented a screen coated with calcium tungstate that fluoresced in response to X-rays about a month later. He named the screen a "fluoroscope," and soon invented a portable fluoroscopic apparatus.

Fluoroscopes were widely used in the early twentieth century, for example in shoe stores so salesmen could check the correct fit of a shoe against the foot bones, resulting in overexposure to radiation and testicular **cancer** among shoe store customers. The first shoe store fluoroscope was patented in 1927. There was no regulation of the amount of radiation emitted by the machines until 1949. The machines were banned by the **Food and Drug Administration (FDA)** four years later.

Additional reading: Kevles, *Naked to the Bone*, pp. 35–38.

Food and Drug Administration (FDA)

The Food and Drug Administration is the U.S. government agency responsible for overseeing the safety of food and medicines.

The federal government first began attempting to investigate adulteration of food in 1867, under the auspices of the Division of Chemistry. Harvey Washington Wiley (1844–1930) became the division's chief chemist in 1883 and raised the agency's profile with a series of reports and experiments, including several in which healthy volunteers consumed various food additives to gauge their safety. Wiley lobbied for a law against adulteration of food and drugs.

Physician and pharmacist groups, women's clubs, and food and drug inspectors joined him in his efforts.

The first federal attempt to control the safety of food and medicine was the Pure Food and Drugs Act of 1906. It was spurred by Wiley's efforts, as well as by *The Jungle*, Upton Sinclair's (1878–1968) 1906 book exposing foul conditions in the Chicago meat-packing industry.

The 1906 law required truth in labeling for all products and banned the shipping of adulterated food over state lines. It also required that products containing 11 potentially dangerous ingredients, including **heroin**, **cocaine**, and alcohol, state their content of these substances on their labels.

Public sentiment grew for a new and more powerful law to ensure the safety of drugs and foods in the 1930s, but no legislation was passed until the Elixir Sulfanilamide disaster of 1937. More than 100 people died after consuming a formulation of the new drug marketed by a Tennessee company. The preparation contained the poisonous additive diethylene glycol, a substance similar to antifreeze. After this incident, the Food, Drug and Cosmetic Act was signed into law in 1938.

This law was the first to require that drugs be tested before marketing. It also banned false advertising for medicines and provided for inspections at factories. Efforts to enforce the new law made it clear that some medications could not be labeled for safe use by the consumer, spurring the development of **prescription** requirements for certain drugs.

Another tragedy brought on the next wave of reform in food and drug safety: the thalidomide disaster of the late 1950s. Thousands of babies with severe **birth defects** were born to mothers who had taken the drug, which had been marketed as a remedy for morning sickness. Because of premarket drug evaluation requirements already in place in the United States, few thalidomide babies were born in this country.

In 1962, in response to the thalidomide tragedy, Congress passed amendments requiring tighter control of drug trials, **informed consent** of patients participating in such trials, and stricter regulation of drug company manufacturing practices. Three years later, the Drug Abuse Control Amendments were passed to restrict the availability of drugs such as hallucinogens, **barbituates**, and **amphetamines**.

Laws were also passed governing pesticides, food additives, and color additives in the 1950s and in 1960. The FDA was made part of the **U.S. Public Health Service (PHS)** in 1973, and subsequently took on some of the PHS's duties, including licensing for biological therapeutics (such as vaccines) and control of radiation emissions from electrical products.

The major recent change in the way food is regulated by the FDA was the Nutrition Labeling and Education Act of 1990, which required that all food products carry detailed labels describing their nutritional content. Four years later, Congress passed a law easing restriction on the sale of and claims for nutritional supplements, which placed the onus for proving such products were adulterated or unsafe on the FDA.

Additional reading: Temin, *Taking Your Medicine;* Kurian, *A Historical Guide to the U.S. Government*, pp. 248–54.

Food Safety and Inspection Service

The Food Safety and Inspection Service, run under the auspices of the U.S. Department of Agriculture, is the agency responsible for monitoring food production.

Congress passed the United States' first food and drug regulation, the Pure Food and Drugs Act, in 1906. One year later, the Meat Inspection Act was passed, requiring that any company slaughtering or processing meat for sale across state lines be inspected continuously by federal officials. It was not until 1957 that a similar law was passed governing poultry.

Officials of the Federal Meat and Poultry Inspection Program examine live animals, supervise slaughter and production, and sample products to screen for contamination with bacteria, pesticides, and other potentially dangerous chemicals.

Tests to check the species of animals being sold as food were initiated in the mid-1980s, after a report of kangaroo meat being sold as Australian beef.

The **Centers for Disease Control and Prevention (CDC)** are responsible for monitoring and reporting any cases of food-related illness. Microbes are the main cause of food-related illness and death in the United States, especially salmonella. The CDC established a national salmonella surveillance program in 1962.

Additional reading: Burros, "U.S. Food Regulation."

forceps

Forceps are pincers placed around a baby's head to aid delivery in difficult births.

The British doctor Peter Chamberlen (1560–1631) invented the first set of forceps, which he and his heirs kept secret for more than a century. When called to assist in a delivery, the Chamberlens would bring the instrument into the room in a box and cover the woman giving birth with a sheet while they used it. Hugh Chamberlen (1664–1726) finally disclosed the secret of the forceps to colleagues.

Since then several modernized versions of forceps have been made as the understanding of the pelvic anatomy and the birth process has improved.

Additional reading: Speert, *Obstetrics and Gynaecology,* pp. 270–73.

fracture repair

Repair of fractured bones is one of the oldest medical techniques. Fossils show that prehistoric humans tried to set bone fractures and were successful about half the time.

Ancient Egyptians used splints made of bark and linen or palm-fiber-cloth bandages to help fractures heal. The **Hippocratic Corpus** describes a device used for setting fractures by mechanically stretching out the limb. The machine, called the Scamnum, probably did more harm than good in general, but the writings include better recommendations for setting fractures in various bones by hand.

Around 1000 A.D., Arab physicians were the first to recommend plaster casts for treating fractured bones. Plaster-of-Paris is in fact an Arab invention and was not used in the West until the nineteenth century. Antonious Mathysen (1805–1878) invented the plaster bandage used in today's casts, describing the invention in 1852. He impregnated a cotton bandage with plaster-of-Paris before applying it. Many of his contemporaries didn't like the new method, because they feared that it compressed the limb too much and restricted circulation.

Avicenna, an Arab physician who flourished around 1000 A.D., developed a method for repairing open fractures—broken bones that pierce the skin. In Hippocrates' (c.460–c.377 B.C.) time, people usually died from these so-called compound fractures.

Guy de Chauliac (1300–1370), a French surgeon, combined past methods of fracture treatment such as traction and open reduction with some success, but he was also incorrect in his reliance on salves applied to the skin.

Native Americans used splints to immobilize joints near the broken limb and made casts by molding wet rawhide to the limb.

Joseph Lister (1827–1912) developed **antisepsis** while he was attempting to improve treatment of compound fractures at the Glasgow Royal Infirmary. He published the results of 11 patients with compound fractures treated during his technique in 1867. Three years later, he treated a patient with a closed fracture of the arm with surgery, opening the wound and reuniting the ends of the bone. Lister performed a number of other surgical repairs of the bones with success using his antiseptic techniques.

Additional reading: Ellis, *Famous Operations*, pp. 63–70.

G

gamete intrafallopian transfer. *See* GIFT.

gamma knife

A gamma knife delivers a highly concentrated dose of radiation to the brain to destroy tumors while leaving healthy **tissue** intact.

Lars Lekskell (1907–1986), a Swedish neurosurgeon and the inventor of radiosurgery, introduced the gamma knife in 1968, using it for the first time to treat a **brain tumor** the following year. Ladislav Steiner of the Karolinska Institute in Sweden and his colleagues discovered four years later that the gamma knife could be used to treat blood-vessel malformations in the brain.

Because Lekskell was only able to treat a few patients, meaning results were hard to evaluate, use of the gamma knife did not catch on worldwide until the 1980s and 1990s. Currently the gamma knife is being investigated for treating **epilepsy.**

Additional reading: Brody, "Device Transforms Brain Surgery."

gastrectomy

Gastrectomy is the surgical removal of part or all of the stomach, usually to excise **cancer** in the organ.

The Austrian surgeon Theodore Billroth (1829–1894) performed the first successful gastrectomy in 1881 in Vienna, to remove a cancer from the stomach of a woman named Therese Heller. Billroth reattached the noncancerous section of the stomach to the duodenum, which connects the stomach to the small intestine. The operation, performed while the patient was anesthetized with chloroform, lasted one-and-a-half hours. Billroth used **antiseptic** techniques.

The patient lived for four months after the surgery, dying because the cancer had spread to her liver. Billroth performed a second pioneering operation three years later, in which he reattached the stomach to the jejunum, or the top of the small intestine.

Though the operation was also performed to treat **ulcers**, this is rarely necessary today thanks to effective drug treatment.

Additional reading: Ellis, *Famous Operations,* pp. 29–35; Schindler, *Gastroscopy.*

gastroscope

A gastroscope is an instrument for viewing the interior of the stomach that is inserted via the mouth and esophagus.

Dr. Rudolf Schindler (1888–1968) conceived of the idea of a semi-flexible gastroscope. Rigid gastroscopes had been built before by German instrument makers in the late 1800s, but these instruments were difficult to use and sometimes dangerous. In 1928, according to his daughter, Schindler sketched out his design for a flexible gastroscope, a series of lenses enclosed in rubber, and sent the sketch to a Berlin instrument maker. The two worked together for four years, ultimately producing a semi-flexible gastroscope that was much safer and easier to use than earlier designs.

Schindler and his family came to the University of Chicago in 1934 after being forced out of Germany by the Nazis. There Schindler, his wife, and his students studied the use of the gastroscope for diagnosing gastritis, training people from around the world to use the instrument. Schindler published *Gastroscopy*, a book on the use of the instrument, in 1937. In 1941, Schindler and his colleagues formed the American Gastroscopy Club, whose name was changed five years later to the American Gastroscopy Society and finally, in 1961, to the American Society for Gastrointestinal Endoscopy.

Building on the capacity for fiberoptics to pass light and images along a curved bundle of glass fibers, Basil Hirschowitz (1925–) designed a prototype for a fiberoptic gastroscope in 1957, using it on himself first and then a patient. He arranged with American Cystoscope Makers to build the device commercially, and the first instrument was delivered in 1960.

A number of advances since then, such as equipping the device with a camera to make photographs and even videotapes of the stomach, as well as to take **biopsies** and remove growths, has made the gastroscope and other endoscopy devices crucial in **cancer** surveillance and prevention. These devices can detect cell changes that herald cancer so these precancerous areas can be removed before the disease develops.

About 2 million gastroscopies are performed in the United States each year.

Additional reading: Cotton and Williams, *Practical Gastrointestinal Endoscopy*; Schindler, *Gastroscopy*.

gene

A gene is the unit, carried on the **chromosome**, through which parents transmit characteristics to their offspring. Genes also carry instructions for proteins used in the body's growth, development, and function, through the process of transcription.

Gregor Mendel (1822–1884), an Austrian monk, first came up with the idea of a unit of inheritance in his work with pea plants. By breeding plants with various characteristics, such as round seeds and wrinkled seeds and tall plants and short plants, and analyzing the way that these traits were inherited, he developed a statistical method for predicting inheritance.

Mendel outlined his work in an 1865 paper that went virtually unnoticed until 1900, when several researchers "rediscovered" what is now known as Mendelian inheritance. In 1903, both Walter Sutton (1877–1916) in America and Theodor Boveri (1862–1915) in Germany, working independently, found that chromosomes were halved in germ (egg and sperm) cells and combined in fertilized eggs, following Mendel's statistical formula exactly.

Wilhelm Johannson (1857–1927), a Danish biologist, coined the word "gene" for these units of inheritance in 1909.

We now know that the sequence of genes on the chromosome constitutes a **genetic code**, by which our **DNA**—which chromosomes are made of—instructs cells to make the proteins we need to live. Mutations in the genes, which may be inherited or may be caused by environmental factors such as exposure to radiation, are responsible for **birth defects**, most types of **cancer**, and probably many other illnesses.

Additional reading: Aldridge, *The Thread of Life,* pp. 137–64.

gene mapping

Gene mapping involves determining the location of specific **genes** on the **chromosome.**

The first genes to be mapped were the sex-linked genes. Females have two X chromosomes, while males have an X and a Y. Since certain inherited diseases, such as **hemophilia,** strike males only, researchers hypothesized that these genes could be found on the X chromosome. Females would have a matching gene to mute the effects of the defective gene, while males would not.

Thomas Hunt Morgan (1866–1945) at Columbia University in New York was the first person to locate a gene on a particular chromosome; he showed in 1910 that fruit flies carried a gene for white eyes on the X chromosome. This method for locating genes by following their inheritance is called linkage analysis. Morgan's colleague Edmund Beecher Wilson (1856–1939) mapped the first human gene, for color blindness, to the X chromosome.

Alfred Henry Sturtevant (1891–1970), one of Morgan's students, published the first linkage map in 1913. The map showed five sites on the X chromosome of a fruit fly.

In 1937, Julia Bell and John Burton Sanderson Haldane (1892–1964) showed that genes for color blindness and hemophilia were inherited together, so they were probably close to one another on the chromosome.

In a 1948 lecture, Haldane set forth the goal of genetics as "the enumeration and location of all the genes found in normal human beings," exactly what the **Human Genome Project** is now seeking to accomplish by 2005. He also suggested the name "Morgan" for a unit of distance on the chromosome, in honor of the Columbia professor.

By 1968, 68 genes had been mapped to the X chromosome but none to the other 45 chromosomes. Roger Donahue (1935–) located a gene for a particular blood type found in himself and his family on chromosome 1, making this the first nonsex-linked gene mapping.

Chromosome banding, invented in the early 1970s, made gene mapping much easier. **Restriction enzymes** and **recombinant DNA** technology, also developed around this time, made it possible to search for specific stretches of genetic material.

David Botstein (1942–) of the Massachusetts Institute of Technology and Ronald Davis (1941–) of Stanford introduced a technique for speedy gene sequencing known as "riflip" technology in the 1980s, making gene mapping much faster and the idea of a complete map of the genome a real possibility.

The catalog of *Mendelian Inheritance in Man,* first published by Victor McCusick (1921–) of Johns Hopkins in 1962, began giving gene locations in its 1971 edition.

Additional reading: Aldridge, *The Thread of Life,* pp. 61–72.

gene therapy

Gene therapy is a strategy for healing disease by repairing a malfunctioning **gene**. Many diseases are caused by genetic defects, which can disable the body's capacity to make an essential protein or cause the body to produce an unusable form of the protein.

The first use of gene therapy in human beings began in 1990, to treat a rare disease called adenosine deaminase (ADA) deficiency. People with ADA deficiency do not make this protein, which is required to change the waste product deoxyadenosine into inosine. When too much deoxyadenosine collects in the body, it combines with phosphorous to produce deoxyadenosine triphosphate, which kills immune system cells—especially T cells. People with this disease basically have no immune system, and usually die young. William French Anderson (1936–), R. Michael Blaese (1932–), Kenneth Culver, and Steven Rosenberg (1940–) devised a therapy in which they extracted white blood cells from the blood of an ADA-deficient individual, incubated them with mouse **leukemia** viruses carrying a functioning human ADA gene, and then infused the doctored cells back to the patients' blood. The team hoped that the cells would then begin making ADA, and remain alive in the patient's body.

The two girls treated with the protocol, who were four and nine years old at the time, responded well. Their immune systems rebounded enough for them to live normal lives. During the therapy, and continuing to this day, both take reduced doses of PEG-ADA, a nongenetic therapy for the disease. Both girls remain healthy, and tests have shown that the engineered cells continue to survive in their bodies and produce the enzyme.

Today gene therapy is being investigated to treat a number of different diseases. In early 2000, President William Clinton called for a national review of gene therapy guidelines. The president and others had raised concerns after a young patient died in the fall of 1999 while undergoing gene therapy for brain cancer at a University of Pennsylvania program. After the patient's death, the **Food and Drug Administration** placed on hold all trials underway at the university's Institute for Human Gene Therapy.

Additional reading: Lyon and Gorner, *Altered Fates,* pp. 232–69.

genetic code

The genetic code is the language in which the four base pairs of **DNA** store directions for constructing proteins. All proteins are made up of a combination of amino acids, of which there are 20 in all, and instructions to make each amino acid are encoded in a particular sequence of three nucleic acids called a "codon." There are four nucleic acids in all: cytosine, guanine, adenine, and thymine. The order in which codons are arranged indicates the protein to be made. Codons that don't denote a particular codon are called "stop" codons, and act like periods at the end of a sentence coding for a particular protein.

In 1943, Austrian Erwin Schrodinger (1887–1961), a Nobel Prize winner for his work in quantum physics, suggested in a series of lectures in Dublin that the **gene** carried a code that carried the information for "a highly complicated and specified plan of development and should somehow contain the means to put it into operation." Schrodinger's lectures, published in a book called *What is Life?*, helped inspire James Watson (1928–) in his search for the structure of DNA. The physicist incorrectly suggested, however, that protein carried the code, not DNA.

Once Watson and his colleagues had discovered the structure of DNA, another physicist, George Gamow (1904–1968), proposed that the four bases of the molecule formed a kind of four-digit code.

Francis Crick (1916–) and Sydney Brenner (1927–) proved by 1961 that sets of three bases were the basic unit of the code, and Brenner named these triplets codons. Marshall Nirenberg (1927–) and Johann Matthei worked out the first correspondence between a set of proteins and an amino acid: three adenines for phenylalanine. By 1967,

Har Gobind Khorana (1922–), Nirenberg, and others had cracked the genetic code of 61 codons for 20 amino acids.

Additional reading: Aldridge. *The Thread of Life,* pp. 29–35.

genetic counseling

Genetic counseling is the discussion of possible hereditary abnormalities with parents planning to have children, and also to assist a person at risk of developing a disease to decide whether or not to be tested for it.

Sheldon Reed (1910–), who was attempting to replace the earlier, eugenics-associated expression "genetic hygiene," introduced the term "genetic counseling" in the 1940s.

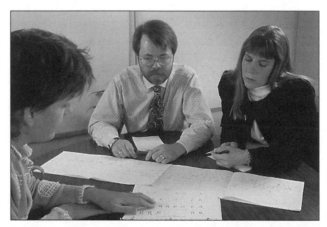

Genetic counselors help prospective parents evaluate their risk of having a child with a genetic disorder. (Courtesy of National Institute for Human Genome Research.)

Genetic counseling became more relevant in the 1950s as understanding of disease inheritance improved. Jerome LeJeune (1926–) discovered the first chromosomal disorder, **Down syndrome**, in 1959. In the late 1960s, it became practical to screen fetuses before birth for certain genetic disorders through **amniocentesis**. In 1975, a committee of the American Society of Human Genetics provided a formal definition of "genetic counseling."

Today, genetic counselors may be doctors (clinical geneticists), nurses (nurse specialists in genetics), or scientists with a doctorate degree in genetics (medical geneticists). There are about 100 programs in the United States that provide graduate training in genetic counseling. (*See also* chromosome; gene)

Additional reading: Kilner, et al., *Genetic Ethics,* pp. 136–55.

germ theory

Germ theory is the understanding that many diseases are caused by microscopic organisms, also called germs.

In 1859, French chemist Louis Pasteur (1822–1895), who began his career working for distilleries, suggested that living organisms caused the chemical process known as fermentation and that similar agents were responsible for spreading disease. His critics still believed that living organisms could arise spontaneously from lifeless matter,

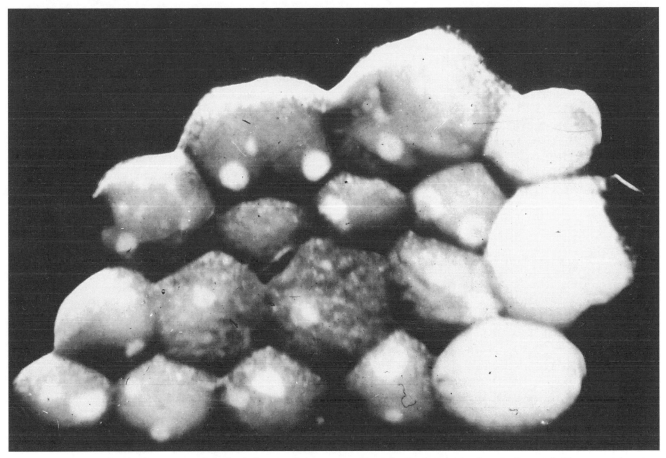

Staphylococcus aureus is a leading cause of infection in humans. Its name comes from the Greek word for "bunch of grapes." (Courtesy of American Society for Microbiology Archives Collection.)

but Pasteur proved this phenomenon was actually caused by impurities in the air.

Inspired by Pasteur's work, researchers including French physician Casimir Davaine (1812–1882), English physician John Burdon Sanderson (1828–1905), and German doctor Robert Koch (1843–1910) began studying microbes and disease. They attempted to isolate an infectious agent from samples of blood or other material from infected animals and people, and then see if this agent would spread the disease to a healthy individual. This system for proving that an agent was responsible for spreading a disease became known as **Koch's postulates**. Using the postulates, these researchers found that **tuberculosis**, **diphtheria**, anthrax, and other diseases were contagious and spread by germs.

Joseph Lister (1827–1912) began advocating **antisepsis** to avoid the spread of infection. He used carbolic spray to treat wounds, and said the dramatic drop in post-surgical infections was proof of the germ theory.

In the 1870s, Koch, Pasteur, and others began to discover the actual organisms responsible for causing disease. The germ theory also contributed to scientific understanding of disease spread, as bacteriologists studied how the germs responsible for illnesses were carried—some by water, some by food, some by insects, some by air, some by other "vectors."

At this point science was not yet able to distinguish between bacteria, viruses, and microscopic parasites, so all of these agents were grouped under the name "germ." Acceptance of the germ theory was widespread by 1900.

Additional reading: Porter, *The Cambridge Illustrated History of Medicine,* pp. 184–85.

German measles. *See* rubella.

GIFT (gamete intrafallopian transfer)

GIFT is a technique for helping women with blocked fallopian tubes to become pregnant. Eggs are collected from the ovary, sperm is injected into the woman's vagina, and then the eggs are reinserted into the end of the fallopian tube closest to the uterus, in hopes that egg and sperm will meet and fertilization and implantation of an embryo will result.

Landrum Brewer Shettles (1909–) was the first to propose the procedure, performing it successfully in 1979. Animal studies followed, as well as attempts to refine the technique. Ricardo H. Asch (1947–), in Texas, suggested using the technique in women with apparently normal tubes who were infertile. Asch reported the first successful pregnancy in such a woman using the technique in 1984, and he coined the name GIFT. He also suggested the possibility of performing the procedure without surgery, by collecting and replacing the egg via an instrument inserted through the vagina and cervix. In 1995, Asch was accused of using an unapproved infertility drug, knowingly implanting embryos in the wrong women without the donor's or recipient's knowledge, and keeping patients' payments without reporting them to the hospital. Asch was indicted on federal mail fraud and tax-evasion charges, and fled to Mexico to avoid trial.

Independently in 1988, Robert P.S. Jansen and W. Wurfel were the first to perform GIFT without surgery, using slightly different techniques. In a related technique, zygote interfallopian transfer (ZIFT), an egg is removed and reinserted after **in vitro fertilization**.

Additional reading: O'Dowd and Philipp, *The History of Obstetrics and Gynaecology,* pp. 373–74.

glaucoma

Glaucoma is a collective name for several diseases in which fluid pressure within the eyeball is abnormally high, leading to damage of the optic nerve and blindness if the condition is left untreated. This usually occurs because the fluid in the eye, known as the aqueous humor, drains more slowly than it is produced. There are currently 1 million Americans who have been diagnosed with glaucoma.

William McKenzie (1791–1868) linked high pressure within the eye to glaucoma in 1835. Five years after the invention of the **ophthalmoscope** in 1852, Albrecht von Graefe (1828–1870) observed the cupping of the optic nerve seen in glaucoma, and classified different types of the disease. He performed an iridectomy on a patient with glaucoma in 1856, the first surgical cure of acute glaucoma. In this operation, part of the iris is removed to allow fluid to drain. Chronic, symptomless glaucoma could not be treated effectively by this method, however, so surgeons developed filtering operations to treat this condition in the late 1800s and early 1900s. By 1896, surgeons understood that high pressure within the eyeball could be controlled by drugs called miotics and with surgery.

In 1916, Edward J. Curran began developing an iridiotomy operation in which an incision is made in the iris to treat glaucoma, eventually finding that it worked best in what he called "acute" glaucoma.

In 1941, Otto Barkan (1887–1958) divided glaucoma into the two types now used for classification: wide angle and narrow angle, or open-angle and angle-closure. In the most common form, open-angle, the drainage channel of the eye remains open so vision loss doesn't occur until the late stages of the disease. In angle-closure glaucoma, the passage between the cornea and the iris through which fluid normally drains is completely closed; there are both acute and chronic forms of angle-closure glaucoma. This is a rare but serious form of glaucoma, which can cause blindness if symptoms are not treated quickly.

Tonography, a method for measuring outflow of fluid from the eyeball, was introduced in 1950, making it possible to learn more about the disease.

Research in the late 1960s revealed that people with glaucoma sometimes had normal pressure within the eye, making it necessary to check patients for certain defects of vision as well as eyeball pressure to screen for glaucoma. This type of glaucoma is called "normal tension" glaucoma.

Treatment for open-angle glaucoma includes eyedrops and oral medications. These work by either increasing liquid flow from the eye or decreasing the amount of fluid produced in the eye. These drugs include miotics, **epinephrine, beta-blockers**, carbonic anhydrase inhibitors and alpha adrenergic agonists. The drug latanoprost, a **prostaglandin** analog, was approved by the **Food and Drug Administration (FDA)** for treating glaucoma in 1996.

There are several types of surgery now used to treat glaucoma: trabeculoplasty, which improves drainage of fluid from the eye; iridiotomy, in which a small hole is made in the iris to promote drainage; and cyclophotocoagulation, in which the ciliary body that produces aqueous fluid is frozen in certain areas to reduce fluid production. All of these surgeries are performed with lasers, which were introduced into glaucoma surgery in 1970. Conventional instruments may be used for filtering surgery, in which a small hole is cut in the sclera of the eye to allow drainage. All of these surgeries can be performed in a doctor's office under local **anesthesia** on an outpatient basis. (*See also* gonioscope)

Additional reading: Saltus, "Out of Sight."

glucose testing

Glucose tests help people with **diabetes** control the disease by keeping track of their blood sugar levels.

Before the discovery of **insulin** in the early twentieth century, Elliot P. Joslin (1869–1962) advised people with diabetes to avoid eating carbohydrates and to have their urine tested frequently for sugar. In 1945, Walter A. Compton (1911–) and Maurice Treneer patented a tablet that greatly simplified sugar testing of urine. The test, in which a tablet was added to a small amount of urine in a test tube, producing a color that indicated the sugar level in the urine, made it possible for people with diabetes to test their own urine at home. Another test, which revealed the presence of ketone bodies in the urine, was invented by Alfred H. Free (1913–) and Helen M. Free (1923–) and reported in 1957. This test was important because the presence of ketones in the urine can be life-threatening. A number of other self-test urine kits became available in the late 1950s.

Physicians and laboratories began using blood tests for glucose in the 1960s. This type of test was particularly helpful for pregnant women with diabetes, who had to maintain their blood sugar at a relatively normal level to avoid fetal damage and stillbirth. Blood tests for glucose became available for self use in the 1970s, and now almost all testing is done at home using a drop of fingertip blood placed on a chemically treated strip of paper allowing a printout of the blood level. **Sensor** technology may soon make it possible for patients to check their blood glucose without puncturing the skin.

Additional reading: Free and Free, "Self-Testing."

goiter

Goiter is a swelling of the **thyroid gland** at the base of the neck caused by deficiency in the mineral iodine. This condition is common in areas where earth and water are iodine-poor and people do not consume the mineral through other sources such as iodized salt. Goiter may be accompanied by either abnormally high or abnormally low thyroid function; the former is a "toxic goiter." Thyroiditis due to viral infection is a common cause of a goiter.

The ancient Greeks treated goiter with seaweed and burnt sponges, both of which are rich in iodine. The Chinese had been using seaweed for this purpose since 2700 B.C.

Bernard Courtois (1777–1838), a Paris nitrate manufacturer, isolated iodine from seaweed in 1811, and Jean Francois Coindet (1774–1834) discovered iodine's effectiveness for treating goiter in 1819. In studies of goiter from 1850 to 1860, the French botanist Gaspard-Adolphe Chatin (1813–1901) linked the iodine content of drinking water, soil, and air with the incidence of goiter.

In 1895, Eugen Baumann (1846–1896) discovered that normal thyroid glands contained goiter, and found that glands with goiter contained less iodine.

David Marine (1880–1976) in Cleveland tried adding sodium iodide to the water supply of brook trout in 1910 and found it prevented thyroid overgrowth in the fish. He then conducted an experiment on schoolgirls from 1917 to 1918 and found that iodine therapy prevented goiter.

In "goiter belt" areas, where iodine was scarce in water and soil, a large percentage of the population had goiter—in some places more than half. One survey of men registered for the draft in Michigan found 30 percent had thyroid enlargement, while another survey found that more than 60 percent did. These findings led to the realization that goiter was a major U.S. public health problem.

David Murray Cowle, a professor of pediatrics at the University of Michigan, suggested adding sodium or potassium iodide to table salt. The state began implementing his program in 1924. Morton Salt Company introduced iodized salt in 1924. The incidence of goiter subsequently fell sharply in areas where iodized salt was used.

Great Britain, the United States, several European countries, and Colombia have iodine prophylaxis programs. Goiter remains common today in iodine-deficient areas in Africa, South America, and Asia. (*See also* Graves' disease)

Additional reading: Kiple, *The Cambridge World History of Human Disease,* pp. 750–55.

gonioscope

A gonioscope is an instrument used to measure the angle between the iris and the cornea, which helps in diagnosing **glaucoma**. Scientists had first visualized this angle in the early 1900s, but had not used this measurement clinically.

In the late 1930s, Otto Barkan (1887–1958) began to use gonioscopy in diagnosing glaucoma, and his findings led to the reclassification of glaucoma from acute and chronic to angle-closure and open-angle.

Additional reading: Albert, *The History of Ophthalmology,* p. 212.

gonorrhea

Gonorrhea is a sexually transmitted disease caused by the bacterium *Neisseria gonorrhoeae.* It is the oldest and most common venereal disease.

Symptoms include burning urination and discharge from the vagina or penis. Women with gonorrhea may have no symptoms, so they may be infected with the disease for months or years, which can lead to pelvic inflammatory disease and sterility. Gonorrheal infection of the eyes at birth was once a major cause of blindness.

Mention of a gonorrhea-like disease appears in an Egyptian papyrus of 3500 B.C. The Greek surgeon Claudius Galen (129–c.199) is believed to have dubbed the disease "gonorrhea," a word meaning "flow of seed." The French called the disease chaude pisse, or "hot piss." In the 1500s, French court physician Jean Fernel (1497–1558) made a distinction between gonorrhea and **syphilis**, but controversy continued. For example, John Hunter (1728–1793) injected himself with discharge from a patient he believed had gonorrhea, and developed syphilis instead. In 1838, Philippe Ricord (1800–1889) proved that syphilis and gonorrhea were separate.

In 1879, German dermatologist Albert Neisser (1855–1916) described the bacterium responsible for gonorrhea, which now carries his name. Ernst von Bumm grew the organism in the laboratory for the first time three years later.

Early twentieth-century treatment of gonorrhea involved flooding the urethra with potassium permanganate. Another popular therapy consisted of heating the patient to kill the germ, which was only sometimes successful. Women had their cervixes painted with Mercurochrome and then underwent a urethral irrigation of silver nitrate solution. These treatments were sometimes successful, but were also often extremely painful and had serious side effects.

In the late 1930s, the drug **prontosil** was found to be successful in treating gonorrhea. However, the medication had serious side effects and some infections resisted it. **Penicillin** became the treatment of choice for gonorrhea when it was introduced in the 1940s. Just after improved production techniques made penicillin widely available, a worldwide pandemic of gonorrhea struck in the late 1950s. It reached its height in the mid-1970s, when penicillin-resistant strains of *Gonococcus* appeared.

In 1880, German gynecologist Karl Sigmund Franz Crede (1819–1892) discovered that giving infants silver-nitrate solution eyedrops shortly after birth would prevent gonorrheal infection of their eyes, and thus blindness. Lucien Howe (1848–1928) urged the American Ophthalmological Society to call for legal requirements for the procedure, known as Crede prophylaxis, in 1887. The National Society to Prevent Blindness finally succeeded in getting this legislation passed in every state. Today, all U.S. newborns receive a weaker silver nitrate solution containing **antibiotics**.

Today, gonorrhea is generally treated with an injection of ceftriaxone or a course of doxycycline taken orally.

Additional reading: Kiple, *The Cambridge World History of Human Disease,* pp. 756–63.

gout

Gout is a painful swelling of the joints caused by an excess of uric acid, which predominantly affects males and has been known since ancient times.

The famous Dutch microscopist Anton van Leeuwenhoek (1632–1723) described a crystal he found in a tophus, which is the accretion of uric acid in solid form found in the joints in gout. In 1776, Swedish chemist Carl W. Scheele (1742–1786) found an acid in urine that he called lithic acid, and 21 years later William H. Wollaston (1766–1828) found that tophi contained lithic acid. The following year, Antoine Francois de Fourcroy (1755–1809) renamed lithic acid *acide ourique.*

In 1847, Alfred B. Garrod (1819–1907) developed a test for detecting uric acid in the blood in people with conditions such as gout where levels of the acid were elevated. He hypothesized, correctly, in 1854 that gout was due to excess production of uric acid or an inability to clear uric acid from the system caused by kidney abnormality

Eating a high-fat diet and drinking alcohol can worsen gout, confirming ancient beliefs that the condition was related to alcohol consumption and gluttony. Heredity may also predispose a person to developing gout.

Extracts of the colchicum plant began to be used to treat gout in the early 1800s, and remained the only effective treatment until 1910, when cinchophen was introduced. This drug turned out to cause liver damage, so colchicum's active ingredient **colchicine** (which was isolated in 1820) came back into favor.

Phenylbutazone was introduced in 1951 to treat gout and was found to treat other forms of inflammation as well. Probenecid, a drug developed to slow the excretion of **penicillin** that was found to increase uric acid excretion, was introduced that same year. In 1963, indomethacin and allopurinal were introduced, the latter for treating chronic gout.

Additional reading: McGrew, *Encyclopedia of Medical History,* pp. 116–18.

Graves' disease

Graves' disease is a condition caused by a malfunctioning **thyroid gland** and was first described by Irish physician Dr. Robert Graves (1796–1853) in 1835. It is also known as toxic diffuse **goiter**. Symptoms of the disease include bulging eyes, goiter, and sometimes raised skin over the shins.

Ancient Greek writers had described cases of exopthalmia, or bulging of the eyes. Byzantine writers noted that goiter and exopthalmia tended to appear together.

Graves' disease is now known to be an autoimmune condition in which the immune system attacks the thyroid-stimulating hormone receptor, so that too much thyroid

hormone is available in the body. Graves' disease is the most common form of hyperthyroid illness, and affects women much more frequently than men.

James Collip (1892–1965) isolated thyroid-stimulating hormone (TSH), or thyrotropin, in 1933. Graves' disease was long considered to be caused by overproduction of TSH, but this theory began to die out when it was found in the 1950s that people with Graves' disease did not have excess TSH in their blood. In 1958, J. Maxwell MacKenzie (1927–) observed that people with Graves' disease had a long-acting thyroid stimulator in their blood. By the 1970s, the autoimmune theory of Graves' disease began to take hold.

Therapy for Graves' disease includes antithyroid drugs and administration of radioactive iodine.

Additional reading: "Overactive Thyroid," *Mayo Clinic Health Letter.*

growth factors

Growth factors are natural substances that stimulate the growth of a variety of different types of cells. They are thought to play an important role in the development of **cancer**, and researchers are currently attempting to harness their powers for use in medicine.

Rita Levi-Montalcini (1909–) discovered the first growth factor, known as nerve growth factor (NGF). Victor Hamburger (1900–unknown) had invited Levi-Montalcini to work at Washington University in St. Louis, after he read a paper she had written on nerve **tissue** development. Levi-Montalcini had been working out of a laboratory in her home bedroom, having been forced out of medical school in 1939 when the Fascist government barred Jews from pursuing academic or professional careers.

In 1951, Levi-Montalcini and Hamburger discovered that mouse tumors release a substance that causes nerve fibers to grow. Levi-Montalcini developed a bioassay for the substance the following year, and named the substance nerve growth factor (NGF) in 1954. Stanley Cohen (1922–) worked with Levi-Montalcini in St. Louis to purify the growth factor in the late 1950s, and isolated epidermal growth factor (EGF) while working there in 1962. He described the structure of the factor 10 years later.

Cohen and Levi-Montalcini shared the 1986 Nobel Prize for their discovery of growth factors.

Other growth factors include fibroblast growth factor, platelet-derived growth factor, brain-derived neurotrophic growth factor, insulin-like growth factor, **vascular endothelial growth factor**, and transforming growth factor. NGF and other nervous-system-related growth factors are currently being evaluated for the treatment of neurological diseases such as amyotrophic lateral sclerosis (ALS, or Lou Gehrig's disease), **Alzheimer's disease**, and neuropathies caused by drugs and **diabetes** and other diseases. Studies are underway in animals to determine whether growth factors can be used to help regenerate nerve tissue (for example, in **spinal cord injury treatment**).

Additional Reading: Heath, *Growth Factors;* Levi-Montalcini, *The Saga of the Nerve Growth Factor.*

H

H. pylori (Helicobacter pylori)

Helicobacter pylori is a bacterium associated with the development of gastric ulcers and other stomach and esophageal problems. Peptic ulcers result from the effects of the enzymes involved in digestion on the mucosal surface of the stomach and esophageal linings. H. pylori is now believed to play a major role in the process of most gastric ulcer formation.

Although most physicians now believe that H. pylori is the cause of most ulcer development, treating this infection may not be sufficient to allow ulcers to heal. Other factors may interact with infection to cause and worsen ulcers and exacerbate pain. Stress and certain types of spicy and acidic foods can worsen the pain of ulcers. Stress management techniques may be helpful in treating ulcers, as well as medications that coat the stomach lining and neutralize stomach acids. **Cimetidine,** a drug that blocks the production of stomach acid, is also used. Surgery may be necessary to repair severe damage to the stomach or intestinal lining from an ulcer.

The bacterium produces large amounts of the enzyme urease, which had been linked to ulcer disease in the 1950s.

Spiral-shaped bacteria were first observed in the stomach glands of animals in 1893, and in humans in 1906, but were thought to be benign. In 1979, a team led by Wye Poh Fung working in Australia found the bacteria in people with chronic gastritis. In the early 1980s, Barry Marshall (1951–) and Robert Warren, also in Australia, observed that the bacteria was found in more than half of patients undergoing gastroscopy, all of whom suffered from ulcers or chronic gastritis. They called the bacteria "Campylobacter-like organisms."

In 1984, to test whether the bacterium was responsible for ulcers and gastritis, Marshall consumed a large amount of H. pylori. He developed gastritis 10 days later.

The first trial of H. pylori eradication to treat ulcers was reported in 1987. **Antibiotic** treatment was found to reduce rates of ulcer relapse and perhaps cure the disease.

In 1994, the H. pylori bacterium was classified worldwide as a **carcinogen,** and the **National Institutes of Health**

(**NIH**) and a European consensus group soon recommended that people with ulcers, gastritis, and gastric **cancer** have extensive therapy to eliminate the infection.

The new genus "Helicobacter" was devised for the bacterium and its relatives in 1989. The entire genome of H. pylori was decoded and reported in 1998.

Additional reading: *H. Pylori and Peptic Ulcer,* National Digestive Diseases Information Clearinghouse.

head-injury treatment

Head-injury treatment is designed to minimize trauma to the brain and prevent brain damage. Control of increased pressure within the skull is an important aspect of head injury treatment, because a rise in pressure can occur after injury and will result in brain damage and death if left untreated.

De Vulneribus Capitus, a writing in the **Hippocratic Corpus,** recommends **trepanation** (cutting a hole in the skull) in head injuries where the skull was not fractured. The writer of this treatise suggested that this surgery was necessary to ease pressure. Trepanning continued to be the recommended treatment for head injuries for nearly 2,000 years.

The battlefield surgeon Ambrose Pare (c.1510–1590) observed symptoms of increased pressure within the skull while attending to Henry II of France, who was dying of a head injury. These symptoms included blurred vision, vomiting, and headache. Pare attributed the symptoms to injury and subsequent "putrefaction" of blood in the brain. Although the surgeon provided a detailed description of these symptoms, he did not understand their significance.

In a 1729 letter, Jean-Louis Petit (1674–1750), another French battlefield surgeon, distinguished between loss of consciousness after a head injury and sleepiness that developed afterwards, and said the first was due to concussion and the second due to compression of the brain. The compression, he wrote, indicated whether a patient required trepanation, not the presence or absence of fracture. Another French surgeon, Henri Francois Le Dran (1685–1770), made a similar observation soon afterwards, and described attempting a trepanation to treat compression. Percival Pott (1714–1788), writing in 1773, supported an aggressive approach, recommending early trepanation after a head injury even if it turned out to be unnecessary.

Benjiman Bell (1748–1806) carefully described the neurological signs indicating brain compression, including the fixed, dilated pupil and paralysis of specific nerves, in his *A System of Surgery* in 1785. He said that trepanation should be performed in the presence of these signs (but not preventively), and that the presence or absence of skull fracture said little about the degree of injury to the brain.

Although several attempts were made to systematically monitor intracranial pressure, surgeons had to continue to rely on the presence of neurological signs to gauge whether pressure was abnormally high. These symptoms could be misleading, suggesting high intracranial pressure where there was none and vice versa. In 1960, researchers at the University of Lund in Sweden described a technique for safe and continuous recording and control of the pressure of the fluid in the ventricles. Although this technique is effective and gives doctors clear information on when and if surgery is necessary to ease pressure on the brain, it is not used universally.

In 1995, the Brain Trauma Foundation and the American Academy of Neurological Surgeons released guidelines for the treatment of severe head injury. Research by both groups had revealed that treatment methods varied widely. The guidelines said that hyperventilating patients to ensure oxygen flow to the brain and treating them with steroids (both common practices) should be avoided, and advised that the intracranial pressure of all patients with severe head injuries be monitored so that pressure could be reduced by draining excess **cerebrospinal fluid**. Mannitol and **barbiturates** could also be given to certain patients to reduce swelling of the brain, according to the guidelines.

Additional reading: Rose and Bynum, *Historical Aspects of the Neurosciences,* pp. 243–53.

health insurance

Health insurance is a system in which a group of people, the government, or their employers (or a combination of these entities) pay into a plan for health care, so that when a person needs care the plan covers the costs partially or in full.

Federally supported health insurance dates back to 1883, when the German government began requiring employees and employers in certain industries to contribute funds for cooperative health care.

The U.S. precursor to modern health insurance was the Marine Hospital Fund, the forerunner to the **U.S. Public Health Service**. Beginning in 1798, sailors were taxed 20 cents a month to fund care for their sick and disabled counterparts.

The first major employer- and employee-funded health insurance program was established in 1868 by the Southern Pacific Railroad in California. The first employee-sponsored mutual benefit plan, the Northern Pacific Railway Beneficial Association, was established in 1882.

In the United States, the first government-funded system for health coverage was the program run by the Federal Emergency Relief Administration from 1933 to 1935, which provided medical care for people receiving unemployment relief during the depression. Participants were allowed to choose their own physician. The Farm Security Administration began offering its own health insurance program because so many farmers had defaulted on their loans due to poor health. In 1944, the program was operating in about one-third of counties in 39 states, but it ended in 1946 when Congress refused to continue paying for it.

During World War II, the Emergency Maternity and Infant Care program was established to cover maternity care for servicemen's wives with the hospital and physician of their choice. The program was closed in 1947, but the Servicemen's Dependents Act of 1956 took its place. Veterans themselves have been eligible for government-funded medical care since the end of World War I.

Early voluntary health care plans run by hospitals became statewide Blue Cross plans after 1932. Around this time medical societies began establishing their own plans, which were called Blue Shield plans. By 1950 there were Blue Shield plans in every state that accounted for about half of physician-service coverage.

Several other health insurance plans were founded by industry and workers groups. The first employee-sponsored group, the Union Health Center, was founded by George Price in 1913 to provide health care for workers in the ladies' garment industry. The United Auto Workers founded the Medical Research Institute in Detroit in 1944; the Kaiser Foundation Health Plan was founded for workers at the Kaiser Company shipyards in 1942; and the Health Insurance Plan of Greater New York was founded in 1947.

Today, **managed care**—often in the form of **HMOs (health maintenance organizations)**—has taken over an increasingly large piece of the health insurance market. The elderly, the poor and the disabled are covered under the federally funded **Medicare/Medicaid** plans.

Additional reading: "Can the Private Sector Help to Put Health Care Right?", *The Economist.*

"Healthy People"

"Healthy People" is a report issued periodically by the U.S. government to promote good health.

As sanitation, vaccination, and **antibiotics** had helped to make infectious disease a less serious problem, Surgeon General Julius Richmond (1916–) launched a "Second Public Health Program" in the 1970s designed to prevent heart disease and **cancer** by promoting healthy eating and regular exercise and encouraging people to quit smoking. In 1979, his Office of Disease Prevention and Health Promotion published "Healthy People: The Surgeon General's Report on Health Promotion and Disease Prevention," setting forth goals for 1990. The report led to the Department of Health and Human Services plan for achieving 226 health objectives in 15 priority areas by 1990.

"Healthy People 2000" was released in 1991, and contained 332 objectives in 22 priority areas. The plan was revised in 1995 and 19 new objectives were added. Since 1993, there have been progress reports on "Healthy People 2000's" goals published annually. About 100,000 copies of "Healthy People 2000" have been distributed.

In 1998, "Healthy People 2010", a considerably larger report, was released, with 521 objectives in 26 priority areas. The stated goal of this version of "Healthy People" is to eliminate disparities in health related to poverty and increase the years and quality of life.

Additional reading: Squires, "Report on Prevention Project is Mixed Bag."

hearing aids

Hearing aids are devices designed to improve hearing by amplifying sound and conveying vibration.

Giovanni Battista Porta (1535–1615) described the first specially designed hearing aids, which were made out of wood in the shape of ears of animals with sharp hearing, in his 1588 book *Natural Magick*. In 1550, Gerolamo Cardano (1501–1576) suggested that bone conduction, in which sound vibrations would be transmitted from outside to the bones of the ear, might help deaf people hear better. Speaking tubes and ear trumpets were developed during the 1700s. Bone conduction devices invented in the 1800s ranged from fans held in the teeth to listening thrones.

In 1898, the Dictagraph Company began making the first battery-powered hearing aid commercially available in the United States. Miller Reese Hutchison (1876–1944), an American inventor, filed the patent for the first electric hearing aid in 1901. In the early 1920s, carbon microphone aids were introduced that featured bone conduction transducers. After World War II, efforts were made to refine hearing aids, but they still required a person to wear two packs—one strapped at the waist, one at the chest—with a wire leading to the ear. Smaller "monopack" aids became available in 1945. Transistors were invented three years later, and the first all-transistor hearing aid, made by Microtone, became available in 1953. "Spectacle" aids were introduced in 1956.

Thanks to miniaturization and microchips, hearing aids now can be made so small that they fit invisibly inside the ear.

Additional reading: Alexander, "Hearing Aids; Now Hear This." University of California Berkeley Wellness Letter.

hearing test

Hearing tests are used both to screen for hearing defects and to gauge the degree and quality of hearing loss.

Instruments that produced a series of clicks to gauge hearing were produced in the early nineteenth century, after researchers had shown that people could lose hearing at certain frequencies and not at others. Tuning forks and whistles were used to test hearing at various frequencies.

Hearing tests were standardized at the seventh International Congress of Otology in 1907 into the "Acoumetric Schema." The tests composing the schema were based on voice, tuning fork, a clicking instrument developed by Adam Politzer (1835–1920) in 1877, and a watch.

In the 1890s, Max Thomas Edelmann (1845–1913) assembled a group of tuning forks and whistles that covered the entire range of audible sound, from 16 to 20,000 Hertz. But these instruments were somewhat unwieldy; the tuning fork producing the lowest tone, for example, was more than a yard long.

Less cumbersome electric audiometers were developed in the late 1800s, but the sound quality of these instruments was far worse than that of the tuning forks and whistles. These audiometers were made with telephone receivers by David Edward Hughes (1831–1900) in England and Arthur Hartmann (1849–1931) in Germany in 1878. Benjamin Ward Richardson (1828–1926) helped popularize the audiometer.

Around the time of World War I, the problem of sound quality was solved when the electric valve was invented. This made it possible to build an instrument that produced pure sounds of any intensity and frequency. The first audiometers using this technology were the Otaudion, made in Germany in 1919, and the 1A audiometer made by Western Electric Company in the United States in 1922.

Today, hearing is tested using two methods: audiometry, in which a person wears earphones and listens to a series of sounds at different pitches and volumes to determine the extent and type of hearing loss; and electrophysiological measurements. The second test uses electrodes and microphones to measure the function of the middle ear, eardrum, and the hair cells of the inner ear, and the transmission of sound from the cochlea to the brain stem. These tests do not require a response from the person being tested, and can be used on young children and others who cannot respond to instructions.

Additional reading: Martin, *Introduction to Audiology.*

heart attack. See angina pectoris; angioplasty; bypass surgery; calcium channel blocker; cardiac catheterization; cholesterol; cholesterol-lowering drugs; coronary care unit; pacemaker

heart transplant

In a heart transplant, a person receives a new heart from a human donor.

Christiaan N. Barnard (1922–) performed the world's first heart transplant in Cape Town, South Africa, in 1967. He implanted the heart of a young woman who had died in a car accident in the chest of a 54-year-old man with congestive heart failure. The man died of pneumonia after 18 days with the new heart.

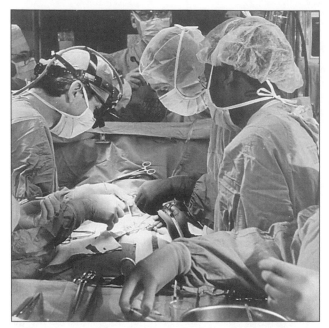

An infant heart transplant. (Courtesy of Archives and Special Collections, Columbia University Health Sciences Division.)

Norman Shumway (1923–) is credited with the first successful heart transplant, performed in 1968 at Stanford University Hospital. Denton Cooley (1920–) of the Texas Heart Institute in Houston also began performing heart transplants around this time.

Initial enthusiasm for the procedure faded because the recipients' immune system would attack and destroy donor hearts, a process known as "rejection." The drug **cyclosporine**, approved by the **Food and Drug Administration (FDA)** in 1983, largely solved the rejection problem by quieting a patient's immune system so that it would not attack the donor heart.

In 1978, a method for preserving the heart safely by chilling it made it possible to keep donor hearts viable for as long as seven hours. The longest-living heart transplant recipient received the organ in 1974, and as of 1998 (the most recent data available), had lived for 23 years, 8 months, and was still alive.

A few patients also have received heart transplants along with **lung transplants** for conditions in which both the heart and the lungs are diseased, such as primary pulmonary **hypertension**. The first such procedure was performed by Shumway and his colleague Bruce Reitz (1944–) in 1981.

Today, heart transplants are the preferred treatment for patients with end-stage heart disease who are otherwise healthy, and about 70 percent of U.S. heart transplant recipients live for four years or longer. According to the United Network for Organ Sharing (UNOS), 2,292 heart transplants were performed in 1997, and currently more than 4,000 people are on the UNOS waiting list seeking a heart transplant. (*See also* immunosuppression)

Additional reading: Acierno, *The History of Cardiology,* pp. 665–69.

heart-lung machine

A heart-lung machine takes over the **circulation** and oxygenation of blood for a person during heart surgery.

John Gibbon Jr. (1903–1973) developed a heart-lung machine that he tested on a human being for the first time in 1952. The first patient to be operated on successfully while the machine sustained her vital functions was Cecelia Bavolek, in 1953. She was connected to the machine for 45 minutes, and for 27 minutes the machine completely replaced the function of her heart and lungs.

Gibbon conceived the idea of a cardiac bypass after watching a patient die from a pulmonary embolism in 1931 when he was a fellow at Massachusetts General Hospital. He theorized that if a machine could have taken over the function of heart and lungs until the danger of blockage with a blood clot passed—or the clot could be removed—the patient would have lived.

He began working on the machine in 1934, at the University of Pennsylvania, with the help of his wife Mary Gibbon (1905–1989), a skilled medical technician. They achieved their first success in an animal experiment in 1935. After World War II, Gibbon moved the project to Jefferson Medical College in Philadelphia, where the IBM Corporation provided free engineering help.

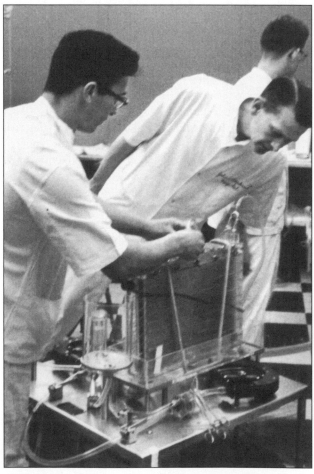

Surgeons and technicians at Johns Hopkins perform a final check on a heart-lung machine in preparation for a 1957 open-heart surgery. (Reproduced with permission of *Johns Hopkins Magazine.*)

In 1932, Texas heart surgeon Michael DeBakey (1908–) invented the roller-pump that Gibbon would use as a blood-oxygenating device in his heart lung machine.

For oxygenation in Gibbon's machine, the blood was passed in a thin film along the center of a revolving cylinder, kept in place by centrifugal force, while oxygen was blown at it as it moved along the cylinder. Two of his assistants had discovered, by accident, that if turbulence was created in the blood flow the blood could be more fully oxygenated. **Heparin** kept blood liquid as it flowed through the machine, which was powered by a roller pump. Two liters of donated blood primed the pump.

The heart-lung machine remains a central part of modern heart surgery. However, advances in heart surgery have made it possible to perform some operations, including **bypass surgery**, on a beating heart, making heart-lung bypass unnecessary.

Another focus of research is the development of strategies for avoiding inflammation after heart-lung bypass. Blood cells are damaged in the machine, leading to inflammation when they are reinfused into the patient. Research in the late 1990s showed that filtering white blood cells dramatically reduces inflammation, resulting in fewer days in the hospital and a quicker recovery. Surgeons have also developed techniques for reducing **red blood cell** damage. Patients may be given a medication such as **erythropoetin** that boosts red blood cell production before surgery. Some centers collect and "wash" the patient's blood after surgery. Another advance involves avoiding transfusion entirely during open-heart surgery by recycling the blood. Usually, a person requires several pints of donated blood during open heart surgery.

Additional reading: Callahan, Keys, and Key, *Classics of Cardiology,* pp. 386–95; Shorter. *The Health Century,* pp. 174–76.

Heimlich maneuver

The Heimlich maneuver is a technique used to expel food from the windpipe to relieve choking and restore breathing. By holding a person from behind and firmly pressing the fist up into the abdomen, it's usually possible to dislodge the obstructing object.

Henry J. Heimlich (1920–), director of surgery at the Jewish Hospital in Denver, developed the technique as an alternative to emergency tracheostomy, in which an incision into the trachea is made to allow breathing. He began testing the method in dogs in 1973, reporting the results of his animal research the following year. In this article, he described how the technique could work in humans and asked for anyone using the maneuver to report it to him. In 1974, almost immediately after his article was published, he received the first report of someone using it to save a choking victim. The American Medical Association endorsed the Heimlich maneuver in 1975.

Additional reading: Glionna, "Heimlich Helper."

Helicobacter pylori. *See* H. pylori.

hemophilia

Hemophilia is a hereditary disease in which the blood lacks a substance necessary for clotting. Symptoms include uncontrollable bleeding and pooling of blood in the joints that can be extremely painful and ultimately crippling. The disease appears mostly only in men.

There are two types of hemophilia, A and B. A lack of coagulation Factor VIII causes A, the most common form, while deficiency in Factor IX causes the B type.

In the early part of the twentieth century, hemophiliacs were treated with ice packs to ease swelling and **blood transfusions** when they became available.

Judith Graham Pool (1919–1975) of Stanford University discovered in 1965 that plasma that had been frozen and then thawed left a residue with a high Factor VIII concentration. This sediment was known as cryoprecipitate, or "cryo," and could be made by freezing a few bags of plasma at a time. It was 10 times more powerful than plasma alone, and patients could store the cryo in their freezers at home.

Later in the decade, Kenneth M. Brinkhous (1908–) at the University of North Carolina, working with scientists at Hyland Laboratories, developed a highly concentrated form of Factor VIII. They used Pool's technique, but with hundreds of units of plasma at a time, and then purified and centrifuged the sediment, resulting in a concentrate that was 100 times richer in the factor than plasma. They began producing lots that contained blood from thousands of donors. Patients could store this form of cryo at room temperature, dissolving the material in water and injecting it when needed.

Although the new highly concentrated Factor VIII was a great advance for hemophilia patients and their families, hemophiliacs often became infected with **hepatitis** because they were injecting themselves with blood material from thousands of donors. The new concentrated Factor VIII set the stage for tragedy in the 1980s when HIV entered the blood supply.

Most hemophiliacs who used Factor VIII during this time became infected with the HIV virus. About 80 percent of severe hemophiliacs, who require more frequent doses of blood products, contracted HIV during the 1980s, while about half of all hemophiliacs became infected with the **virus**.

The German laboratory products company, Behringwerke AG, developed a method for treating Factor VIII so it could be heated and sterilized safely, and in 1983, Hyland (a division of Baxter) became the first U.S. company to hold a patent for heat-treating Factor VIII. Other techniques for creating Factor VIII without viral contamination include monoclonal purification and Factor VIII produced by cells altered with **genetic recombination** techniques.

In 1998, President William Jefferson Clinton (1946–) signed legislation establishing the Ricky Ray Hemophilia Relief Fund, named in honor of a boy with hemophilia who died after contracting HIV from contaminated blood. The

$750 million fund will provide a $100,000 settlement to each person who contracted **AIDS** from tainted blood.

Additional reading: Massie, *Journey;* DePrince, *Cry Bloody Murder.*

heparin

Heparin is a substance produced by the mammalian liver that prevents blood clotting and is used as an **anticoagulant** drug.

In 1916, Baltimore medical student Jay McLean discovered a substance in stored liver extracts with anticoagulant properties that his professor William Howell (1860–1945) called heparin. Howell discovered a different and more effective anticoagulant in liver extract in 1922. Clinical tests of the substance failed, however, because it was so impure.

Charles Best (1899–1978) at the Connaught Laboratories in the University of Toronto succeeded in purifying small amounts of heparin in 1933, and clinical use of heparin to prevent clotting began two years later.

Heparin played a vital role in the development of both kidney **dialysis** and the **heart-lung machine**, as it stopped blood from clotting as it passed through these machines. It continues to be important in cardiac and vascular surgery today.

Additional reading: Comroe, *Exploring the Heart,* pp. 64–68.

hepatitis

Hepatitis is a general term for a group of viral diseases that cause liver damage. The three main types are hepatitis A, hepatitis B, and hepatitis C. Hepatitis A is spread by fecal-oral contamination, while B and C are transmitted by infected serum, contaminated needles, blood transfusions, and sexual intercourse. Hepatitis A is usually mild; B can be mild as well, but in its severe form it can lead to cirrhosis and liver **cancer**. Hepatitis C virus infection (HCV) is the most common bloodborne infection in the U.S. and can cause critical liver damage. In fact, HCV-associated end-stage liver disease is the most frequent indication for liver transplantation among adults.

About 143,000 people in the United States and as many as 10 million worldwide contract hepatitis A each year, while 200,000 people are infected with hepatitis B in the United States annually.

The disease was likely recognized in prehistoric times. In the 700s, Pope Zaccharias, is believed to have been the first to observe that hepatitis was contagious. From the late 1700s onward, hepatitis was well known to strike soldiers during wartime, and was called "campaign jaundice." Until the twentieth century, hepatitis was not distinguished from jaundice, in which the skin and eyeballs become yellow. Jaundice is now known to occur because the body is not adequately clearing digestive byproducts such as bile from the blood, and is a symptom of liver damage or malfunction but not a disease in itself.

After Rudolph Virchow (1821–1902) observed one patient with mucus blocking the bile duct in 1865, hepatitis and jaundice were long thought to always occur because of such blockage.

When a number of soldiers developed hepatitis after receiving **yellow fever** vaccinations during World War II, while others appeared to have caught hepatitis from person-to-person contact or contaminated food, it became clear that there were at least two kinds of infectious hepatitis. Research began to find the infectious agent responsible, and in 1947, Richard M. McCallum of the University of Virginia Health Science Centers named infectious hepatitis "hepatitis A" and hepatitis that could be spread by blood serum "hepatitis B."

Baruch Blumberg (1925–) of the Institute for Cancer Research in Philadelphia and his colleagues at the **National Institutes of Health (NIH)** discovered an **antigen** carried by the hepatitis B virus in 1965, which was also called the "Australia antigen" because the team found the virus in the blood of an Australian aborigine. Blumberg won the 1976 Nobel Prize in Medicine and Physiology for this discovery, which made it possible to develop a blood test for hepatitis B.

In 1967, a doctor working at Willowbrook State School, an institution for people with mental disabilities in Staten Island, New York, confirmed the existence of two distinct kinds of hepatitis, calling them MS1 (infectious) and MS2 (serum). The doctor, Saul Krugman (1911–1995) was later criticized because he and his colleagues had intentionally infected inmates of the school in their studies of hepatitis.

In 1970, D.S. Dane of Middlesex Hospital Medical School in London and colleagues described hepatitis B virus particles after observing the infectious agent with an **electron microscope**. One year later, June D. Almeida and colleagues from Wellcome Research Laboratories in Kent, United Kingdom, showed that it was possible to check donated blood for hepatitis B infection by screening for the Australia antigen. The American **Red Cross** began screening for hepatitis B in 1971, and screening at all blood collection centers was mandated in 1972.

The hepatitis A virus was described in 1973, and Maurice Hilleman (1942–) of the drug company Merck and his colleagues were able to grow the virus in culture in 1979.

Krugman prepared a crude **vaccine** for hepatitis that was somewhat, but not completely, effective in protecting the Willowbrook inmates from hepatitis B infection. Hilleman developed a vaccine that was tested on a large group of gay male volunteers, who were at high risk for the disease, and found to be safe and effective in 1980.

Hepatitis B and C can be treated with doses of **immunoglobulin** containing **antibodies** to the virus. The first vaccine approved in the United States against hepatitis A was released in 1995. A vaccination is also available against hepatitis B.

Hepatitis C was long called "non-A-non-B" after it was first recognized as a distinct disease in the 1960s. Scientists at Chiron Corporation in Emeryville, California, cloned parts of the hepatitis C virus and developed an antibody test for the disease in 1989.

Additional reading: Radetsky, *The Invisible Invaders,* pp. 255–95.

herbal medicine

Herbal medicine is the ancient technique of treating disease and promoting health with plant material. The popularity of herbal medicine has mushroomed at the end of the twentieth century, along with the growing use and acceptance of other forms of **alternative medicine.**

In the United States, herbal medicine is estimated to be a $1.5 billion market. In Europe, where herbal medicine is more broadly accepted and has been extensively investigated in clinical trials, especially in Germany, sales are thought to total $6 billion.

Some popular herbs are St. John's wort, for treating **depression**; garlic, for cardiovascular health; echinacea, for strengthening the immune system; saw palmetto for easing the symptoms of benign prostate enlargement; and ginseng, for boosting energy. Some doctors recommend these herbs for their patients. In the past 20 years, according to experts on botanical medicine, more and more Americans have been using these products to maintain health as well as to treat illness.

In 1991, the **World Health Organization (WHO)** published "Guidelines for the Assessment of Herbal Medicines," intended to help nations set up regulation for testing the safety and quality of these preparations. The first U.S. government funded conference on herbal medicine was sponsored by the **National Institutes of Health's (NIH)** Office of Alternative Medicine and the **Food and Drug Administration (FDA)** in 1995.

Herbal medicine has been essentially unregulated in the United States since 1994, when Congress passed the Dietary Supplement Health and Education Act. The law bars the FDA from regulating these products, allows manufacturers to make "structure and function" claims about herbal medicine's benefits, and requires the FDA to prove that an herbal medicine is harmful before its sale can be restricted. Advocates of botanical medicine are urging the U.S. to adopt a system for regulation of herbal medicines.

Additional reading: Porter, *Medicine,* pp. 68–92; Okie, "Herbal Relief."

Herceptin

Herceptin is the first monoclonal **antibody** approved by the **Food and Drug Administration (FDA)** for treating **breast cancer**.

Herceptin is named for the HER-2 **gene**. Normally, a person has two copies of the gene and a few receptors for proteins made by the HER-2 gene on the surface of his or her cells. But 25 to 30 percent of women with breast **cancer** have extra copies of the gene and an abnormal proliferation of HER-2 receptors. These receptors receive signals from proteins that encourage cell proliferation, which are called **growth factors**. Scientists believe that the cells of people with extra HER-2 receptors may be more susceptible to cancerous growth, and that cancers in these individuals may be more difficult to treat than in those without them. Herceptin is also being tested in men with **prostate cancer**.

Dr. Dennis Slamon (1948–) of the University of California at Los Angeles discovered the role of the HER-2 gene in breast and prostate cancer.

Herceptin works by attaching itself to HER-2 protein receptors so that cells cannot respond to these signals. The drug is given to patients along with **chemotherapy**, not by itself.

The FDA approved Herceptin, which has the generic name trastuzumab, in October 1998 for treating breast cancer patients whose disease had spread and who had failed one course of chemotherapy. However, in May 2000, the drug's maker, Genentech, reported that Herceptin had been linked to adverse reactions and deaths in 62 of an estimated 23,000 people who had taken it. Genentech was working with the FDA to amend the drug's label to prevent such events in the future.

Additional reading: Bazell, *HER-2.*

heroin

Heroin, a highly addictive derivative of **morphine**, was introduced by the German drug company Friedrich Bayer & Company in 1898 as a cough suppressant and treatment for patients with lung disease. The drug, also known by the chemical name diacetylmorphine, has not been used in the United States as a medicine since 1924. But heroin continues to be used illegally, and some policy analysts believe it became more popular in the 1990s, partly because the heroin sold is cheaper and purer than it had been in the past.

While investigating morphine derivatives, Charles Alder Wright synthesized heroin in 1874. Animal tests of the drug, and similar substances Wright had synthesized, began in the late 1880s. In 1890, David Dott and Ralph Stockman, a chemist and physician working at the University of Edinburgh, reported that diacetylmorphine was more effective than morphine for depressing spinal cord and respiratory function in animals, but had a weaker narcotic action.

Felix Hoffman, a chemist at Bayer, synthesized diacetylmorphine in 1897. Heinrich Dreser, the new head of the company's pharmacology laboratory, began studying the effects of the compound in rabbits. His main goal was to evaluate whether it could be used as a cough suppressant, to replace codeine. Dreser found that diacetylmorphine made animals breathe more deeply and slowly, and his experiments with human volunteers seemed to confirm the finding. He concluded that the drug would be an effective treatment for respiratory disease. Researchers at Bayer believed that the drug had a uniquely specific action on the lung.

Soon after the introduction of heroin, cases of abuse of the drug were reported. One 1912 account described addicts as using the drug by inhaling it through the nostrils (the same way that **cocaine** is used). Heroin at the time was available over the counter, and was not thought to be as addictive as morphine or codeine.

In 1914, Congress passed the Harrison Act, which limited the amount of heroin that patent medicines could contain to less than 10 milligrams per gram. The United States banned the use of heroin as a medicine in 1924. Morphine, a less potent and thus less addictive **opium** derivative, became the pain-killing medication of choice, and remains in use today.

There were an estimated 50,000 heroin users in the United States in the 1950s; today, there are thought to be approximately 250,000. Most users inject the drug with a **syringe**, although some users sniff it into the nostrils and others smoke it, a practice known as "chasing the dragon." Recent reports have shown that smoking heroin can lead to permanent brain damage.

For heroin addicts, getting off the drug is extremely difficult because of the painful symptoms of withdrawal, which include **depression**, vomiting, diarrhea, and aches, pains, and cramps throughout the body, as well as excess mucus production. Addicts actually must continue to take heroin in order not to get sick. In fact, it is possible for people to die from respiratory failure during withdrawal.

Methadone maintenance, in which a patient takes this opiate derivative as a substitute for heroin, is one effective treatment method for heroin addiction. **Opiate antagonists**, which oppose the action of heroin and other drugs, can also be used; patients who take opiate antagonists as maintenance medication will not "get high" if they take heroin. Finally, a relatively new technique called **rapid opiate detoxification,** which involves putting the person under general **anesthesia** and then speeding-up the withdrawal process with the administration of opiate antagonists, is helpful for some people but expensive (and generally not paid for by **health insurance**).

Additional reading: Fernandez, *Heroin.*

HGH. *See* human growth hormone.

hip replacement

In a hip replacement, the joint between the femur and pelvis is replaced surgically with artificial material. Hip replacements are generally used to replace joints painfully immobilized by arthritis.

Replacing the natural ball-and-socket arrangement requires material that is both strong and slippery, so the joint will continue to move freely without working its way out of the bone. Most importantly, the material must not react with human tissue.

In the 1890s, Thomas Gluck, a German, experimented with ivory joint replacements, using grout to attach the implant to the bone. In London in the 1930s, John Wiles tried several total hip replacements using stainless steel, performing the first in a human in 1938, but the implants wore out too quickly and also tended to react with the body.

Such early attempts involved replacing either the socket of the joint or the tip of the femur, but not both. Various metals met with various results, but even with the most suc-

cessful implant patients needed to walk with a cane and required another operation within five to ten years.

A team in Norwich, England, led by George Kenneth McKee (1906–1991), began experimenting with artificial joints that included both the ball and the socket. About half of the patients who received these new joints in the late 1950s had fair to good results. After trial and error, the Norwich group learned that the ball and socket should be made of two different materials—those made of identical materials tended to begin welding themselves together. Briton John Charnley (1911–1982) developed a technique for attaching the femoral component in which the bone marrow cavity was hollowed out and filled with acrylic cement and the **prosthesis** was forced into the cavity while the cement was still soft. This resulted in much better attachment, and McKee began using this technique in 1961 with greatly improved results.

Both McKee and Charnley experimented with different designs, methods for lubricating the joints, and plastics and metals for building the joints. The best turned out to be high molecular weight polyethylene, a type of plastic, which proved both durable and, with design modifications, slippery enough to keep the joint moving.

Now that hip replacement has become a relatively common operation in older people, device manufacturers continue to look for better designs, better techniques for implanting the artificial joints, and better materials that will last longer, making it practical in some cases to perform hip replacements in younger people.

Additional reading: Baurac, "Joint Exchange"; McBeath, "Total Joint Replacement." "New Life for Old Hips," *Consumer Reports on Health.*

Hippocratic Corpus

The Hippocratic Corpus is a group of about 70 works, from fragments to essays, written between 420 and 370 B.C. by several different authors. A few may have been written by Hippocrates himself, who lived from 460 to 380 B.C. The collection may come from the library of his medical school at the Greek island of Cos.

Hippocratic medicine is based on the idea that the body contains four humors: blood, yellow bile, black bile, and phlegm. For a person to be healthy, according to the philosophy of **humoralism,** the humors must be in proper balance with one another.

Some more long-lasting contributions of Hippocratic medicine include **cauterization, auscultation**, wound drainage with a tin tube, bandaging, and the use of wine and vinegar as **antiseptics**. Hippocratic medicine was also fairly advanced in terms of surgery.

Unfortunately, the corpus's advocacy of bleeding and purging to treat disease led to these often harmful treatments being relied upon by doctors for nearly 2,000 years afterwards.

Writings included in the corpus recommend careful observation of patients, describe case histories, and challenge the idea that disease is caused by evil spirits. For this reason some historians consider the corpus to be the foundation of scientific medicine.

Additional reading: Heidel, *Hippocratic Medicine;* Smith, *The Hippocratic Tradition.*

hirudin

Hirudin was the first substance used medically to stop blood clotting, and the first naturally occurring **anticoagulant** discovered.

Leeches produce hirudin to keep blood flowing from their host. Hirudin works by stopping the blood chemical thrombin from acting on fibrinogen to produce fibrin threads, which form the basis of blood clots.

John Berry Haycraft (1857–1922) first reported that leeches produced an anticoagulant material in 1884. A preparation made from dried, ground-up leech heads was introduced at the turn of the century. However, hirudin was generally only used in the lab because a live leech remained the best way of administering the anticoagulant substance to a living patient.

John Jacob Abel (1857–1938), who built an experimental artificial kidney in 1914, used hirudin to keep blood flowing through the device.

Hirudin continues to be used as a medication today. Recent studies have shown it is a safer blood-thinner than **heparin** when taken long-term. A synthetic form of the drug, made by genetic recombination, is used today.

Additional reading: Comroe, *Exploring the Heart,* pp. 61–62.

histamine

The body releases many inflammation-producing substances after injury or during an allergic reaction, and histamine was the first of these substances to be discovered.

The British scientist Henry H. Dale (1875–1968) first isolated histamine in 1911, while searching for uterine-stimulating drugs. However, because histamine's effects in the body were so widespread, the drug wasn't suitable as medicine. Dale and Patrick Playfair Laidlaw (1881–1940) observed in animal studies that the effects of histamine were similar to those of anaphylactic shock. Dale and his colleagues recognized that histamine also had something to do with allergic reactions, and published their findings in 1919.

Charles Best (1899–1978), famous for his role in the discovery of **insulin**, worked with Dale to investigate the physiological effects of a liver extract that reduced **blood pressure**, and found its effects were due to histamine, which opened blood vessels. Their work and that of others confirmed that histamine was found naturally in the body.

There are now known to be three types of histamine receptors in the body. The first group, those that are inhibited by the early **antihistamine** drugs, were classified as H1 receptors in 1966. These histamines are the type generally involved in inflammation and allergic reactions. Six

years later, James W. Black (1924–) identified H2 receptors and some H2 receptor blockers. H2 receptors control stomach acid secretion, but most likely also play a role in immune-system reactions. This research ultimately resulted in the development of **cimetidine**, a drug that blocks stomach acid production and was the first effective nonsurgical treatment for ulcers.

H3 receptors were identified in 1983. H3 receptors may modulate activity of nervous and cardiovascular systems, but their exact function remains unclear. (*See also* allergy; anaphylaxis)

Additional reading: Shorter, *The Health Century,* pp. 230–31.

HIV. *See* AIDS.

HMO (health maintenance organization)

HMOs are **health insurance** plans that provide all of a person's medical care for a preset fee, and place an emphasis on preventive care.

The first prepaid health maintenance organization was established in California by the Ross-Loos Medical Group in 1929. California steel magnate Henry J. Kaiser (1882–1967) founded the Kaiser Permanente Medical Care Program in 1942, and today it is the largest HMO in the United States. Other pioneering HMOs include the Health Insurance Plan of Greater New York and the Group Health Cooperative of Puget Sound, in Washington state.

The U.S. government began advocating HMOs in the 1970s as a method for controlling health care costs. Today, HMO-type Medicare (largely voluntary) and Medicaid (largely compulsory) plans have been established in several states (*see* **Medicare/Medicaid**).

Although HMO supporters say this type of health insurance provides better preventive care, critics argue that the plans restrict access to care to a dangerous degree. As the debate continues, HMOs and other **managed care** plans have taken up a larger and larger share of the health insurance market.

Additional reading: Anders, *Health and Wealth.*

Hodgkin's disease

Hodgkin's disease is a **cancer** of the lymphatic system that is now curable in more than 70 percent of cases. It is named for the British physician who first described it, Thomas Hodgkin (1798–1866).

In the United States, there are roughly 7,200 new cases of Hodgkin's disease and 1,300 deaths from the disease annually.

Hodgkin presented his study of seven cases of people with enlarged lymph glands and spleens in 1832. Sir Samuel Wilks (1824–1915) named the disease Hodgkin's disease in a paper he published nearly 30 years later. Wilks also provided the first microscopic study of the disease.

In 1902, Dorothy Reed (1874–1964) observed that giant white blood cells often appeared in people with

Hodgkin's. Karl Sternberg (1872–1935) had seen these cells four years earlier, although in less detail. The cells are named "Reed-Sternberg" cells in their honor.

The first effective treatment for Hodgkin's disease was **radiation therapy**, introduced by William Allen Pusey (1865–1940) and Nicholas Senn (1844–1908) in 1902 and 1903. This therapy didn't cure Hodgkin's, but did help shrink tumors in some cases. Radiation therapy became more effective in the 1950s, when mega-voltage equipment was introduced that made it possible to deliver higher doses of radiation to tumors without harming patients.

The first **chemotherapy** for Hodgkin's disease was **nitrogen mustard**, which continues to be used as therapy for this disease today along with vincristine (one of the **vinca alkaloids**), procarbazine, and prednisone, a drug related to **cortisone**. (*See also* lymph system)

Additional reading: Kaplan, *Hodgkin's Disease.*

homeopathy

Homeopathy is a school of medical thought founded in the nineteenth century by German doctor Samuel Christian Hahnemann (1755–1843). The basic concept of homeopathy is that "like cures like": substances that produce a particular effect in people will cure diseases that have similar symptoms, when given to the patient in tiny doses. Hahnemann published his ideas in 1810 in his *Organon of Rational Healing.*

Homeopathic physicians would conduct "proving" sessions in which they tested the effects of various substances on themselves and then on others. Homeopathic physicians also advocated exercise, a healthy diet, fresh air, and good hygiene.

Because much medical treatment at the time involved massive **bloodletting** and dosing patients with poisonous and purgative medicines that often hastened death, and because homeopathy was based on relatively scientific methods of experimentation, the school of thought developed a wide following.

Constantine Hering (1800–1880), a German homeopath, established the first college of homeopathic medicine in the United States, in Allentown, Pennsylvania, in 1835.

Homeopathy has made some significant contributions to medicine, including pointing the way toward the discovery of **nitroglycerin** as a useful treatment for **angina pectoris**. But allopathic or conventional physicians have forced homeopaths out of the mainstream.

Today many people use homeopathic remedies. Although these therapies are considered to be quackery by most practitioners of organized medicine, they are probably never harmful in themselves.

Additional reading: Ullman, *The Consumer's Guide to Homeopathy.*

hormone

Hormones are substances released by glands that travel through the bloodstream to produce certain specific actions.

In 1877, Emil du Bois Reymond (1818–1896) suggested that some type of "stimulatory secretion" excited activity in the body. Scientists also observed a number of different small organs, such as the **thyroid gland** and the pituitary, that had no ducts and appeared as if they released material directly into the bloodstream or lymph glands. In the 1850s, Thomas Addison (1793–1860) and Charles-Edouard Brown-Sequard (1817–1894) suggested, that the **adrenal glands** had some sort of vital function.

Upon reading an 1890 report on a woman with myxoedema who recovered after being treated with implants of a sheep's thyroid gland, George Murray (1865–1939) concluded that her rapid recovery was most likely due to some substance in the gland. He prepared an extract of sheep thyroid and gave a patient with myxoedama injections of the extract, and she subsequently recovered. Several other experiments around this time showed that other glands released powerful and specifically active substances. **Epinephrine** was the first hormone to be isolated and identified, by John J. Abel (1857–1938), in 1903.

Ernest Henry Starling (1866–1927), who studied substances involved in digestion, coined the name "hormone" for chemicals released from the glands and transported by the bloodstream, in 1905. The name comes from the Greek word "to urge on" or "set in motion." The system of glands that release hormones into the bloodstream was named "endocrine" in 1913.

Throughout the twentieth century, as hormones such as **insulin, human growth hormone,** and **cortisone** were discovered, methods for producing commercial quantities of these substances made it possible to easily treat many diseases caused by hormone deficiency. Another major advance in hormone research was the introduction of the **birth control pill** in 1960, which uses artificial hormones to block conception.

Genetic recombination, a technique invented in the 1970s for producing pure proteins in unlimited quantities, has superseded the practice of treating people with hormones collected from other people and from animals, thus eliminating the risk of infection.

Designer **estrogens,** including the drug **tamoxifen,** became available in the 1970s and 1980s and are used to prevent and treat **cancer.** They also may be used to prevent **osteoporosis** and other conditions related to menopause without increasing a woman's risk of **breast cancer.**

Many mysteries remain about the production and purpose of hormones, and how these substances regulate body processes. The hormones melatonin (produced by the **pineal gland**) and DHEA became popular in the 1990s as a jet-lag treatment and an anti-aging preparation, respectively, but doubts about the effectiveness and safety of taking these hormones remain.

One major concern of researchers today is whether **estrogen**-like substances found in the environment and in foods may increase a woman's risk of certain cancers. The interaction between hormones and cancer in general continues to be a vital area of research. (*See also* androgens)

Additional reading: Angier, *Woman,* pp. 177–92.

hormone replacement therapy (HRT)

Hormone-replacement therapy is the use of artificial **hormones** to treat people whose glands no longer produce hormones on their own. Most commonly, HRT describes a combination of **estrogen** and **progesterone,** or estrogen alone, given to menopausal and postmenopausal women to ward off some of the degenerative processes associated with menopause, such as **osteoporosis,** as well as symptoms such as "hot flashes."

Samuel Geist and Frank Spielman at Mt. Sinai Hospital in New York first discussed the idea of treating menopausal symptoms with estrogens in 1932. Robert Wilson popularized hormone replacement for women experiencing menopause in Europe and the United States with his book *Feminine Forever,* published in the United Kingdom in 1966. He called menopause "Oestrogen Deficiency Syndrome," and proposed treating it with estrogen. The first scientific meeting on hormone replacement therapy was held in Geneva in 1971.

Now, millions of menopausal women use HRT to prevent heart disease, osteoporosis, urinary incontinence, and ovarian **cancer.** The main risk of HRT is its association with **breast cancer.** Researchers are now developing specially tailored estrogens, such as **tamoxifen,** that do not stimulate breast-tissue growth, allowing women with a history of breast cancer to take estrogen safely.

Additional reading: O'Dowd and Philipp, *The History of Obstetrics and Gynaecology,* pp. 319–23.

hospice

Hospice is a system of providing holistic care for dying people. The word "hospice" comes from the same root as hospital, and today's hospices have much in common with the first hospitals, established in early Christian times to provide comfort and care for the dying.

Cicely Saunders (1918–) founded the modern hospice movement, which focuses on making patients comfortable and fulfilling their spiritual as well as physical needs. Saunders founded St. Christopher's Hospice in Sydenham, England, in 1967. The hospice was a descendant of those established around the late 1800s to early 1900s by orders of nuns such as St. Luke's House and St. Joseph's Hospice, both in London.

Today in the United States hospices may be freestanding institutions, or they may employ nurses and doctors to care for the patient in his or her home; the philosophy is more important than the place. Hospices provide palliative care and pain treatment, and attempt to meet the spiritual needs of the dying patient.

The first freestanding hospice in the United States was the Connecticut Hospice in New Haven, founded in 1973. In 1983, **Medicare** began paying for hospice care.

Additional reading: Siebold, *The Hospice Movement.*

hospital

A hospital is an institution where sick or injured people receive care and treatment. The forerunners of today's hospitals stem from ancient Greek and early Christian times.

In ancient Greece, sick people went to temples of the god Asclepius for healing. At these temples, the patient was expected to have a dream about the god, who would prescribe treatment. The patient would then receive treatment at the shrine, offering sacrifices to the god as payment. These shrines, known as Asclepieia, were often built in wooded valleys near springs or caves. During Roman times, baths became the focus of these temples, and sick people came to be cured with **hydrotherapy.** The Romans also created institutions dedicated to caring for sick and wounded soldiers, the first of which dates back to about 9 A.D. These valetudinaria, as they were called, also eventually began providing medical care to slaves.

The Emperor Constantine (306–337), the first Christian Roman emperor, decreed in 335 A.D. that nosocomeia, or infirmaries, must be built in Rome. Bishop Basil and Ephraim the Syrian established similar institutions several decades later in Caesarea in Cappadocia and Edessa, respectively. This region, a crossroads between Europe and Asia, was a hotbed of disease and famine. It was also during this era that city populations had become dense and large enough to sustain epidemics of infectious disease.

Fabiola, a wealthy Roman widow living in the fourth century, learned about the nosocomeia during a visit to the East and went home to establish two similar institutions in Italy. Several Christian religious orders, such as the Benedictine monks, also established **hospices** and hospitals in Europe during the Middle Ages. Prayer and meditation was part of the treatment regimen.

These early hospitals were for poor people. The well-to-do received care at home from private doctors. Hospitals also were often used to confine people with contagious diseases such as **leprosy** and the plague and to warehouse the mentally ill.

During the late Middle Ages and into the Renaissance, governments became involved in providing and distributing charitable care and in running hospitals and asylums (the forerunners of **mental hospitals**). Hospitals also increasingly became centers for training doctors and surgeons and for performing clinical research. "Teaching hospitals," ones that treated patients but were dedicated to teaching medical students, were established in Europe during the 1700s.

With the development of **anesthesia** and **antisepsis** in the 1800s, it became possible to plan and perform operations systematically, rather than using surgery as a last-ditch effort. Caring for patients before, during, and after surgery thus became a major role of the hospital by the 1880s.

It was at this time, as understanding and acceptance of the **germ theory** of disease became complete, that the importance of controlling the spread of infection within the hospital became clear. Hospitals still currently struggle with this issue.

The focus of hospitals today is to provide medical treatment to patients and save them, rather than to provide comfort in dying; institutions called hospices have sprung up to serve this need. Throughout the 1900s and into the 21st century, U.S. hospitals have also been faced with the struggle of keeping costs down. Some attempt to do so while continuing to provide charitable care. Other forces that have changed the way hospitals provide care have been the rise of **ambulatory surgery** and the spread of **managed care.**

Additional reading: Risse, *Mending Bodies, Saving Souls.*

HRT. See hormone replacement therapy.

Human Genome Project

The Human Genome Project is a worldwide effort, launched in 1988, to map the location of every **gene** on each **chromosome** (there are 50,000 to 80,000), and sequence the three billion base pairs that form the genome.

Part of the project includes mapping the genome of other forms of life, such as mice and flies. In the United States, the project is largely being funded by the Department of Energy (DOE) and the **National Institutes of Health (NIH)**, although some private companies also are

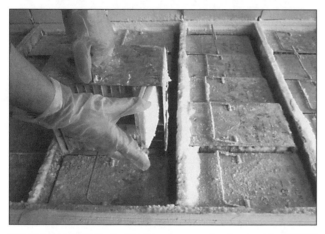

Scientist places fragments of the human genome in a freezer at the NHGRI. These fragments are being stored as part of the Human Genome Project, which seeks to map the entire human genome. (Courtesy of National Institute for Human Genome Research.)

involved. The National Science Foundation and the Howard Hughes Medical Institute have provided grant support. About half of the work is being done in the United States and roughly 30 percent in Europe by the United Kingdom, Germany, and France. Several other nations are involved in the research including Japan, Australia, South Africa, and Canada.

Robert Sinsheimer (1920–) organized the first conference on mapping the human genome in 1985. Nobel Prize winner Walter Gilbert (1932–) began promoting the idea as well. The DOE became interested at this time also, largely as part of its efforts to determine the effects of radiation on

human **DNA**. The first section of the project was launched by the DOE's Charles DeLisi (1941–) in 1987.

In 1989, the Human Genome Organization (HUGO) was incorporated to coordinate international genome sequencing efforts. Norton Zinder (1928–) of the NIH said HUGO would be a "U.N. for the human genome."

The project, expected to be complete in the year 2005, has already yielded a great deal of new information on human genetics. It has also raised a number of ethical issues, such as whether it should be legal for a company to patent a particular gene sequence.

Knowing the language of our chromosomes will allow us to learn whether a person is likely to develop certain diseases, and to invent molecularly targeted drugs that could prevent such diseases. The first such drug for treating **breast cancer**, **Herceptin**, is already on the market. Assembling the components of the genome will also allow for unprecedented understanding of normal fetal development, growth, cellular metabolism, and other physiological processes, and help us to recognize and treat problems caused by malfunctions in these mechanisms. (*See also* gene mapping)

Additional reading: Speaker and Lindee, *A Guide to the Human Genome Project.*

human growth hormone (HGH)

Human growth hormone, a substance released by the **pituitary gland**, stimulates growth in children and adolescents and may also contribute to the maintenance of muscle strength in adults.

Since the nineteenth century, scientists had suspected that the pituitary gland influenced growth, because people with growth disorders such as acromegaly or dwarfism often had tumors near or within the gland. The specific substance responsible was not known, however, until Choh Hao Li (1913–1987) and Herbert Evans (1882–1971) isolated human growth hormone from ox pituitary gland extract in 1944. Li and Harold Papkoff (1925) made the first purified preparation of human HGH in 1956, and the first clinical use was reported in 1958. The **hormone** quintupled the 17-year-old patient's rate of growth during the 10-month trial.

Although pituitary extract was an effective treatment for stunted growth, it was also very scarce, since it had to be harvested from the pituitary glands of human cadavers.

A number of trials of human HGH were conducted in slow-growing children from the late 1950s until the early 1970s, with some success. But the trials came to a halt when some HGH recipients developed Creutzfeldt-Jakob disease, a fatal brain malady transmitted by infected nerve tissue. This problem was resolved in 1986 when researchers used recombinant techniques to make HGH, ensuring a steady, sterile supply of the hormone.

Today, researchers are investigating HGH's possible therapeutic effects beyond growth, such as speeding healing and building lean muscle mass.

Additional reading: Kuczynski, "Anti-Aging Potion or Poison?"

humoralism

Humoralism is the idea that the body contains four elements known as humors: blood, phlegm, black bile, and yellow bile. These substances correspond to the elements of fire, air, earth, and water, as well as to the four temperaments, or types of personality: sanguine, phlegmatic, melancholic, and choleric.

Adherents to humoralism believed that disease resulted from an imbalance in the four humors, which could be caused by climate, poor diet, or poor digestion. Humoralism was used as a rationale to explain mental illness and a basis for stereotyping people depending on the climate in which they lived.

Humoralism dates back to ancient Greece, and was endorsed by the influential Greek physician Claudius Galen (129–c.199), whose ideas held sway until the sixteenth century. The Swiss alchemist Paracelsus (1493–1541) first challenged humoralism, but the doctrine persisted in certain circles into the late nineteenth century.

The stress humoralism places on balance is similar to the philosophies underlying **Ayurveda** and **Chinese medicine**. (*See also* Hippocratic Corpus)

Additional reading: Majno, *The Healing Hand*, pp. 178–80, 417–18.

hydrocephalus

Hydrocephalus, or "water on the brain," occurs when the **cerebrospinal fluid (CSF)** fails to drain properly from the ventricles of the brain, causing the brain and eventually the skull to swell. It can be caused by congenital malformations, brain tumors, or injury. This condition, which usually appears shortly after birth, once guaranteed that a child would have mental disabilities and die an early death, but it is now possible to treat this condition surgically, often leaving mental function intact.

The Greeks and other ancient peoples tried to treat hydrocephalus with incision and drainage, and attempts at surgical drainage continued with varying success.

Giovanni Morgagni (1682–1771) confirmed that hydrocephalus was caused by fluid accumulating in the ventricular system. Compression therapy for hydrocephaly—basically squeezing the skull with bandages—enjoyed brief popularity in the beginning of the nineteenth century. This treatment was intended to encourage drainage, but often produced convulsions and skull fractures.

Carl Wernicke (1848–1905) advised in 1881 that a permanent open drain be installed in the skull to treat hydrocephalus. Five years later, Johann von Miculicz-Radecki (1850–1905) first employed a drainage system that emptied fluid inside the body.

In 1914, Walter Dandy (1886–1946) and Kenneth Daniel Blackfan (1883–1941) provided the first detailed description of the CSF circulation, which increased understanding of hydrocephalus and paved the way for improved treatment.

Silicone shunts for drainage were introduced in the 1950s. Ventroarticular shunting, in which the excess CSF fluid is drained into the heart, was first used in 1955 and became the most commonly used hydrocephalus treatment in the 1960s.

Today children with hydrocephalus can often be successfully treated with a shunt that drains inside the body, but they still face many complications, including infection and possible intellectual impairment.

Additional reading: Toporek, et al., *Hydrocephalus.*

hydrotherapy

Hydrotherapy is the use of water—especially in bathing—for healing purposes.

The belief in the therapeutic powers of water is ancient, and hydrotherapy has come in to and gone out of fashion since the beginning of history. Physicians of Hippocrates' (c.460–c.377 B.C.) time recommended bathing to encourage the passage of urine, and in 1924 researchers showed that water immersion has many physiological effects, including producing diuresis after two hours. Therefore, the advocacy of bathing to treat edema and "dropsy," an excess of fluid in the body, since Greek times did have some actual therapeutic merit. Of course, bodily cleanliness also has healthful effects.

The ancient Egyptians, Babylonians, and the proto-Indian Zoroastrian civilization all took medicinal baths, which were closely linked with religious practices. Chinese physicians of the second century B.C. recommended cold baths for fever. The therapeutic effects of bathing were also important to the Romans, who established bathing sites across Europe, including Bath in England and Aachen in Germany.

After the fall of Rome in the Middle Ages, bathing was no longer popular, largely because the Roman Catholic Church associated bathing with decadence and weakness. Baths came back into popularity in the late Middle Ages, but public baths were also often sites for the unsanitary medical treatments of the time, such as **bloodletting**, which contributed to the spread of disease and led to the closure of these baths. In the early 1700s, bathing again returned to favor.

The most recent period of bathing-mania began in the 1800s. The Austrian farmer Vincenz Priessnitz (1799–1851) began advocating ancient healing techniques including bathing beginning in the 1820s. Sebastian Kneipp (1821–1897), a German priest, published a book called *Meine Wasserkur* in 1887 and established the Central Kneipp Association three years later. He recommended application of cold water along with herbs to improve general health, and his ideas spread from Germany through Europe to the United States. The water cure was also popular for Europeans suffering from "nervous," or psychiatric, problems.

In the United States, public baths were established in many urban areas in the late 1800s so that people who weren't wealthy enough to have running water in their homes could pursue cleanliness. Spas also sprang up around mineral springs that had been frequented by Native Americans.

Today, spas, the modern-day hydrotherapy, remain popular in many areas of the world, especially Europe. In Italy, Britain, France, and many formerly Communist nations, governments subsidize spa treatment for their citizens.

Additional reading: Campion, *Hydrotherapy.*

hyperbaric oxygenation

Hyperbaric oxygenation involves placing a person in a high-pressure chamber that makes it possible for the body to absorb more oxygen through the respiratory system than is possible under normal pressure.

This is useful for treating **tissue** damage caused by injury or infection, a type of bone inflammation called osteomyelitis, smoke inhalation, carbon monoxide poisoning, and other maladies.

Henshaw, whose first name has been lost to history, is believed to have been the first person to suggest that changes in air pressure might help treat illness. He had an airtight room in which it was possible to produce different pressure conditions, and in his 1664 writings he recommended pressure treatments for breathing, digestion, and lung problems.

The first therapeutic compression chamber in North America was built in Canada in 1860. A fad for hyperbaric chambers and oxygen therapy subsequently arose in the United States and Europe in the late nineteenth and early twentieth century. Orval J. Peterson (1880–1937), a Kansas City physician, claimed to be able to treat **influenza**, **syphilis**, **cancer**, and **diabetes** with compressed air. In 1928, he built the largest compression chamber in the world, with five stories and twelve bedrooms on each floor.

Two researchers working in the 1950s spurred a renaissance of hyperbaric therapy by showing that it had therapeutic effects: Henry Cunningham Churchill-Davidson, who focused on **radiation therapy** applications, and Ite Boerema (1902–1980), who studied the use of hyperbaric therapy during cardiac surgery. Boerema had suggested saturating the body with oxygen before stopping circulation for heart surgery, which increased the amount of oxygen kept in the tissues and made it possible to safely halt circulation for twice as long. He later showed that hyperbaric oxygen was an effective treatment for certain infections, circulation problems, and even for some types of cancer when combined with radiation.

Additional reading: Fischer, et al., *Handbook of Hyperbaric Oxygen Therapy.*

hypertension

Hypertension, or high **blood pressure**, is a chronic condition that is now understood to contribute to heart disease and to increase a person's risk of **stroke**.

British physician Frederick Mahomed (1849–1884) was one of the first doctors to systematically measure blood pressure as part of his evaluation of patients, beginning in the late 1800s. He observed that people with high blood pressure usually remained healthy until they got older, after which they began to suffer symptoms such as lung disease and apoplectic seizures—which are now known as stroke.

Theodore Janeway (1872–1917), who began studying hypertension in 1903, saw high blood pressure as a disease of the circulatory system. In 1931, Franz Volhard (1872–1950) described two types of hypertension: "red," in which a person has high blood pressure for a long time and remains healthy until organ damage began to take its toll; and "white," in which the kidneys are involved and death results quickly.

Irvine H. Page (1901–1991) announced the first reversal of malignant—or "white"—hypertension in 1937, using an antimalarial drug called pentaguine that dilated the blood vessels. This drug could not be given long-term, so it couldn't be used for chronic hypertension.

Diuretics were also among the first therapies to be used to treat hypertension; they had been used to treat dropsy, a condition related to heart failure in which excess fluid collects in the tissues. Physicians also recommended low salt diets for their patients with high blood pressure.

The earliest drug treatment for hypertension involved medications that suppressed the sympathetic nervous system, which is responsible for speeding the up heartbeat and raising the blood pressure, such as phenobarbitol. Leonard Rowntree (1883–unknown) and Alfred Adson (1887–1951) performed a sympathectomy, in which certain nerves were removed in order to reduce blood pressure, in 1925, with good results. This type of operation, along with removal of the adrenal cortex to eliminate the production of **epinephrine** (which became safe in the 1930s because synthetic adrenal **hormones** were developed that could be given to patients whose adrenal glands were removed, which would otherwise be fatal), remained the main treatment for hypertension for about a decade.

The discovery of the **renin-angiotensin system** of the kidneys, along with growing understanding of the function of the nervous system in blood pressure, opened the door to better treatments for hypertension, such as **ACE inhibitors** and beta blockers.

Launched in 1949 by William Kannel (1923–) and his colleagues, the Framingham study, an investigation of hypertension and risk factors in 5,200 men and women in this Massachusetts town, firmly established that hypertension is a risk factor for stroke, heart failure, and death.

Today public health is moving in the direction of recommending antihypertensive drugs for even mild hypertension, which is controversial given the fact that some of these drugs can be dangerous. Several controllable factors, including obesity, lack of exercise, cigarette smoking, stress, and poor diet all are known to contribute to hypertension, so treatment of the condition also focuses on exercise, weight loss, quitting smoking, and behavior modifications that reduce stress. Hereditary factors may also influence whether or not a person develops high blood pressure.

Additional reading: Comroe, *Exploring the Heart,* pp. 48–64.

hyperthermia

Hyperthermia is a technique for treating **cancer** by heating the tumor. Some studies have shown that heating a tumor can double the effectiveness of radiation and **chemotherapy**. The challenge of hyperthermia is to deliver the heat to the tumor without damaging normal **tissue**.

Renato Cavaliere and colleagues in early 1970s confirmed that heat could kill tumors. In 1976, Harry LeVeen (1916–) of the Medical University of South Carolina suggested using localized radiofrequency. Microwaves worked well but could only be used near the surface of the body. In the late 1970s Paul Turner invented a microwave array that could safely heat deep tumors, while William Harrison of UCLA invented a technique called human magnetic induction heating.

Meanwhile, investigators around the country found that the effectiveness of heat might be due to the fact that blood vessels supplying tumors were primitive and could not respond to thermal stress effectively. Dozens of **clinical trials** of hyperthermia were conducted in the 1980s, with inconclusive results. Hyperthermia has largely fallen out of favor in the United States, although European, Japanese, and Canadian scientists are still investigating the procedure.

Additional reading: Galton, *Med Tech,* pp. 249–52.

hypnotherapy

Hypnotherapy is the use of hypnosis to treat certain **mental illnesses, addictions,** and other health problems. A person in a hypnotic state, which is similar to sleep, is thought to be open to suggestion. Hypnosis is considered by some medical historians to be the earliest form of **psychotherapy**.

Franz Anton Mesmer (1734–1815), a Viennese physician, first developed hypnotherapy in the 1770s, calling it "animal magnetism." His theory was that the universe was filled with magnetic fluid, and that health depended on the amount and distribution of this fluid. He produced cures by laying on of hands and physical contact with objects.

In 1784, his pupil, Marquis de Puysegur (1751–1825), published observations of a sleep-like state that occurred during the course of this treatment that he called "somnambulism," what we would now call hypnosis. In 1815, French mesmerists realized that the laying on of hands wasn't necessary to produce this effect, which they defined as psychological. In the height of mesmerism's popularity, operations were performed painlessly on mesmerized people.

In 1850, Dr. A.A. Liebeault (1823–1904) attributed the success of mesmerism to suggestion. In 1884, Hippolyte Marie Bernheim (1837–1919) established "suggestion therapy." He theorized that anyone could be hypnotized, and that the state was related to normal sleep. Under hypnosis, Bernheim proposed, brain control is diminished, and automatic and suggested responses take over. He successfully treated neuroses, rheumatism, menstrual disturbances, and gastrointestinal problems with hypnosis. Pierre Janet (1859–1947) believed traumatic memories could be recalled under hypnosis, and founded the cathartic method of treatment. He believed only hysterics or intoxicated people could be hypnotized.

Today, hypnosis is often used to treat phobias and anxiety, to help people quit smoking and, controversially, to help people recover past memories of abuse that critics say are not memories of real events but products of the therapist's suggestion.

Additional reading: Owen, *Hysteria, Hypnosis and Healing,* pp. 170–211; Silvers, ed., *Hidden Histories of Science,* pp. 1–35.

I

ibuprofen

Ibuprofen is a pain-relieving, fever-reducing drug that is marketed as Advil, Motrin, and Nuprin. It belongs to a class of medications known as **nonsteroidal anti-inflammatory drugs (NSAIDs)** that are helpful for treating rheumatoid arthritis and osteoarthritis. Ibuprofen also is helpful for treating menstrual cramps.

In the 1950s, scientists from the Boots Company in the United Kingdom began looking for an aspirin-like drug for rheumatoid arthritis that would have fewer side effects, and discovered ibuprofen. Boots introduced its new product as Brufen in the United Kingdom in 1969. The Upjohn Company introduced the drug to the United States in 1974.

Although the complete mechanism by which ibuprofen works is unclear, the drug is known to interrupt the inflammation process by blocking the production of **prostaglandins**.

Additional reading: Bindra and Lednicer, eds., *Chronicle of Drug Discovery, Vol. I*, pp. 149–72.

ICU. *See intensive care unit.*

immune tolerance

Immune tolerance is a phenomenon in which an animal tolerates exposure to another animal's tissue, such as a skin or organ graft or blood transfusion, because it has been exposed to the animal's tissue prenatally or shortly after birth.

Ray David Owen (1915–) first observed this phenomenon in nonidentical twin cows. He theorized that blood cells and embryonic precursors to these cells had passed between the animals before birth, so that each twin could tolerate the tissues of the other even though they were not genetically identical.

Owen published his observations in 1945. Four years later, Frank Macfarlane Burnet (1899–1985) and Frank Fenner (1914–) wrote extensively on Owen's work in their book *The Production of Antibodies*. In 1951, Peter Medawar (1915–1987) showed that nonidentical twin animals accepted skin grafts from one another, and two years later

demonstrated that such tolerance can be induced by exposing an animal to another's tissue before or shortly after birth. Burnet and Medawar shared the 1960 Nobel Prize for discovering acquired immune tolerance, which would eventually point the way to techniques for manipulating the immune system to prevent rejection of donated organs and also give researchers a basis for understanding why **autoimmune disease** occurs.

Additional reading: Clark, *At War Within*, pp. 117–20.

immunoglobulin

Immunoglobulins are a family of proteins that act as **antibodies**. The first immunoglobulin-like protein discovered—actually part of an immunoglobulin—was the Bence Jones protein, in 1845.

In 1921, Carl Prausnitz (1876–1963) and Heinz Kustner (1897–1963) demonstrated that an injection of serum from an allergic person into a nonallergic person would transfer the **allergy**. The pair named the responsible material "reagin," but this substance wasn't characterized until the late 1960s when Japanese researchers suggested that reagin was actually a class of immunoglobulins they named IgE.

The **World Health Organization (WHO)** adopted the Roman letter method for naming the immunoglobulins in 1965. Officially accepted as an immunoglobulin in 1968, IgE is important in allergic reactions; people with certain inherited allergic diseases such as **asthma** have high levels of IgE in their blood.

IgG, or gamma globulin, discovered in 1939, is the chief immunoglobulin in the human body, and plays the most important role in fighting viruses and bacteria. Gamma globulin made from donated plasma is used for treating patients with immune diseases, and may also be helpful in treating certain types of neuromuscular disease.

IgA, discovered in 1959, is secreted by the mucous membranes, in tears, and in breast milk, and helps protect mucous surfaces from invasion by bacteria and viruses.

IgD, characterized in 1965, is given to Rh-negative mothers who have borne Rh-positive children to prevent the mother's immune system from attacking the fetus.

IgM, characterized in 1944, is formed early in the immune response, and helps activate other components of the immune system.

Additional reading: Clark, *At War Within,* pp. 89–106.

immunosuppression

Immunosuppression is an attempt to weaken the immune system with drugs or radiation so the body will accept transplants of foreign **tissue**. It may also be used to treat **autoimmune diseases**, which are caused by an overactive immune system. Treatment to suppress the immune system is always risky, because it makes the body more vulnerable to infection.

When a person receives a tissue transplant from a person who is not genetically identical, even if he or she is closely related, his or her immune system will attack the foreign tissue, a process known as rejection. Selecting a donor who is a close tissue match will help, but immunosuppression is still necessary for the graft to be accepted unless it comes from a twin.

The first attempts to suppress the immune system were made along with kidney grafts, using total body radiation, which was known to suppress **antibody** formation. But radiation also damaged bone marrow function, sometimes permanently.

In the 1950s, Gertrude Belle Elion (1918–1999) and George H. Hitchings (1905–1998) developed the immune-suppressing drug **six-mercaptopurine**, which revolutionized transplants. The next series of immunosuppressive drugs are believed to suppress the immune system's **T cells**. The first of this generation is **cyclosporine**, approved by the **Food and Drug Administration (FDA)** in 1983.

Several drugs have since been developed that interrupt communication among immune system components by various methods. Today transplant surgeons generally use a combination of immunosuppresant drugs to increase tolerance. (*See also* bone marrow transplant; kidney transplant; lung transplant)

Additional reading: Clark, *At War Within,* pp. 185–94; Gutkind, *Many Sleepless Nights,* pp. 34–41.

impotence treatment

Impotence occurs when a man cannot achieve or sustain an erection. This can be caused by injury, disease, certain medications, drug or alcohol abuse, or psychological issues.

One of the first treatments developed for erectile dysfunction was the vacuum pump. A patent for this type of vacuum pump was issued in 1917. A version was approved by the **Food and Drug Administration (FDA)** for marketing. Several others are now available. The vacuum pump is safe and fairly effective.

The first effective surgery for erectile dysfunction, which involved tying off the vein that drains the penis, was reported in 1902. The procedure is still used for certain patients who have problems with venous drainage of the penis. Surgeons at the Institute for Clinical and Experimental Medicine in Prague had the first success with surgical revascularization of the penis to correct erectile dysfunction in 1972.

Surgeons began attempting to use "splints" inserted in the penis to treat impotence in the 1950s, and silicone inserts became the preferred treatment in the late 1960s and 1970s. By 1973, these implants were generally accepted as effective treatment for men whose impotence had an organic cause. In the 1970s and 1980s, implants were introduced that were hinged or inflatable so the penis could be maintained in both flaccid and erect states.

During the 1980s, injecting the penis with phenoxybenzamine or papaverine was found to produce an immediate erection. This combination was effective and remained the preferred treatment until the end of the 1980s. Another drug, alprostadil, was found to produce erection by penile injection and was approved by the FDA in 1995 as Caverject. A delivery system called MUSE, with which drugs can be injected via the urethra rather than into the penis, was released in the 1990s.

The major milestone in erectile dysfunction treatment has been the release of sildenafil citrate, or Viagra, a drug (in pill form, taken orally) approved by the FDA in March 1998 for treatment of impotence. The drug is made by Pfizer. Its main side effects include headache, flushing, visual disturbances, and indigestion. It can lead to dangerous heart problems if it is taken with nitrate medications, such as **amyl nitrate** and nitroglycerine.

The drug marks a major advance in impotence treatment, as it is taken orally rather than by injection into the urethra or flesh of the penis, works quickly, and only produces an effect in conjunction with sexual stimulation. It is effective for 70 percent of the men who take it.

The drug increases the sensitivity of the penis. Nerves release nitric oxide in response to sexual stimulation, and this in turn triggers the formation of cyclic guanosine monophosphate (GMP), an enzyme that promotes relaxation of smooth muscle and blood vessels within the penis. This relaxation produces an erection by allowing the organ to fill with blood. Sildenafil increases levels of GMP within the penis by blocking the action of a chemical that normally breaks it down.

Pfizer chemist Nick Terrett and colleagues initially began developing the drug as a treatment for heart disease, because of its ability to improve blood flow.

Some preliminary studies have shown that Viagra is effective for women with difficulty becoming sexually aroused. Although the FDA has not approved the drug for female use, many women take it.

Additional reading: Mestel, "Sexual Chemistry;" Sternberg, "Impotence Treatment Keeps Urologists Busy"; Alberts, "When Sex Get Sidelined."

in vitro fertilization (IVF)

In vitro fertilization is a technique for uniting sperm and egg outside the body

IVF allows women whose fallopian tubes have been blocked by disease or injury to become pregnant and bear children. Patrick Steptoe (1913–1988), a leading laparoscopic surgeon and gynecologist, along with scientist Robert Edwards (1925–), engineered the conception and birth of the world's first IVF or "test tube" baby, Louise Brown, born in 1978.

Edwards and Steptoe began working together in 1969. Steptoe would collect eggs from the hopeful mother-to-be using laparoscopic techniques (an operation that took minutes), fertilize the egg with the hopeful father's sperm, allow the embryo to mature to the eight-cell stage, and reimplant it in the mother's uterus. During the course of their work, Steptoe and Edwards made many other discoveries important for human infertility treatment. At first, they had used drugs that caused women to produce multiple eggs at once—or "superovulate." But these drugs, they found, also made the uterus shed the embryo. After working for several years and having only one unsuccessful pregnancy (the embryo lodged in the stump of the patient's fallopian tube and had to be removed), the team decided to try allowing patients to go through a normal cycle. They would use a diagnostic test to determine when the egg was near-ripe and ready for collection. On the pair's second attempt using this method, Lesley Brown became pregnant and delivered a healthy baby girl by **cesarean section** just as Steptoe retired.

Before Steptoe's death in 1988, he saw the delivery of the one-thousandth baby conceived in vitro at Edwards' facility. Today, thousands of couples have used IVF and related techniques to conceive.

Additional reading: Edwards and Steptoe, *A Matter of Life.*

inborn errors of metabolism

Inborn errors of metabolism are genetic defects in which the body fails to break down a potentially harmful substance, resulting in build-up of that substance. Some inborn errors of metabolism, such as phenylketonuria (PKU), can easily be treated with dietary restrictions, while others are untreatable and result in eventual brain damage and death.

Sir Archibald Garrod (1857–1936) first developed the idea of inborn errors of metabolism and their genetic nature. In a 1908 lecture, he noted that alkaptonuria (incomplete metabolization of the amino acids phenylalanine and tyrosine), albinism (absence of pigment), cystinuria (excretion of cystine, lysine, arginine, and ornithine), and pentosuria (excretion of pentose) all had features in common.

Asbjorn Folling (1886–1972) discovered the disease that came to be known as PKU, the most common inborn error of metabolism, in 1934. A dentist had consulted him about the strange odor of the urine of his two children with mental disabilities. Folling analyzed the urine, finding that it contained phenylpyruvic acid. He subsequently analyzed the urine of hundreds of individuals with mental disabilities and found nine, two of whom were siblings, who had the chemical in their urine. He concluded that the disease was caused by a hereditary defect in phenylalanine metabolism.

About one in 14,000 children are born with PKU. A simple blood test for PKU was developed in the mid-1960s. Now, some states require PKU testing for newborns, and food labels include warnings if a product contains phenylalanine. Infants with PKU can develop normally as long as they do not eat foods containing this substance.

Additional reading: Clarke, *A Clinical Guide to Inherited Metabolic Disease.*

industrial hygiene

Industrial hygiene is the study of the health effects of the workplace.

The need for industrial hygiene arose with the Industrial Revolution of the late nineteenth century, when more and more men and women were working in factories.

One of the first occupational diseases to be recognized was "phossy jaw," a necrosis of the jaw bone striking people who worked in factories where phosphorous matches were made. The first such factories were built in 1833 in Germany and Austria, and these nations issued decrees regulating exposure to phosphorous fumes in 1846.

The United States was relatively slow to adopt regulation of phosphorous or to take any other steps to protect workers' health. The International Association for Labor Legislation was formed in Basel, Switzerland in 1900, and by 1912 all the European nations had joined but the U.S. had not.

However, individual U.S. companies were making efforts to protect the health of their workers. For example, workers at Chicago's Crane Company began using protective goggles in 1897. Two years later, the McCloud Lumber Company in California established a hospital on company property as well as a preventive medicine program. The Wheeling Corrugating Company, in West Virginia, set up an in-plant health care system in 1907 to care for injured workers and also to promote plant safety. Other Wheeling companies developed similar programs. In 1912, the Association of Iron and Steel Engineers set up a group of industry leaders and government officials to promote worker safety. This organization eventually became the National Safety Council.

The Wheeling Steel Corporation, formed in 1920, set up a Safety First Department that distributed safety equipment to workers and in some cases redesigned machinery to make it safer for workers to use.

The First National Conference on Industrial Diseases was held in the United States in 1910. During that year, the first survey of workers' health was conducted in Illinois. In 1911, the Triangle Shirtwaist Fire in New York tragically exposed dangerous working conditions in the garment industry. After a fire broke out in the factory, 142 women were killed in the blaze or jumped to their death because the factory's owners had locked the doors to the stairs and there was no functioning fire escape system. The New York Investigating Commission was set up to study and remedy these conditions.

In 1912, the Hughes Esch Act placed a prohibitive tax on the makers of phosphorous matches that basically put them out of business. The United States Department of Labor was founded the following year, and the ladies garment industry founded its Union Health Center. The **U.S. Public Health Service** formed a Division of Occupational Health in 1914.

The health dangers of silicosis, or dust inhalation, were brought to public attention in 1935 with press coverage of the Gauley Bridge episode. Beginning in 1929, work began on a water power tunnel dug through quartz and sandstone in West Virginia. Workers did not wear protective gear. Dynamite blasts used to break the stone forced the dust into the workers' lungs, and they began to die of pneumonia, tuberculosis, and silicosis. This incident, along with research by a number of industrial physicians on silicosis, brought the danger of dust inhalation to public attention. There were so many claims filed across the country by workers claiming to have been injured by dust inhalation that according to historians a "racket" of false claims sprang up, abetted by crooked doctors and lawyers.

The silicosis scandal led to the formation of the Air Hygiene Foundation in 1936 to study the problem of silicosis and learn how it could be prevented. The foundation was established by the U.S. Public Health Service, the Bureau of Mines, the Mellon Institute, and representatives of several industries. The name of the foundation was changed to the Industrial Hygiene Foundation in 1941, as its scope had broadened to cover a number of other work-related health problems.

Dr. Alice Hamilton (1869–1970) was a leading figure in the development of U.S. workplace safety programs. She investigated carbon monoxide poisoning in steelworkers, mercury poisoning in hat makers, and "dead fingers syndrome" in workers who used jackhammers. She was named an assistant professor of industrial medicine at Harvard Medical School in 1919, and was the first woman on the university's faculty.

Although mining remains the most dangerous occupation for U.S. workers today, death rates among people in this industry have declined dramatically, thanks in part to the 1969 Federal Coal Mine Health and Safety Act, which established mandatory health and safety standards for mines. The Occupational Safety and Health Act, which was passed one year later and created the Occupational Safety and Health Administration (OSHA) and the National Institute for Occupational Safety and Health (NIOSH) within the **National Institutes of Health (NIH)**, was modeled on the new mines law. NIOSH investigates workplace hazards, researches injury prevention methods, and develops educational materials for workplace safety. OSHA is authorized to develop safety standards and inspect workplaces for compliance with these standards.

Other recent focuses of U.S. industrial hygiene include investigating fatalities among firefighters, efforts to prevent agricultural injuries in children, and efforts to study and prevent workplace violence. The first National Occupational Injury Symposium was held in 1997.

Additional reading: Sellers, *Hazards of the Job.*

infant feeding

The understanding of the best method for infant feeding, breastfeeding or giving a baby a bottle with a formula or other type of milk, has changed dramatically throughout history. Cultural and social preferences have also played a major role in how a woman will feed her baby.

It is now known that breastfeeding is the best approach to infant nutrition in nearly every case. Breastfed babies have fewer infections, are less likely to suffer from **asthma** and **autoimmune disease**, and may also be more intelligent. Mothers who breastfeed reduce their risk of **breast** and **ovarian cancer** and **osteoporosis**.

Throughout recorded history women called "wet nurses" have breastfed babies for other women. From 1750 on, traditional practice in Europe involved feeding the infant colustrum (breast secretions that occur in the first two or three days after delivery, before the onset of true lactation) and breastfeeding for at least 18 months. Breastfeeding declined in the nineteenth century and mothers or wet nurses typically breastfed babies for seven months. The glass feeding bottle and the rubber nipple were developed during this century.

Commercial baby foods were invented in the 1860s. Women began feeding their infants commercial formulas and cow's milk in the 1870s, some because it was necessary for them to work outside the home and others because they had a difficult time finding a wet nurse. When the science of chemistry made it possible to analyze the composition of milk, doctors began modifying cow's milk to make it more like human breast milk, for example by diluting it and adding sugar and cream. Commercial laboratories soon opened in many cities to provide specially prepared milk for infants.

Dried milk became available in the United States in 1898, and this invention, along with electrical refrigeration, made it safer to feed babies formula because dried or refrigerated milk was less likely to spoil. Early in the twentieth century, infant formula makers began marketing their products to doctors, hoping that these physicians would recommend the preparations to their patients. The American Medical Association (AMA) began giving certain products its Seal of Approval.

In the 1920s, formula's approximation to human milk became more scientific (for example, vegetable fats were added to milk rather than butter fat), and in the 1930s formula makers began adding vitamins and iron to infant formula.

In the United States, breastfeeding continued to decline; about 75 percent of women bottle-fed their babies after leaving the hospital by the 1940s. Women were even given injections to suppress lactation. However, along with the move toward natural childbirth, breastfeeding became more popular among U.S. mothers in the 1970s. More women began breastfeeding their babies, and they breastfed them for longer.

Changes in breast feeding in less developed countries, similar to those that occurred in the late nineteenth century in Europe and North America, have occurred in the twentieth century.

Additional reading: Angier, *Woman*, pp. 144–61.

influenza (flu)

Influenza is a viral infection that can vary greatly in severity, but usually produces fever, chills, cough, and aches and pains. There are three basic types of flu **virus**: A, B, and C. Type A viruses infect animals as well as humans, while the other types infect humans only.

The word "influenza" (which means "influence" in Italian) to refer to the illness was first used in Italy in the sixteenth century. The Italians—and most other Europeans of the time—believed that epidemics were caused by the influence of the movements of the planets and the weather.

The type A virus was first isolated from a human in 1933. Two years later, the discovery that viruses can multiply in chicken eggs paved the way for the development of a flu **vaccine**. A type B virus was isolated in 1940, and nine years later researchers isolated a type C virus.

Edwin Kilbourne (1920–) showed that viruses change slightly from year to year, a process known as antigenic drift. A more substantial change in the virus is called antigenic shift. Major epidemics and pandemics of flu occur when many people are exposed to a virus that is very different from ones they had been exposed to previously—when a virus undergoes an antigenic shift, or when people are exposed to flu virus from a foreign country. In 1918, an epidemic of "Spanish flu" killed 20 to 40 million people worldwide and at least 500,000 in the United States. A lesser epidemic of Asian flu struck in 1957, killing about 70,000 in the United States.

The first mass flu-vaccine program was launched in 1976 in an attempt to protect Americans against the swine flu after a soldier at New Jersey's Fort Dix was found to be infected with this potentially lethal virus. The swine flu vaccine increased the incidence of Guillian-Barre syndrome four- to eight-fold among the 45 million people who received it in 1976. The cause of this syndrome, which is characterized by fever and paralysis from which people usually recover, is unknown. Later epidemiologic studies have found that nonswine-flu influenza vaccines carry a miniscule risk of causing a person to develop this disease. About one person per million who receives the vaccine will develop Guillian-Barre syndrome. Because people who have suffered Guillian-Barre in the past are at greater risk, the danger may be reduced by not giving the vaccine to anyone within a year of his or her recovery from neurologic illness.

Today older people and people with suppressed immune systems are urged to get flu shots during flu season. **Medicare** began paying for flu shots in 1993. Companies make up new batches every year in an attempt to replicate the type of virus that will strike. The drug amantadine can be used to prevent influenza type A, but it is ineffective against B and C.

In 1998, **clinical trials** of two new drugs began—Relenza, an orally inhaled medication made by the drug company Glaxo-Wellcome; and a pill, GS4104, made by Hoffman-LaRoche and Gilead Sciences. Early evidence suggests that both drugs are effective in relieving symptoms of flu and speeding recovery from infection.

Both drugs inhibit the action of a substance called neuraminidase which the flu virus uses to break itself away from an infected cell so it will be free to infect others. The drugs strand the virus on a cell so that infection cannot spread.

Additional reading: Gadsby, "Fear of Flu."

informed consent

Informed consent is a patient's agreement prior to receiving to any medical procedure, test, or medication. For informed consent to be valid, a patient must be competent and well-enough informed to understand the risks involved. One of the first legal statements outlining informed consent was the **Nuremburg Code**, a statement of ethics produced by the judges who tried Nazi doctors for atrocities they committed during World War II.

Until the mid-twentieth century, physicians often thought informing patients fully would interfere with their ability to treat them; the doctor knew best. But there were isolated cases of patients who protested their doctors' actions. In the eighteenth century, an English patient sued his doctor for rebreaking a fracture without his consent. In 1898, the German doctor Albert Neisser (1855–1916) injected patients, many of them prostitutes, with serum from **syphilis** victims as a means of "vaccinating" them. But the patients receiving the potentially infectious injections—some of whom developed syphilis—were never told what the injection contained or asked for their consent. Most of Neisser's colleagues supported his actions, but some, including psychiatrist Albert Moll (1862–1938), said Neisser's actions were unethical. Moll wrote a book called *Physicians' Ethics* that contained 600 cases of unethical research.

In 1900, the Prussian government issued a directive requiring physicians to inform patients of "possible negative consequences" of any intervention, and that patients had to provide "unambiguous consent." The directive also said that no person who was incompetent, or a minor, could have any intervention that wasn't for diagnostic or treatment purposes. Unfortunately, the directive wasn't law, and did little to restrain Nazi doctors a few decades later.

U.S. legal cases addressing this issue began appearing in the early twentieth century. The Supreme Court ruled, in 1914, that "every adult patient of adult years and sound mind has the right to determine what shall be done with his body." The writers of the decision considered verbal consent to be adequate.

After the Nuremburg Trials, the world began thinking more deeply about consent in medicine, especially as it applied to prisoners and mentally ill or otherwise mentally impaired people whose ability to provide true, uncoerced consent was in question.

The term "informed consent" first appeared in a U.S. district court decision, which actually ruled that physicians could withhold disturbing information from patients. This definition of informed consent has changed, however; now, it means that patients should be informed of all possible dangers.

After a **Centers for Disease Control and Prevention** worker exposed the Tuskeegee study, in which more than 400 black men with advanced syphilis were purposely left untreated without their knowledge, an outside panel called for the termination of the program and reported that the U.S. system for protecting human experimental subjects was seriously lacking.

The American Hospital Association (AHA) put out a document in 1972 called "A Patient's Bill of Rights," which states that patients have the right to all the information about their diagnosis, treatment, and prognosis from physicians in terms they can understand. The Declaration of Helsinki, an elucidation of the principles of informed consent, was set forth in 1964 by the World Medical Association, a physician group formed during World War II. The definition of informed consent continues to be shaped in the courts.

Additional reading: Annas and Groden, *The Nazi Doctors and the Nuremberg Code*, pp. 227–39.

insulin

Insulin is a **hormone** secreted by the islets of Langerhans (clusters of specialized cells) in the pancreas. It helps the body use and store sugar. People who do not secrete insulin can't break down glucose for fuel, so sugar builds up in their blood and they become weak and tired, a condition called **diabetes mellitus**. Without treatment, a person with diabetes may fall into a coma and die.

A team of Canadian researchers isolated insulin in 1922, making it possible to treat diabetes for the first time. Previously, children with diabetes died soon after diagnosis. Those who developed diabetes later in life lived longer, but usually died prematurely from infection or from complications related to the deterioration of the small blood vessels.

Frederick Banting (1891–1941) conceived of the experiments that would lead to insulin's discovery in 1920. Having read about the connection between the islets of Langerhans and diabetes, he proposed trying to isolate the islets' secretion in dogs and use this secretion to treat diabetes. Banting brought the idea to John Macleod (1876–1935), who provided him with space at the University of Toronto and assigned Charles Best (1899–1978) to work with him. The two performed a series of experiments in dogs. James Collip (1892–1965) later joined the team and purified the pancreatic extract used in the first test of insulin on a human, in January 1922. By the following year,

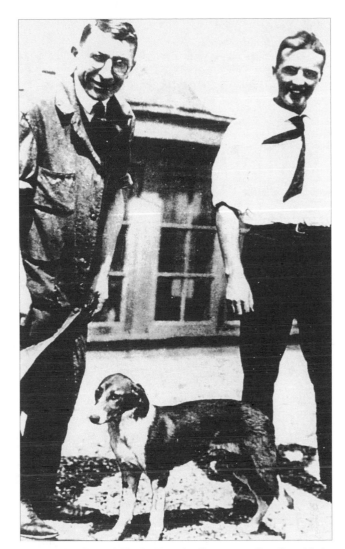

Frederick Banting and Charles Best, the discoverers of insulin, with the dog who played a crucial role in their experiments. (Courtesy of Eli Lilly and Company Archives.)

Best had established an insulin mass-production facility at Connaught Laboratories in Toronto, making it possible for thousands of diabetic patients to receive insulin therapy. The Canadian researchers provided information on insulin production to the American drug company Eli Lilly, which was within a year able to supply insulin to every person with diabetes in the United States.

Banting and Macleod won the Nobel prize in medicine in 1923 for the discovery of insulin; Banting split his share of the prize money with Best, and Macleod gave half of his award to Collip.

John Jacob Abel (1857–1938) of Johns Hopkins University in Baltimore isolated pure insulin in 1926. Subsequently, preparations of the drug were developed with additives that made it possible for diabetic patients to keep their blood sugar in control with fewer injections. During the 1970s, techniques were developed for purifying insulin to make the drug safer.

In 1977, the San Francisco company Genentech released insulin made by genetic recombination that was thus free from impurities. Eli Lilly licensed the technology. Insulin was one of the first biological substances to be made with recombinant techniques.

Additional reading: Bliss, *The Discovery of Insulin*.

intensive care unit (ICU)

Intensive care units are areas within a hospital set aside to care for patients whose vital signs must be monitored constantly. ICUs have helped make it possible to keep a person alive during an intense health crisis, such as a heart attack or a severe **head injury**, so they eventually recover.

ICUs became necessary in the late 1950s, due to changes in health care payment. Patients were increasingly being put in private or semi-private rooms, rather than housed together in large rooms called "wards" that had made it easy for nurses to monitor their health. This occurred because more and more people had private health insurance that would pay the extra cost.

One of the first ICUs was organized at the North Carolina Memorial Hospital in 1953. By 1958, there were 25 ICUs in U.S. hospitals; by the mid-1960s there were 250 ICUs and 250 additional **coronary care units (CCU)**.

In the 1960s, technology developed by the space program to monitor body functions of astronauts, along with computers, made sophisticated, real-time monitoring of patients' vital signs feasible. Special ICUs for premature infants were also developed during this decade.

The Society for Critical Care Medicine was formed in 1970, and began issuing certificates to critical care physicians in 1987.

Additional reading: Park and Saunders, *Fighting for Life*.

interferon

Interferon is a substance the body produces to fight infection. White blood cells and fibroblasts pump out interferon when a **virus** attacks, which can stop the virus from infecting cells and spreading through the body. Interferon enhances the action of the immune system in other ways, and may also fight tumors. Interferon is one of dozens of chemicals known as **cytokines** that cells produce to communicate with one another.

Alick Isaacs (1921–1967) and Jean Lindenmann (1924–) first described interferon in 1957. Although worldwide efforts ensued to test interferon for treating **cancers** and viral infections, so little of the substance could be produced that large **clinical trials** were impossible until the early 1980s.

There are several different types of interferon. Interferon alpha is produced by some white blood cells; fibroblasts release interferon beta during viral attacks; and interferon gamma is released by **T cells** when they are stimulated by several different **antigens**. Interferon gamma also heightens the phagocytic activity of macrophages.

The structure of interferon alpha was described in 1980, and starting in the early 1980s, recombinant **DNA** technology made it possible to produce large amounts of pure interferon for trials.

The early promise that interferon would turn out to be a "magic bullet" against many diseases hasn't been realized. However, interferon does help boost the power of other medications for treating cancer and infection. It is a useful drug for fighting viral infection and possibly tumor growth. Interferon beta has helped to slow the progress of disease in some patients with **multiple sclerosis**.

Additional reading: Shorter, *The Health Century*, pp. 140–50.

intrauterine device (IUD)

An IUD is a contraceptive device inserted into the uterus that prevents pregnancy by making it impossible for an egg to attach itself to the uterine wall. Ancient peoples probably used IUDs made of various substances for **contraception**. The first modern IUDs were ring-shaped devices invented in the 1920s and 1930s in Germany and Japan.

When their use became widespread, IUDs brought on infections and pelvic injury in some patients—perhaps because the devices were inserted improperly—and this method fell out of favor until the 1950s, when interest in finding a relatively easy and inexpensive birth control method was renewed. U.S. physicians Lazar C. Margulies (1895–1982) and Jacob Lippes (1924–) invented the first flexible plastic IUDs, both of which were inserted through the cervix. Marketing for the product began in the 1960s. Also in the 1960s, work began on making IUDs with copper, because ions of the metal released into the uterus were found to increase contraceptive effectiveness. Several versions of these devices went on the market in the 1970s. Later in that decade, the second type of medicated IUD, which released **progesterone**, went on the market.

One type of IUD, the Dalkon shield, was linked to pelvic inflammatory disease—a serious condition that can cause sterility—and was pulled off the market in 1974. Studies found that bacteria had probably traveled up the string (attached to the device for easy removal) into the uterine cavity, causing infection. Further developments of copper- and **hormone**-releasing IUDs have been successful.

Today, IUDs are generally an effective, safe method of contraception, although they are not widely used in the United States. Some experts believe that doctors and patients erroneously see all IUDs as dangerous, after the well-publicized problems of the Dalkon shield.

Additional reading: Rosenthal, *The Gynecological Sourcebook*, pp. 130–33.

ipecac

Ipecac, a drug that induces vomiting to rid the body of poisons, is derived from the ipecacuanha root, a plant native to South America.

In Peru and Brazil, the root was used to induce vomiting by natives. Wilhelm Piso (1611–1678), a Dutch doctor who had spent years in Brazil, described ipecacuanha in his 1684 *Natural History of Brazil*, and said it was a remedy for **dysentery**.

The root became a popular remedy for dysentery in Spain and Portugal, but its use fell out of favor because it was ineffective. It later became popular in France after a merchant's assistant treated the court of Louis XIV (1643–1715) with the root. The active substance of ipecacuanha was isolated by the French chemist Pierre-Joseph Pelletier (1788–1842) and the physiologist Francois Magendie (1783–1855) in 1817, who named it emetine.

Today, many families keep ipecac in their medicine cabinets as an emergency treatment for poisoning.

Additional reading: Mofenson and Caraccio, "Benefits/Risks of Syrup of Ipecac."

iron lung. *See* **Drinker respirator.**

IUD. *See* **intrauterine device.**

IVF. *See* **in vitro fertilization.**

K

kidney transplant

Kidney transplants, in which a donor gives one of the paired organs to another person who needs it, were the first type of organ transplants to be performed and the first to be perfected.

The first kidney transplant, from one identical male twin to another, was performed in 1954 at Peter Bent Brigham Hospital in Boston.

The surgical team included John Merrill (1917–1984), Joseph Murray (1919–), Hartwell Harrison (1909–1984), and Warren Guild (1926–). The patients were age 24 at the time of the operation. Before the operation, the surgeons gave the sick twin a skin transplant from his brother, which "took" completely, suggesting that the kidney also would be accepted. Then the surgeons proceeded with the removal and transplant of the kidney, with the twins in adjacent operating rooms. The operations took about three-and-a-half hours and were successful.

This was also the first successful human organ transplant. The Boston doctors proceeded to perform a transplant on a set of twins each year throughout the decade. In 1959, the team transplanted a kidney from one nonidentical twin to another, after performing total body irradiation on the recipient twin to weaken his immune system and prevent rejection. The recipient survived for 25 years. Murray shared the 1990 Nobel Prize for his work with organ transplants.

The drug **six-mercaptopurine (6-MP)**, developed as an anticancer drug by George Hitchings (1905–1998) and Gertrude Elion (1918–1999), was found to help suppress the immune system, paving the way for transplants between less closely related individuals.

In 1962, after years of experimentation with animals, the first kidney transplant from an unrelated donor was given to a man in kidney failure, along with the 6-MP relative azathioprine. He lived for a year. Three years later, 80 percent of people who received a kidney from a relative lived for at least a year afterwards, while 65 percent who received an organ from a nonrelated dead person lived that long.

The introduction of **cyclosporine** in 1983 made immunosuppressant therapy more effective.

Today, kidney transplants are the most common form of transplant and the most successful; about 85 to 95 percent of people survive for four years or more, and some people have survived with the transplants for more than 30 years.

According to the United Network for Organ Sharing (UNOS), there were 11,409 kidney transplants performed in 1997, with 3,628 from living donors. There are currently about 41,000 people waiting for a kidney transplants. (*See also* immunosuppression)

Additional reading: Ellis, *Famous Operations,* pp. 37–42.

Koch's postulates

Koch postulates, developed by the German bacteriologist Robert Koch (1843–1910) and his teacher Friedrich Gustav Jacob Henle (1809–1885), are a system of rules for evaluating whether an infectious agent causes a disease.

The postulates are that the parasite always occurs in the disease; it does not appear in any other disease; and when it is isolated and grown in the laboratory, the parasite can infect another organism and induce the same disease, or as Koch said "induce the disease anew." Henle described the principles of causation in an 1840 book, *On Miasmata and Contagia,* which were further developed by Koch and described in two lectures in 1884 and 1890.

One difficulty with Koch's postulates occurred with the discovery of the role of **viruses** in human disease in the 1930s, because viruses are difficult to grow in the laboratory. Viruses must be grown in living cultures, such as eggs or tissue. In 1937, Thomas Milton Rivers (1888–1962) proposed rules for linking a virus to a disease: A specific virus must be found to be associated with the disease with a degree of regularity; and the virus must be shown to occur in the sick individual not as an incidental or accidental finding but as the cause of disease under investigation. In 1957, Robert J. Huebner (1914–) later added that epidemiological evidence was needed as well when attempting to establish a virus as the cause of a disease.

Microbiologists continue to use Koch's postulates to identify the cause of an infectious disease.

Additional reading: Bynum, *Science and the Practice of Medicine in the Nineteenth Century,* pp. 129–30.

kwashiorkor

Kwashiorkor is a disease of malnutrition characterized by water retention, wasting of the limbs, diarrhea, sores, lightened hair, sores of the mucous membranes, a fatty liver, and **immunosuppression**. The condition only appears in the tropics and it mainly strikes children.

Kwashiorkor is believed to be caused by protein deficiency. If the condition isn't treated soon enough, by gradually providing more protein in the diet and also treating symptoms such as diarrhea, a child can suffer permanently retarded mental and physical growth. The name kwashiorkor comes from a word in the African Ga language meaning "the sickness the older child gets when the next baby is born."

Kwashiorkor was first described by British physician Cicely Williams (1893–1992), writing in the 1931–1932 Annual Medical Report of the Gold Coast. She identified it as a disease occurring in young children of both sexes who were living on a diet of corn. She said it occurred in children who were either no longer breast feeding or were being breast fed by a grandmother or aunt with insufficient milk.

Williams didn't learn the name "kwashiorkor" until three years later, because the Ga women considered it bad luck to speak the word out loud.

Although the prevalence of the disease has decreased somewhat since the 1960s, probably because of relief programs and improvements in agricultural production, kwashiorkor countinues to take a major toll on people of the developing world.

Additional reading: Kiple, *The Cambridge World History of Human Disease,* pp. 950–55.

L

Lamaze method

The Lamaze method is a technique with which women prepare for labor by learning breathing and relaxation exercises. Although the method is known by his name, Dr. Fernand Lamaze (1890–1957) was not its inventor.

In the early twentieth century, J.S. Fairbairn (1868–unknown) emphasized the importance of a relaxed state of mind for the pregnant woman and taught women exercises to help restore their bodies to their pre-pregnancy state after labor. He compared this training to a military drill, and said it was vital for women approaching labor to have confidence in themselves as "physically strong and healthy" women. Grantly Dick Read (1890–1959) also stressed the importance of self-confidence.

In the early 1950s, Russian obstetricians developed methods for "conditioning" women not to feel pain during labor, based on the ideas of Ivan Petrovich Pavlov (1849–1936). They argued that women felt pain during childbirth because they had been "conditioned" to expect it. The training would "decondition" women, teaching them how to use their muscles properly and how to remain calm during labor. In the early part of labor, women were supposed to keep their brain active to block the sensation of pain. The system quickly became popular. In Europe, Lamaze began training patients in the system. Adherents called the training "active" relaxation.

Although the Lamaze method certainly does not obliterate pain during labor, it can help to raise a woman's threshold for pain tolerance. The method remains popular today; about one-quarter of American women prepare for childbirth by learning Lamaze techniques.

Additional reading: Bing, *The Adventure of Birth.*

laparoscopy

Laparoscopy is a technique for viewing the inside of the body through a small incision in the abdomen. Surgery performed using laparoscopic techniques is generally an improvement over conventional open surgery, provided that the surgeon has sufficient skill and experience, because patients recover much more quickly. These operations are also cheaper, and produce fewer complications.

In 1805, Philip Bozzini (1773–1809), was one of the first people to attempt laparoscopy. He examined the interior of a patient's urethra and bladder using light reflected from a candle. Throughout the nineteenth century, researchers attempted to use various illumination techniques to visualize the interior of the body. In 1877, Max Nitze (1848–1906) used a platinum wire heated with electricity and cooled with a continuous flow of ice water for illumination.

The invention of the incandescent light bulb by Thomas Edison (1847–1931) in 1880 actually may have set laparoscopy back. Because the great majority of energy produced by this new invention was heat rather than light, **endoscopes** using the bulbs burned many patients. This problem was solved by the invention of instruments with the ocular components sheathed separately, which allowed esophagoscopy, laryngoscopy, and proctoscopy to become routine by the end of the 1800s.

Hans Christian Jacobaeus (1879–1937) at Sweden's Karolinska Institute performed the first laparoscopic procedure in humans, publishing his work on 109 laparoscopies in 69 patients in 1912.

Flexible fiberoptic instruments were introduced in 1957, which made viewing around sharp angles possible and also produced cool light. Patrick Steptoe (1913–1988), a British gynecologist, became a leading laparoscopist and published the first textbook on using laparoscopy for gynecological diagnosis and surgery in 1967. He and his colleague Robert Edwards (1925–) helped to produce the world's first "test-tube baby" by **in vitro fertilization.**

By the 1960s and 1970s, gynecologists were using laparoscopy regularly for diagnosing and treating their patients. Other medical specialties were slow to accept the technique. In 1986, a video computer chip made it possible to magnify laparoscopic images and project them onto video screens, which in turn made more complex surgery possible.

The first laparoscopic gallbladder removals were performed in 1987 and 1988. Laparoscopic gallbladder removal is now the gold standard for this procedure; this also paved the way for the use of laparoscopic techniques for other types of abdominal surgery.

Today laparoscopy is used for hernia repair, removal of abdominal adhesions, organ removal, and bowel surgery, and experts believe improvements in technique and instrumentation will make it possible to perform more types of surgery laparoscopically in the future. Surgery of other parts of the body, such as the chest and the brain, is being performed more and more frequently using laparoscopy-like techniques. These operations, including laparoscopy, are known collectively as **minimally invasive surgery.**

Additional reading: O'Dowd and Philipp, *The History of Obstetrics and Gynaecology,* pp. 417–22.

laser surgery

Laser surgery is the use of highly concentrated light beams to cut **tissue** and to destroy abnormal tissue. There are several types of laser of various wavelengths, each with different effects.

In 1917, Albert Einstein (1879–1955) first suggested that molecules in a higher state of energy would emit radiation rather than absorbing it. The principle of the laser was developed in 1958 by Charles Townes (1915–) and Arthur L. Schawlow (1921–) of Columbia University. Laser is an acronym for "Light Amplified by Stimulated Emission of Radiation," and Townes and Schawlow suggested that mirrors be used to amplify the light.

Theodore H. Maiman (1927–) of Hughes Aircraft built the world's first working laser in 1960. It consisted of a ruby crystal with mirrors for amplification. Chandra Kumar Naranbhai Patel (1938–) at Bell Laboratories invented the carbon dioxide laser in 1963. Several types of lasers using the noble gases, including argon, krypton, and xenon, were invented soon afterwards.

Experiments soon showed the carbon dioxide laser could be used as a scalpel for cutting tissue, and a surgical version was built and described in 1970. M. Stuart Strong (1924–), a surgeon at Boston University, used the instrument in treating patients with **cancer** of the larynx and for other types of otolaryngolic surgery. Today the carbon dioxide laser remains the preferred type for surgery on the larynx, throat, and trachea.

The carbon dioxide laser was first used to destroy abnormal precancerous cells in the cervix in 1974. The laser, combined with **colposcopy,** is now commonly used to treat both such abnormal growths and also genital warts.

Excimer lasers, which are used in **refractive surgery** of the cornea to correct nearsightedness, were invented at AVCO Incorporated in 1975. These lasers use rare gases such as argon fluoride, krypton fluoride, xenon chloride, and xenon fluoride.

The neodymium:yttrium aluminum garnet (Nd:YAG) laser was introduced in 1985, and has broader applications than other types of lasers because it can cut, coagulate and vaporize tissue, and can also be placed in contact with tissue. Nd:YAG lasers have many surgical applications, including surgery of the gastrointestinal tract or respiratory tract, performed during **endoscopy**; eye surgery; **plastic surgery**; and neurological surgery.

In 1991, the Q-switched ruby laser was approved for use in the United States after being investigated in Scotland in the previous decade, and soon came into use for removing tattoos and other types of pigmented tissue.

Today, lasers are commonly used in cardiovascular surgery and to close off arteries to prevent bleeding during surgery. Lasers are also frequently used in dermatologic procedures, for example to remove port-wine birthmarks, to "resurface" the skin to remove wrinkles, to destroy excess hair, and to eradicate spider veins and other blemishes.

Additional reading: Galton, *Med Tech,* pp. 267–71.

leprosy

Leprosy is a bacterial infection that strikes the skin and nerves, causing numbness and ulceration. *Mycobacterium leprae* is the responsible organism. Leprosy is also called Hansen's Disease after A.G.H. Hansen (1841–1912), the Norwegian microbiologist who isolated the bacterium in 1873. This was the first bacterium determined to be the cause of a specific human disease.

People with leprosy lose sensation in the hands, feet, face, and other parts of the body, which can lead to infection and tissue damage. The eyebrows and eyelashes of person with leprosy eventually disappear, and his or her face will lose expression and movement. Leprosy progresses slowly, with symptoms not appearing until three to five years after infection.

The Arab doctor Avicenna (980–1037) provided the first clinical description of leprosy in the tenth century A.D., but the disease has been known for much longer. In the Old Testament, victims of leprosy were "cast out" from their communities. Leprosy was stigmatized in Judeo-Christian, Indian, and East Asian societies. During the Middle Ages in Europe, priests or other spiritual leaders declared people with leprosy to be dead to society, sometimes even performing "last rites" with the leper standing at a grave.

The drug dapsone, introduced in the early 1940s, was the first effective treatment for leprosy. Unfortunately, strains of *M. leprae* resistant to the drug became widespread. Research on leprosy was long hampered by the fact that no animal aside from humans was known to be susceptible to leprosy, but scientists found in the 1960s that armadillos could be infected with the bacterium.

Alternative treatment became available in the early 1980s with the introduction of multi-drug therapy for leprosy. People with the disease now receive treatment with dapsone and the **tuberculosis** drug rifampicin. Patients with more severe disease also receive the antibiotic clofazamine.

Today leprosy is most common in sub-Saharan Africa, southeast Asia, and parts of the Americas. In 1997, there were approximately 1.2 million cases of leprosy worldwide, and roughly 500,000 new cases appear each year. The **World**

Health Organization (WHO) is seeking to eliminate leprosy, which means bringing prevalence of the disease down to an extremely low level.

Additional reading: Kiple, *The Cambridge World History of Human Disease,* pp. 834–39.

leukemia

Leukemia is a disease in which the blood-cell producing cells of the bone marrow proliferate out of control but do not mature, eventually replacing normal cells. This overgrowth results in blood-cell abnormalities that can be fatal.

In 1841 the first detailed study of a case of leukemia was performed by David Craigie (1793–1866), in Edinburgh. The patient was a 30-year-old man with an enlarged spleen and general weakness. Upon death, his veins were found to contain a pinkish fluid. Craigie saw another patient with the same disease three years later, and when he died, John Hughes Bennett (1812–1875) performed the autopsy of this patient, writing it up in the *Edinburgh Medical Journal.* Bennett suggested that the disease was caused by an accumulation of pus cells.

At about the same time, Rudolph Virchow (1821–1902) autopsied a 50-year-old woman who died from a similar disease. He said the condition was a disease of the spleen and lymph glands that resulted in the overproduction of white blood cells that he named "leukemia," which is Greek for "white blood."

The role of bone marrow in producing blood was discovered in 1868. In 1879, Paul Ehrlich (1854–1915) published a technique for classifying types of blood cells that made it possible to distinguish between leukemia and elevated white blood cell counts caused by infection as well as various forms of **anemia**.

Leukemias were among the first **cancers** to succumb to chemotherapeutic drugs. The first remission of leukemia was produced by the **antimetabolite drugs** methotrexate and aminopterin in 1948.

Leukemias are divided into two types: myelogenous and lymphocytic, based on the type of cells that proliferate in the disease. Both types occur in acute and chronic forms.

Acute myelogenous leukemia is the most common type of leukemia, accounting for 90 percent of all leukemias in adults. Chronic myelogenous leukemia almost always appears in people with a genetic abnormality known as the Philadelphia **chromosome**. This was the first genetic defect definitively linked to a type of cancer, and was discovered in 1960 by Peter Nowell (1928–) and David Hungerford. Both Nowell and Hungerford were working at the University of Pennsylvania in Philadelphia, and the chromosome was named after the city for this reason.

In children, the most common form of this disease is acute lymphocytic leukemia. Nine in 10 children with the disease once faced death; now most can be cured with **chemotherapy.**

Chronic myelogenous leukemia usually strikes people in their 40s, while chronic lymphocytic leukemia usually occurs in older people. This type of disease is not generally fatal, although it does put people at higher risk of dying from infection or bleeding.

There are approximately 30,200 new cases of leukemia in the United States each year and 22,100 deaths annually.

Today a variety of chemotherapeutic drugs, along with radiation, are used in combination to treat leukemia, and often produce remission of the disease. **Bone marrow transplants** are also often successful.

Additional reading: Kiple, *The Cambridge World History of Human Disease,* pp. 843–48.

lithium

Lithium is a drug used for treating the manic phase of manic-depressive illness, and also for preventing the development of mania.

Lithium's first medical application, in the mid-1880s, was as a treatment for stones in the urinary tract. The idea that many ailments were caused by uric acid imbalances, which could be treated with lithium, led to the first treatments of mania and **depression** with lithium salts in the late 1800s. Bottled mineral waters, including Lithium Beer and 7-Up, were advertised as containing lithium. But these beverages contained only tiny amounts of the mineral.

In 1949, lithium again appeared in the public eye with two discoveries: a "miracle" and a "debacle." The bad news was that lithium chloride, used experimentally as a salt substitute for cardiac patients, killed some people. The good news, discovered by John Cade (1912–1980), was that lithium had antimanic effects. Cade, working in an Australian mental hospital, was investigating whether mania was caused by a toxic substance in the body. In experiments in which he injected guinea pigs with the urine of manic patients (which killed the animals), he determined that mixing uric acid with lithium made it safe for injection. He then tried injecting the guinea pigs with lithium alone, and found it made them lethargic. He injected himself with lithium to test its safety and then tried it in a series of manic patients, reporting his results in 1949. He found that lithium made the patients better, and could also be used as a maintenance medication.

In the 1950s, Danish psychiatrist Mogens Schou (1918–) began investigating lithium for manic depressive illness, which ran in his family and which he himself suffered from. He tried it on himself, family members, and others with the illness and found it relieved the symptoms of the illness.

However, lithium was not approved for treating manic depressive illness by the **Food and Drug Administration (FDA)** until 1970. This was partly because of skepticism among the psychiatric establishment and partly because the pharmaceutical industry had no financial interest in backing lithium since it was a naturally occurring, inexpensive substance.

Today, lithium is still used widely and safely for treating manic depressive illness, and has helped many with the disease. It can be toxic, so patients taking it must have regular blood tests.

Additional reading: Lickey and Gordon, *Drugs for Mental Illness*, pp. 205–217; Shorter, *A History of Psychiatry*, pp. 255–58.

lithotomy

Lithotomy, a surgery for removing stones from the bladder and urinary tract, is one of the world's oldest operations. The name comes from the Greek word for stone cutter, "lithotomus." Hippocrates (c.460–c.377 B.C.) described bladder stones, admonishing physicians not to use a knife to remove them but to leave the operation to specialists. (For this reason, urology could be considered the first medical specialty.)

The first known person to have performed the surgery is Ammonius of Alexandria. Working in about 200 B.C., he invented a tool to break up stones that were too large to pass through surgical incisions. The first-century Roman physician Aulus Cornelius Celsus described a lithotomy operation requiring only a knife, to make two incisions between the rectum and bladder, and a hook, to remove the stone. Greek and Alexandrian surgeons employed the method Celsus outlined, which remained in use until the mid-1700s.

In the nineteenth century, urological surgeons developed techniques for crushing stones and removing them from the bladder by washing them out through the urethra. Henry Bigelow (1818–1890), a U.S. surgeon, invented a large caliber tube that made it possible to break and remove the stone in a single operation. The cystoscope, a type of endoscope that allowed the user to view the inside of the bladder, became available in the 1890s and greatly refined the technique of lithotomy. This instrument is still used today to examine the interior of the bladder and urethra.

As recently as the early 1980s, open surgery was necessary to remove kidney stones, requiring a 25-centimeter incision and two weeks of recovery in the hospital. Surgeons began using **endoscopy** to remove stones from the renal tract in 1979, and by 1983 the operation had become relatively common. In 1980, external shockwave lithotropsy, a technique in which **ultrasound** waves are used to break up kidney and bladder stones, was first performed in humans. Second-generation versions of the shockwave machines, introduced in 1985, made the operation virtually painless, so it could be performed on an outpatient basis. Today, about 85 percent of urinary tract stones can be removed using this technique. In nearly every other case, the stones can be removed using a type of **minimally invasive surgery** called percutaneous endoscopic lithotomy.

Doctors now remove bladder stones by breaking them up with an electrohydraulic instrument, which is inserted into the bladder through the urethra. Open surgery is necessary only when the stones are especially large.

Additional reading: Rutkow, *American Surgery*, pp. 583–98.

liver transplant

People receive liver transplants because the organ has been damaged by **hepatitis** infection, poisoning, **cancer** and other causes. Thomas Starzl (1926–) performed the first liver transplant in a human in 1963, but it took decades for the surgery to be truly feasible.

The first liver transplants were performed on dogs in the 1950s. These operations failed both because the animals' immune systems rejected the donated organ and because surgeons had not fully worked out the liver's complex blood supply. Drugs such as steroids and total body irradiation slightly improved organ survival. Better success using azothioprine and prednisone (a type of **cortisone**) with animals in the early 1960s led to trials of liver transplants in humans. Only two of the first three patients to have liver transplants, in 1963, survived, and both lived for less than a month.

The development of a third drug, antilymphocyte globulin, along with better methods for preserving donated organs, led to a number of patients surviving longer after receiving liver transplants in the late 1960s. Starzl performed the first successful liver transplant in 1967, at the University of Colorado Health Sciences Center in Denver.

The world's first liver transplant programs, at UCLA and Cambridge University, opened in 1967 and 1968, respectively. Programs in Germany and Paris were established in the early 1970s.

When the **immunosuppressant** drug **cyclosporine** became available in 1983, liver transplants—along with transplants of other organs—became much more feasible.

Today, approximately 70 percent of people who have liver transplants survive for four years or longer. The longest-living liver transplant recipient has survived more than 29 years since receiving the transplant, at age 3, in 1970.

A continuing concern about liver transplants is whether individuals who have developed cirrhosis (extensive scarring of the liver) as a result of alcoholism should receive liver transplants. Organ transplant experts agree that the number of people who need liver transplants is climbing and will continue to do so because of the growing prevalence of **hepatitis** C infection. People with hepatitis C, which is difficult to cure, often develop cancer of the liver several years after first being infected.

In the late 1990s, an operation in which part of a living donor's liver is removed and given to a person who needs the organ was being performed with increasing frequency and may eventually help solve the shortage problem. A small piece of donated liver can be taken from an adult donor for use in an infant or small child with success. The first such operation was performed at the University of Chicago Medical Center in 1989. Surgeons at Virginia Commonwealth University and a team at Mount Sinai Hospital in New York have performed the most living-donor liver transplants to date. So far, there have been no deaths and no serious complications among donors or recipients.

Although the procedure has raised concerns among some medical ethicists, it appears to be safe for both donor and recipient when performed by experienced surgeons.

Additional reading: Gutkind, *Many Sleepless Nights;* Grady, "Live Donors Revolutionize Liver Care."

lobotomy

Lobotomy is a surgical procedure, now rarely performed, that was widely used to treat psychiatric disorders in the 1940s and 1950s. In lobotomy, a surgical instrument is introduced into the frontal lobe of the brain to sever the nerves connecting the hypothalamus to the prefrontal cortex.

Gottlieb Burckhardt (1836–1907), a Swiss asylum psychiatrist, first suggested the use of brain surgery to treat mental disorders. At the mental hospital he supervised, he removed brain sections from six patients and reported his results in 1891. His work was discredited because one patient died and two suffered seizures.

About 40 years later, John Fulton (1899–1960) reported on work he and his colleagues had done on chimpanzees, who apparently lost their violent tempers after sections of their prefrontal cortexes were surgically destroyed. Antonio Egas Moniz (1874–1955) attended the conference and decided to try a similar operation on humans, performing the first lobotomy in 1935. He first injected alcohol into the section of the brain to be destroyed; he later developed a "leukotome" for surgically severing the nerves. Although his results were equivocal, because there was no other treatment available for mental disorders, the operation was widely adopted, especially in U.S. state hospitals where its effects in making patients more tractable were useful to administrators.

Two Americans, Walter Freeman (1895–1972) and James Watts (1904–1990), played a major role in popularizing lobotomy. They refined the procedure, using it mainly on patients with **depression**. Freeman developed a different procedure called transorbital lobotomy in which an ice-pick-like instrument was inserted under the eyelids of the patient and moved back and forth to destroy brain tissue; patients were "anesthetized" with **electroconvulsive therapy** beforehand. Freeman promoted this operation extensively, after first performing it in 1946, eventually breaking with Watts over its merits.

During the 1940s, the popular press trumpeted the surgery as a way to cure "sick minds," and Moniz shared the 1949 Nobel Prize for developing the surgery. In the heyday of lobotomy, 5,000 such surgeries were performed in the United States every year. Researchers knew that the operation made patients more tractable and less emotional, but they began to see that it also caused them to lose initiative and autonomy.

Once the first **antipsychotic drug**, chlorpromazine, became available in 1954 and **antidepressant drugs** soon afterwards, lobotomy became less popular.

In rare cases, such as **cingulotomy**, surgery is still performed to treat some intractable **mental illness**, but technology including stereotactic techniques and **CAT scanning** has made such operations much more precise and less damaging, and psychiatric drugs have made them a true last resort.

Additional reading: Valenstein, *Great and Desperate Cures.*

LSD (lysergic acid diethylamide)

LSD is a hallucinogenic drug derived from the natural substance **ergot**.

Albert Hofmann (1906–), director of research at the Swiss pharmaceutical company Sandoz, synthesized LSD in 1938 while working on ergot derivatives. In animal tests, it was found to stimulate the uterus and excite some animals while making others catatonic. In 1943, while investigating the compound, Hofmann became dizzy and restless and then began hallucinating. He believed he had consumed some of the lysergic acid compound by accident, and resolved to take some of the substance experimentally. On his first try, with a tiny amount, he experienced wild hallucinations—his later experiments proved he had actually used five times the effective dose.

Hofmann reported his findings on LSD in 1947, noting that the chemical produced changes in perception similar to those of **schizophrenia**.

After LSD was investigated more fully, a number of attempts were made to find use for it in treating **alcoholism** and **drug addiction**, acute psychosis, as a therapeutic agent for dying patients, and for a number of other purposes, but no clinical applications were found. Meanwhile, Timothy Leary (1920–1997) and other counterculture leaders of the 1960s called on people to "trip" with LSD to expand their minds, and a psychedelic culture sprang up around the use of this and other hallucinogenic drugs.

The U.S. government began to tightly control use of LSD with the Drug Abuse Control Act of 1965. The following year, the world's only authorized maker of LSD, Sandoz withdrew the drug from the market. However, contraband LSD is still used recreationally today.

Additional reading: Stevens, *Storming Heaven.*

lung cancer

Lung **cancer**, usually caused by smoking or less frequently by occupational exposure to **carcinogens** such as asbestos, is one of the most difficult cancers to treat.

Beginning in the 1870s, a handful of surgeons attempted to treat lung cancer by removing the cancerous section of the lung. Hugh Morriston Davies (1879–1965) performed the first lobectomy for lung cancer in 1912; however, the patient died soon after the operation because an effective method for dealing with the space left after the lung was removed had not yet been developed. Harold Brunn reported some successful lobectomies in 1929; he inserted a tube into the pleural space to allow the area to drain.

Evarts A. Graham (1883–1957) performed the first removal of an entire lung to treat lung cancer in 1933. The patient survived for many years, apparently cured. The operation became the standard treatment for lung cancer, along with removal of the nearby lymph nodes. However, Edward Churchill (1895–1972) of Harvard reported in 1950 that it was equally effective and also safer to remove just the affected lobe of the lung.

The first remission of lung cancer was reported in 1948, in patients given **nitrogen mustard**. The patients' symptoms improved, and some experienced a remission a few weeks long.

In the first half of the twentieth century, there was a large increase in the incidence of lung cancer, making it the most common type of cancer among men. Scientists had first suggested that smoking might cause lung cancer in the late 1800s.

Ernest L. Wynder (1922–) and Graham provided the largest study to date of lung cancer and cigarette smoking in 1950, concluding that "excessive and prolonged use of tobacco, especially cigarettes, seems to be an important factor in the induction of bronchiogenic carcinoma." That year Richard Doll (1912–) of Great Britain issued a similar report, finding that heavy smokers had a 50 times greater risk of developing lung cancer and concluded that "smoking was an important cause of carcinoma of the lung."

Many doctors and scientists did not accept the findings, but several other studies supported them, including a report on 200,000 men released by the American Cancer Society in 1954.

Small-cell lung cancer (SCLC) was determined to be distinct from other types of lung cancer in the 1970s. SCLC, which accounts for approximately 25 percent of lung cancers, responds well to **chemotherapy** and radiation. Treatment of nonsmall cell lung cancer (NSCLC) with cisplatin, beginning in the 1970s, produced some modest benefit.

On average, patients with SCLC survive for 10 months, and about half respond to chemotherapy. From 10 to 40 percent of patients with NSCLC survive for a year. The overall one-year survival rate for lung cancer is 41 percent while the five-year survival rate is 14 percent, according to the American Cancer Society.

The number of people diagnosed with lung cancer has grown steadily in the United States from the 1930s to the 1980s, following an increase in the number of people who smoke, but 1992 marked the first decline in that rate. There are currently 171,600 new cases of lung cancer annually and 158,900 deaths from the disease each year in the United States.

Additional reading: Roth, et al., *Lung Cancer.*

lung transplant

Lung transplantation is most commonly performed on people with **cystic fibrosis** or other types of obstructive lung disease, who may need a transplant of a single lung, two lungs, or even a heart and both lungs.

The first transplant of a human lung was performed in 1963 by Mississippi physician James D. Hardy (1918–) and his colleagues on a 58-year-old convict who had **cancer** in one lung. The donor had died of a heart attack. The recipient lived for 18 days, dying of kidney failure, but did not reject the lung. After the first lung transplant, a handful of other operations were performed with most patients dying shortly afterwards.

The Toronto Lung Transplant Group developed a surgical technique for improving the regrowth of blood vessels around the lung after transplantation, and proposed avoiding steroid drugs for immunosuppression until several days after the procedure to promote healing. A 58-year-old man was the first to receive a lung transplant using this technique in 1983; he remains alive and active today. The team performed the first successful double-lung transplant in 1986. The recipient, a 42-year-old woman with end-stage emphysema due to a metabolic deficiency, remains alive and healthy.

The success of lung transplantation, because of the complexity of the blood-vessel structure in the pulmonary area and the scarcity of suitable donors, has lagged behind the transplantation of other organs. However, transplants of one or two lungs and even heart and lungs together are becoming increasingly successful.

Bruce Reitz (1944–) of Stanford University performed the first heart-lung transplant in 1981. The procedure became much easier after Robert Hardesty (1940–) and his colleagues at the University of Pittsburgh developed a system for removing the heart and lungs together from the donor's body and preserving them with the heart still beating and the lungs still "breathing" oxygen. The heart-lung "box" is basically an aquarium kept at body temperature. The team used the apparatus they designed for the first time in 1985.

In the early 1990s, Vaughn Starnes (1951–) and his colleagues at the University of Southern California School of Medicine performed transplants in which a lobe of the lung was removed from the donor and placed in the chest of the recipient. In 1994, he reported the results of the surgery on two newborns, three children, and one adult. The babies received the lobes from cadavers, while the other patients were given a section of lung from a living, related donor. Five of the patients survived. In 1993, after several experimental operations in dogs, surgeons at the Hospital Broussais in Paris transplanted two sections of a donor's lung into the chest of a 40-year-old patient with respiratory failure. The operation was successful.

Although these procedures offer hope that the lack of donor organs could be supplemented by partial lungs donated by living people, especially for children who need lung transplants, only a handful of surgeons know how to perform the operation. It is currently used only in emergency situations.

Today, lung transplantation is a relatively routine procedure after which most patients can expect to live several years, but it still has limited applications. (*See also* immunosuppression)

Additional reading: Gutkind, *Many Sleepless Nights*, pp. 66–69, 125–34.

Lyme disease

Lyme disease is caused by a bacterial infection transmitted by deer tick bites, and is common in the Northeast and northern Midwest United States. Researchers believe Lyme disease has appeared because of new construction in woodland areas where these ticks live.

The disease is named for the town of Lyme, Connecticut, where cases of a mysterious disease marked by arthritis and flu-like symptoms first appeared in the early 1970s. Allan Steere (1943–), then a postgraduate medical student at Yale University in nearby New Haven, saw the first cases and suspected that they might be caused by a vector-borne (carried by an insect or animal) infectious agent.

Dr. Andrew Spielman (1930–) of Harvard pinpointed the species of tick responsible for spreading the disease in 1979. Populations of this tick had grown dramatically in towns along the Connecticut River Valley before the disease began to appear. The infectious agent, a spirochete, was identified in 1981 by Willy Burgdorfer (1925–) on Shelter Island, New York. Two years later, researchers proved that the spirochete caused Lyme disease, and the bug was named *Borrelia burgdorferi* in honor of its discoverer.

Although Lyme disease is difficult to diagnose because the symptoms mimic other diseases, characteristically a flat or slightly raised red lesion occurs at the site of the bite, oftentimes spreading several inches into a rash. Lyme disease can be cured with **antibiotics**, but if left untreated it can cause neurological damage, heart problems, and arthritis-like symptoms.

Lyme disease vaccines have been developed, with the first being approved by the **Food and Drug Administration (FDA)** in 1998. Such vaccines will be helpful for preventing the infection in people living in Lyme disease–ridden areas, but are not 100-percent effective. **Public health** officials urge people in areas where Lyme disease is endemic to carefully check their clothes and skin (and pets) for ticks, and also to wear light-colored long sleeves and long pants to protect their skin against tick bites, even if they have been vaccinated.

Additional reading: Henig, *The People's Health*, pp. 41–45; Kiple, *The Cambridge World History of Human Disease*, pp. 852–55.

lymph system

The lymph system is a network of vessels and nodes that produces immune-system cells known as lymphocytes and monocytes, and also serves to filter bacteria from the blood. Lymph forms in the tissues of the body and eventually drains from these tissues back into the blood stream. Although lymph nodes can be protective, they can also be the originating site of tumor growth.

Lymph is derived from the Greek word "nymph," a creature associated with clear streams. Gaspar Aselli (1581–1625) discovered the lymphatic system in 1623, after observing that the lymph glands in the intestines of humans and dogs fill with a milky looking substance called chyle that contains digested food (mostly fats) after eating. He suggested that the intestines secreted lymph as the breasts secreted milk, and proposed that the liver changed lymph into blood.

William Hewson (1739–1774) suggested that lymph, produced by the thymus and lymph glands, contained particles essential to normal growth and tissue repair. In 1878, Claude Bernard (1813–1878) deduced that lymph comes from all body cells, and forms the circulating plasma in order to sustain homeostasis.

Additional reading: Clark, *At War Within*, pp. 44–49.

lysergic acid diethylamide. See LSD.

magnetic resonance imaging (MRI)

Magnetic resonance imaging is a technique for obtaining cross-sectional "pictures" of the inside of the body that is especially useful for examining soft **tissue** structures.

During an MRI, the patient's body is surrounded by a giant ring-shaped magnet, or several magnets arranged in a ring. This magnet aligns the body's magnetic field, and then a radiofrequency pulse is sent through the aligned atoms. Variations in the way the atoms respond to the energy provide an exquisitely detailed image of the composition of the body, because different elements reflect different parts of the energy spectrum. The MRI can also reveal tumors.

MRI is harmless to the body, but it is expensive and requires a person to sit still for a lengthy amount of time as the image is made.

MRI began with nuclear magnetic resonance (NMR), a technique for measuring the magnetic moment of a nucleus. Isidor Isaac Rabi (1898–1988), a physicist, made this measurement for the first time in 1937, and won the 1944 Nobel Prize for his discovery. Edward M. Purcell (1912–) and Felix Bloch (1905–), two American physicists working independently, discovered a method for measuring the magnetic moment of the proton in bulk material in 1946, and shared the 1952 Nobel Prize.

NMR first was used to analyze chemical samples. Jay Singer (1921–) at the University of California first used the NMR on a living creature; he showed in 1959 that he could measure blood flow in a mouse without hurting the animal.

Raymond Damadian (1936–), a physician at the Downstate Medical Center in Brooklyn, proposed that NMR could be used to detect tumors in tissue. In 1970 he used an NMR machine to examine rats with tumors, and proved that the tumor tissue produced readings different from those of the healthy tissue. He patented a device for detecting tumors in 1972, and built a full-body machine that he called the "Indomitable" in 1977. He also founded a company for producing his NMR devices that he named FONAR.

In 1971, Paul Lauterbur (1929–), a chemist at the State University of New York at Stonybrook, developed a mathematical method for producing images from NMR that was a precursor to MRI. He called his technique "zeugmatography," and an article he wrote including the first NMR image taken—of a test tube containing capillary tubes full of water—was published in the journal *Nature* in 1973.

The first NMR image of an animal, a mouse, was taken in 1974 in Aberdeen, Scotland. A couple of years later Damadian published images he had taken of a mouse with a device he designed. The process of making images with the machines of this time was extremely slow because they were collected one point at a time.

A group working in Nottingham, England, using a slightly speedier method that produced better images, published the first recognizable image of the human brain in 1980. Richard R. Ernst (1933–) suggested some modifications that made MRI scanning more practical, and won the 1991 Nobel Prize in Chemistry for these contributions.

MRI scanners became available commercially in the mid-1980s.

In the early 1990s, researchers learned it was possible to use MRI to detect changes in blood oxygenation within the brain by taking a rapid series of images, providing a valuable tool for the study of brain function. This technique, pioneered by AT&T Bell Laboratory physicist Seiji Ogawa (1934–), is referred to as fast or functional MRI, fMRI for short. Ogawa's technique makes it possible to pinpoint and measure metabolic activity within the brain without injecting a contrast agent, as is required in **PET scanning.** MRI is also useful for targeting **radiation therapy** of **cancers,** by helping radiologists pinpoint tumor location.

During the 1990s, surgeons began using MRI machines to guide them in taking **biopsies** and removing brain tumors, and these machines may soon be used to help surgeons perform more complex operations using **minimally invasive surgery** techniques.

Additional reading: Kevles, *Naked to the Bone,* pp. 173–200.

major histocompatibility complex (MHC)

The MHC is the section of the **chromosome** responsible for producing molecules on the surface of the cell that serve as identity markers. When the immune system scans the body, it will recognize "nonself" markers and mount an attack against the foreign organism, which could be bacteria or a virally infected cell, while leaving healthy "self" cells alone.

Baruj Benacerraf (1920–), Jean Dausset (1916–), and George Snell (1903–1996) won the 1980 Nobel Prize for identifying and locating the various immune-system regulating factors on the chromosome in animals.

While investigating viral infections in mice in Australia in the 1970s, Peter Doherty (1940–) and Rolf Zinkernagel (1944–) discovered the mechanism by which the MHC defends an individual against a **virus**, for which they won the 1996 Nobel Prize.

The MHC in humans is called the histocompatibility locus **antigen** complex, or HLA complex for short.

Additional reading: Hall, *A Commotion in the Blood*, pp. 271–73.

malaria

Malaria is a parasitic infection transmitted by mosquitoes. The *Plasmodium* parasite infects the **red blood cells**. Toxic substances are released into the body at the end of each parasitic reproductive cycle, when the parasite destroys these cells, and the malaria sufferer experiences chills and fever.

About 200 million people are infected with malaria each year. Four different species of the genus *Plasmodium* cause malaria infection, and the disease usually is spread from person to person by the bite of a female Anopheles mosquito.

The word "malaria" is Italian for "bad air," which had been thought to be the cause of this disease. An essay from the **Hippocratic Corpus**, "Airs, Waters, Places," written around 400 B.C., made the first connection between swamps—where mosquitoes breed—and malaria.

The first successful treatment for malaria was Peruvian tree bark, or cinchona, which was introduced to Europe in the early 1600s. In 1820, Joseph Bienaime Caventou (1795–1877) and Pierre-Joseph Pelletier (1788–1842) isolated the active ingredients **quinine** and cinchonine from the cinchona bark, and the substance was soon synthesized by laboratories throughout Europe.

Many drugs used for malaria are quinine-based. These drugs can often be used to prevent as well as treat malaria. Plasmoquinine was introduced in 1924. A related compound, quinacrine, was introduced in 1932. Chloroquine was synthesized in 1934 and replaced quinacrine as the antimalarial drug of choice. As resistance to chloroquine has grown, quinine has become popular again. These drugs are all effective, although their side effects vary. Also, certain strains of malaria may be resistant to one but not to others.

New drugs for malaria include mefloquine (Lariam) and halofantrine (Halfan), both developed by the U.S. Army,

and compounds extracted from the herb qinghaosu, which has been used in **Chinese medicine** to treat fever since 341 A.D. and was found in 1971 to be antimalarial.

Even though successful malaria treatments had been developed well before the nineteenth century, the cause of the disease remained a mystery.

Alphonse Laaran (1845–1922) discovered the parasite that causes malaria in 1880. Cuban doctor Carlos Finlay (1833–1915) and American doctor Walter Reed (1851–1902) worked out the connection between the mosquito and the parasite in 1901, and determined that the spread of malaria could be halted by getting rid of uncovered pools of water where mosquitoes breed.

Efforts to eradicate malaria by draining swamps and wiping out mosquitoes with pesticides began in the 1950s with the invention of dicholorodiphenyltrichloroethane (DDT). Beginning in 1995, the **World Health Organization (WHO)** sponsored such campaigns in several countries. By the mid-1970s, *A. egyptii*, the major carrier of malaria, had been squeezed back into a quarter of its original worldwide habitat. But malaria prevention efforts lost support around this time, as many groups that had been funding this work—including the Rockefeller Foundation—became convinced that wiping out malaria was an impossible goal. They had a point: several different types of mosquito can carry the **virus**; pesticides are harmful to people; and pesticides toughen mosquitoes as successive generations develop resistance to them.

In 1980, the World Health Organization recommended that malaria eradication efforts be combined with primary health care.

Additional reading: Altman, *Who Goes First?*, pp. 129–58; Kiple, *The Cambridge World History of Human Disease*, pp. 855–62.

mammography

Mammography is a **cancer**-screening technique in which the breast is X-rayed. If a tumor is suspected, a **biopsy** of the **tissue** is done and checked for malignancy.

Albert Salomon (1883–unknown), a German surgeon, was the first to describe the ability of roentgenography to detect cancers in the breast, in 1913. In a 1938 article, Jacob Gershon-Cohen (1915–) at the Jefferson Medical College in Philadelphia urged that healthy breasts be studied in order to make it easier to recognize and treat breast disease, such as cancer.

Stafford Warren (1896–1981) at UCLA developed a system for identifying changes in breast tissue with **X-rays** in the 1930s. He published the first reliable data on the clinical use of mammography. An X-ray machine specifically designed for breast examination was invented in France by Charles Gros in the mid-1960s. The Compagnie Generale de Radiographie began selling the device in 1967. The electronics companies Siemens, Philips, and Picker followed with their own mammography devices in the 1970s.

In 1960, Dr. Robert L. Egan (1920–) at M.D. Anderson Cancer Center in Houston, Texas, reported on a new technique using high-resolution film that provided mammograms of a much higher quality than previously available. Two years later, he reported that he had been able to detect 53 cases of cancer in 2,000 women screened using his method.

The Health Insurance Plan of New York, one of the first **HMOs**, ran the first controlled trial of mammography in the early 1960s, and found that women who received mammograms were one-third less likely to die of **breast cancer**.

Despite these findings, as well as positive results from a subsequent national study of mammography in 250,000 women by the National Cancer Institute and the American Cancer Society, doctors were hesitant to adopt mammography because of concerns about exposing women to radiation.

Technical developments during the 1970s by Xerox and Kodak corporations and others made it possible to produce clear mammograms with much less radiation. Magnification was added in the late 1970s, further improving image quality.

In 1974, First Lady Betty Ford's battle with breast cancer brought the previously taboo disease into the public spotlight, increasing women's awareness of the disease and the necessity of breast cancer screening. The American Cancer Society and the American College of Radiology organized an accreditation program for mammography technicians in 1986. Three years later, 11 health organizations urged all women to begin having regular mammographies after age 40.

Training techniques similar to those devised to help Air Force pilots spot camouflage have helped technicians to spot irregularities in mammograms, as have computer-assisted searches. Congress passed the Mammography Quality Standards Act, which created a system of federal regulation for ensuring the quality of the test, in 1992.

Additional reading: Kevles, *Naked to the Bone,* pp. 250–60.

managed care

Managed care is a system of health care in which a person's use of resources is "managed" to cut costs. Managed care seeks to control expenses with preventive care, such as careful management of chronic diseases such as **diabetes mellitus** and smoking cessation and weight-loss programs. In a typical managed-care plan, a person can choose among providers contracted by the company to provide care at reduced cost, and his or her use of medical care is controlled by a "gatekeeper," the primary care physician. Managed care seeks to shift financial risk from the health plan to the health care provider.

There are several types of managed care health plans: **HMOs (health maintenance organizations),** preferred provider organizations (PPOs), and managed fee-for-service plans.

During the 1800s, forerunners of managed care in the form of prepaid health services were organized by companies for their employees, particularly for work forces in isolated areas such as lumber camps and railroads. Some immigrants formed cooperative health systems. **Health insurance** plans became available in the United States in the early twentieth century. After World War II, indemnity plans such as Blue Cross/Blue Shield that provided fee-for-service care dominated the market. Beginning in the 1960s, as costs rose, the U.S. government began to advocate HMOs and other managed care systems to cut costs. Corporations backed these efforts, because an increasing amount of their pretax profits were being spent on employee health care. The Health Maintenance Organization Act of 1973 provided grants and loans to companies seeking to establish HMOs.

To further manage the cost of health care paid for by the government, the federal government introduced diagnostic-related groups in 1983. Under this system, a hospital receives a fixed payment from **Medicare/Medicaid** based on a patient's diagnosis, rather than the amount of money actually spent on his or her care. A similar system for physician payment was put in place in 1992. Medicare and Medicaid are also increasingly shifting beneficiaries into privately run managed care programs.

Although a number of private companies enrolling Medicare patients in managed-care plans have gotten out of the business recently, citing declining reimbursement, enrollment in these plans continues to grow. As of June 1999, there were more than 6.8 million seniors in these programs. Concerns have been raised about whether these programs, which are charging higher premiums and reducing their prescription drug coverage, are providing adequate care to older people.

Advocates for the poor and disabled have similar questions about managed-care Medicaid plans, and fear that for-profit companies may cut corners in the care they provide in order to preserve profits. While Medicare patients can opt for or out of managed care, a growing number of Medicaid managed-care programs are mandatory for most patients.

Additional reading: Anders, *Health and Wealth.*

marijuana

Marijuana is a drug, made from the female marijuana plant, that has been used for millennia. The *cannabis*, or hemp, plant can be easily grown in subtropical and temperate climates. Users typically smoke the drug.

Reference to marijuana has been found in Greek, Roman, Assyrian, and ancient Egyptian literature. The first mention appears in a Chinese list of medications from 2737 B.C. The drug spread to Europe in around 1800, and has been known in South and Central America for centuries.

In 1913, Sir William Osler (1849–1919) recommended marijuana as the best treatment for **migraine**. It has also been used to ease labor pains, stimulate the appetite, and fight nausea. Marijuana became popular in the United States around 1920. The Marihuana Tax Act of 1937, designed to ban nonmedical use of the drug, made it so difficult to obtain that medical use stopped as well.

However, recreational use of marijuana continued, despite efforts to enforce the laws making it illegal. The LaGuardia Report, commissioned by New York City Mayor Fiorello LaGuardia and released in 1944, found that marijuana was not linked to criminal behavior, and that the drug was not addictive. Marijuana use continued to be common among the lower economic classes, and the drug was popular among the "Beatniks" of the 1950s. During the 1960s, use among young people became widespread.

Israeli chemists discovered tetrahydrocannabinol (THC), the active ingredient in marijuana and hashish, in 1963 and synthesized it in 1964.

THC became commercially and legally available in the United States in capsule form in 1985, as Marinol. Some studies have found Marinol to be less effective than smoked marijuana. It's believed that the natural form probably contains other components that contribute to its effects. It also may be easier for marijuana cigarette smokers to control the amount of the drug they consume.

Today marijuana is used as a recreational drug by many, as well as for medical purposes, often illegally. **Cancer** patients may use it to fight nausea, **AIDS** patients to stimulate appetite, and people with **glaucoma** to ease pressure on the eye. Medical marijuana became legal in a handful of states in the 1990s.

Additional reading: Abel, *Marihuana.*

measles

Measles is an extremely infectious viral disease that causes a rash of red bumps to arise on the skin. The disease is usually mild in healthy children, but can produce severe illness in people with weakened immune systems.

Measles was long confused with **smallpox,** another disease characterized by rash. In 1758, Francis Home (1719–1813) first proved that measles is an infectious disease. In 1911, John Anderson (1874–1958) and Joseph Goldberger (1874–1929) showed that measles was caused by a **virus**.

John Enders (1897–1985) and his colleagues at Harvard Medical School isolated the measles virus in 1954, and Enders and Samuel Katz (1929–) developed an attenuated strain for use as a vaccine in 1958. An attenuated "live" **vaccine** was licensed by the United States for general use in 1963.

Children generally receive a measles vaccine at 15 months of age, sometimes as part of the combination measles-mumps-rubella **immunization**. The first measles-mumps-rubella vaccine was licensed in 1971.

Since the **World Health Organization (WHO)** established its Expanded Programme on Immunization in 1974, most nations now have a measles vaccination program in place.

Additional reading: Williams, *Virus Hunters,* pp.377–400; Kiple, *The Cambridge World History of Human Disease,* pp. 871–75.

medical journals

Medical journals publish studies, new findings, opinions, and other information of interest to doctors. There are currently approximately 15,000 biomedical journals in publication worldwide. Medical journals are an important forum for publicizing clinical advances and studies, and are the main way that physicians keep informed about news in medicine.

The first scientific journals, the *Journal de Scavans* in Paris and the *Philosophical Transactions of the Royal Society* in Britain, were published in 1665. Physicians of the time would release their findings in general scientific journals like these, or in books or pamphlets they published themselves. At this time, most scientific journals were published in German.

Journals focusing on medicine alone began to appear in the 1800s, with the *Transactions of the Medical Society* of London in 1810, the *New England Journal of Medicine* in 1812, the *Lancet* in 1823, and the *Gazette des Hopiteaux* and the *Midland Medical and Surgical Reporter* in 1828. All are still in publication today although some appear under different names, such as the *Journal of the Royal Society of Medicine* (formerly *Transactions of the Medical Society*) and the *British Medical Journal*. Around this time, specialist medical journals began appearing.

By the start of the twentieth century, most countries were publishing general medical journals, and by World War I, most medical specialties had their own journals. English overtook German as the language of science, with complete predominance in journals by the 1930s.

Increasingly specialized journals began to appear, focusing on specialties within specialties. The number of new scientific journals now grows by 7 percent a year.

About three-quarters of journals in print follow peer review, meaning that articles they publish have been reviewed by other scientists in the same discipline. Peer review does not guarantee correctness of information or quality of research, however.

Additional reading: Bynum, et al., eds., *Medical Journals and Medical Knowledge.*

Medicare/Medicaid

Medicare and Medicaid provide affordable health care for the elderly and for disabled and low-income people. The elderly are covered by Medicare, while Medicaid covers disabled and low-income people. The United States Congress passed legislation establishing these programs in 1965.

The Medicare law has two parts: Part A, which covers hospital care for people over 65; and Part B, which provides for Supplementary Medical Insurance (SMI). Under this program, a person is eligible to buy SMI that will cover nonhospital medical costs, such as visits to a doctor.

Every working American pays into Medicare, and then hopes to enjoy the benefits of coverage when he or she reaches the age of 65. Today the future of Medicare is in doubt, since the proportion of the nation's population 65 and older is increasing greatly, meaning that many more people will depend on fewer, younger working people. Several proposals for restructuring Medicare are being debated, such as increasing the eligibility age and requiring wealthy recipients to contribute more extensively to their care.

Efforts in the late 1990s to turn management of Medicare benefits over to HMOs were not universally successful; many of these managed care companies soon left the Medicare market because it was not profitable enough.

Medicaid falls far short of providing health insurance to all poor Americans. Minimum income requirements, which are set individually by states, may be well below the poverty line, and poor people who do not have dependent children may not be eligible.

Additional reading: David, *With Dignity*.

melanoma

Melanoma is a **cancer** of the pigment cells in the skin. It is much more deadly than the two other, more common types of skin cancer, basal cell and squamous cell carcinoma. In 1998, 1 million new cases of skin cancer were diagnosed, 41,600 of them malignant melanomas, and about 9,200 people died of skin cancer.

The incidence of melanoma has risen steeply since the 1950s, and mortality from the disease has climbed as well. Melanoma is related to sunlight exposure, and occurs more frequently in light-skinned people who do not tan.

Rene Laennec (1781–1826), the inventor of the **stethoscope,** first described melanoma as a disease in 1806, and used the name "melanoma" for the first time in a paper six years later. William Norris, in 1820, described for the first time a case of melanoma that had spread to the internal organs. In 1857, Norris published a paper in which he made several observations of the epidemiology and pathology of melanoma. He observed a link between moles and melanoma, and also noticed that the disease was more common in pale, fair-haired people and those living in industrial areas. He also noted that the disease appeared in some cases to be hereditary. Norris's recommended treatment was to surgically remove the tumor and the surrounding tissue, but he noted that once the disease had spread widely it could not be treated effectively.

In 1865, James Paget (1814–1899) was the first to note that moles could become malignant.

Mohs micrographic surgery, a technique for removing melanomas and other types of skin cancer layer by layer after chemical treatment until microscopic investigation of the **tissue** shows that cancerous growth has been completely eradicated, was developed in the 1930s by Frederic E. Mohs (1910–1979). The technique is still used today for surgical removal of melanoma lesions.

Wallace Clark, Jr. (1924–1997), a pathologist at Tulane University in New Orleans (who later taught at Harvard Medical School, Temple University in Philadelphia, and the University of Pennsylvania) made several important discoveries about melanoma. In 1958, he first used the **electron microscope** to study melanoma, and published the first description of the melanosome. This is an organelle

characterizing melanoma cells that manufactures the pigment melatonin. He also developed a system for classifying the stages of growth of malignant melanoma.

It was during the 1970s that scientists first noticed that the incidence of melanoma was on the rise around the world, particularly in Australia and the United States. Public health campaigns urging people to use **sunscreen** and other methods for protecting themselves against ultraviolet light began in 1980. During this decade, researchers confirmed a link between sunlight exposure and melanoma, and found that tanning beds and other artificial sources of ultraviolet light also increased skin cancer risk.

Melanoma can now be diagnosed at an extremely early stage by examining the skin with a microscope immersed in oil, a technique known as epiluminescence microscopy (ELM).

Scientists began investigating **cancer vaccines** and other types of immunotherapy for treating melanoma in the late 1980s, but so far these techniques have not been proven effective. Surgery remains the main treatment. Sentinel-node **biopsy** has helped surgeons locate the spread of melanoma and avoid extensive lymph-node removal in some patients.

Additional reading: Poole, *Melanoma*.

mental hospital

A mental hospital is an institution where the mentally ill are confined and given therapeutic care. An earlier term used to describe these institutions, "asylum," has fallen out of favor.

The first asylums were built in the Middle East around 700 to 800 A.D. and in Europe from 1100 to 1300 A.D. These asylums were most likely just warehouses for the mentally ill, and remained so until the 1700s when some European physicians began to revolutionize care of the mentally ill.

William Battie (1704–76), the head of St. Luke's Hospital in London, was the first to suggest that confinement of the mentally ill could be therapeutic in his 1758 "Treatise on Madness." Following his lead, Vincenzio Chiarugi (1759–1820) established a special hospital for psychiatric patients in Florence in 1788.

Philippe Pinel (1745–1826), director of the Bicetre Asylum and Salpietre in Paris, was famous for "striking off the chains" of asylum patients, although he wasn't the first to do it. His 1801 *Traite medico-philosophique sur l'Alienation mentale* outlines his more humane approach to caring for the mentally ill. He saw the hospital as the main therapeutic agent, and recommended physical exercise and work for patients. He also rejected beating, although he did consider short periods of restraint in a strait jacket to be useful treatment.

Pinel emphasized clinical findings and statistics, and believed that **mental illness** came from hereditary and environmental causes, as well as an irregular way of life and possibly a conflict between instinct and religious dogma. His student, Jean Etienne Dominique Esquirol (1772–1840), carried on his work.

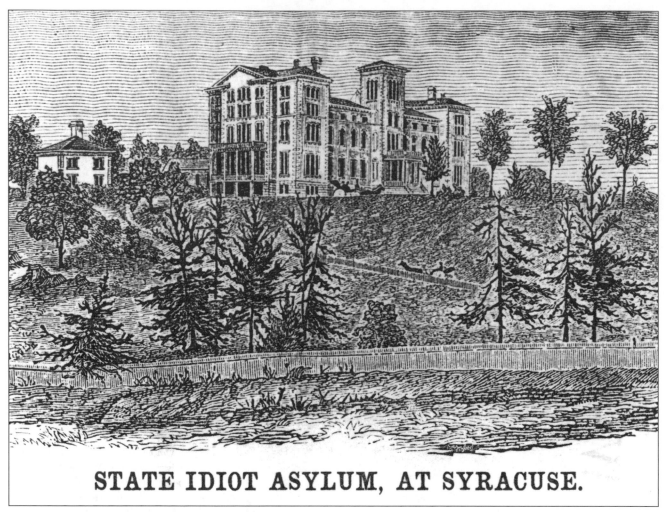

STATE IDIOT ASYLUM, AT SYRACUSE.

Frontispiece of the Seventh Annual Report of the New York Asylum for Idiots to the New York State Legislature, 1858. (Courtesy of Department of Historical Collections, Health Sciences Library, SUNY Health Science Center at Syracuse.)

A leader in reforming the U.S. asylum system was Dorothea Dix (1802–1887), who drew attention to the horrible conditions experienced by mentally ill people who were being kept in poorhouses and jails. The first new-style public asylum in the United States was established in Worcester, Massachussets, in 1833.

Unfortunately, unbearable crowding of these institutions meant that by the end of the nineteenth century most asylum directors had given up trying to provide therapy for the patients housed there. There have been many different causes proposed for this overcrowding: growing intolerance of deviance in families; people being shifted to asylums from home and poorhouse; an increase in **alcoholism** and **syphilis** (which in its later stages can cause insanity); greater frequency of mental illness (the cause of such an increase is unknown); and the general stressfulness of modern life.

Many mental hospitals were closed for good in the 1950s, when **antipsychotic drugs** allowed psychiatrists to believe it would be possible to release mentally ill people into the community. President John F. Kennedy's Community Mental Health Centers Act of 1963 was intended to provide community care for the people who were leaving

mental hospitals, but these centers wound up being devoted to caring for people with milder psychiatric problems and not for the seriously mentally ill.

The number of patients in U.S. mental hospitals declined from 559,000 in 1955 to 338,000 in 1970 to 107,000 in 1988. In 1994, there were 72,000 people in state-run psychiatric hospitals. In the 1980s, more private mental hospitals opened to provide care, but lack of treatment for mentally ill people remains a grave problem in the United States. Increasingly, mentally ill people are being confined in jails and prisons where they may or may not receive treatment; according to current figures, there are 200,000 mentally ill people in jail and 61,700 in state hospitals. Some researchers estimate that 600,000 to one million mentally ill people are admitted to jails each year. Men in large urban jails have two to three times the rate of major psychiatric illness found in the general population, while only 20 percent of jails offer discharge planning for mentally ill inmates. Spending by states, which have the primary legal responsibility for caring for the mentally ill, is a third of what it was in the 1950s.

A 1998 study found that fewer than half of people suffering from **schizophrenia** in the United States receive adequate care. And while research has shown that mentally ill people are no more violent than other people when they receive proper treatment, people with schizophrenia who receive no treatment may frequently strike out violently at others.

The National Alliance for the Mentally Ill, founded in 1979, is leading the effort to improve care for mentally ill people in the United States.

Additional reading: Porter, *The Cambridge Illustrated History of Medicine,* pp. 286–97; Porter, ed., *Medicine,* pp. 147–49.

mental illness

Mental illness is any disorder of the mind or behavior.

The ancient Greeks were among the first to study mental illness. The Greek physician Soranus of Ephesus, writing in approximately 100 A.D., recommended that patients be isolated in a light, warm, airy room, with high windows so that they couldn't jump out. Other treatments included playing chess, traveling, and giving speeches to a friendly audience. Melancholia was seen at the time a disease of the esophagus.

The Roman philosopher Celsus (25 B.C.–50 A.D.), writing in 30 A.D., recommended menacing, torturing, whipping, and ducking those afflicted—treatments that remained popular for more than 1,000 years.

The Greeks and Romans were relatively advanced in their assumption that mental illness was a physical disease, and not caused by demonic possession or an evil spirit. But the more primitive conception of mental illness held sway throughout the Middle Ages, and only began to change during the Renaissance.

Paracelsus (1493–1541), in a book published in 1567 and written in about 1520, titled *Diseases Which Lead to a Loss of Reason,* said mental illnesses were natural diseases and not caused by spirits. He explained that many such illnesses were caused by vapors that rose and lodged in the head, and could change into worms. "True insanity," he said, was a permanent state related to the stars that was caused by diseased semen or being affected by the moon while in the womb.

A revolution in caring for people with mental illness came in the late eighteenth century, when in Europe (and later, the United States) physicians began "striking the chains" from the mentally ill people kept in **mental hospitals** and recommending kinder, more reasonable treatment.

This revolution spread throughout the nineteenth century, but by the early twentieth century asylums were so packed with people that it became impossible to treat them there.

This century has seen a variety of treatment attempts, some more successful than others, from **psychoanalysis** to **lobotomy** to **convulsive therapy** to drug treatment, or psychopharmacology.

During the 1960s and 1970s, Thomas Szasz (1920–) and Ronald Laing (1927–1989) denied that there was such a thing as mental illness, and said that this was a label given to deviant individuals to control them.

Although people who hold this view are in the minority, mental illness is indeed difficult to define. The success of many medications in treating **schizophrenia**, manic depression, and **depression** since 1950 has given foundation to the idea that mental illness may be caused by innate, biological factors. Scientists now tend to see parental behavior or environment as contributors to mental illness, but not causes.

Additional reading: Ackerknecht, *A Short History of Psychiatry;* Shorter, *A History of Psychiatry.*

methadone

Methadone is an opiate first synthesized in 1946 in Germany that is used as a maintenance treatment for opiate addicts.

Researchers began using methadone to treat opiate withdrawal in the late 1940s. Vincent Dole (1913–) and his colleagues launched the first effort to use oral methadone as a continuous treatment for **heroin** addicts in 1964. In 1966, they reported that addicts who took daily doses of methadone were able to lead normal lives; they didn't experience the "highs" and withdrawal sicknesses that they would have while taking heroin, but instead maintained a relatively normal emotional state. Also, if they took heroin while on methadone, the illicit drug would have little effect.

Methadone maintenance treatment enjoyed a "honeymoon period" in the first five years after its introduction. However, it has always been controversial, because critics say it replaces one **addiction** for another. Methadone treatment is not a cure for an addiction but could be likened to maintenance treatment for chronic disease.

Methadone is still an accepted method for treating heroin addiction and many addiction experts believe it should be used more broadly.

Additional reading: Hentoff, *A Doctor among the Addicts.*

MHC. See major histocompatability complex.

microscope

A microscope is an instrument used to magnify tiny objects to make them visible.

Single-lens microscopes were used as early as the fourteenth century. Zaccharias Jannsen (1580–c.1638), his father Hans, and Hans Lippershey (1570–1619) are all considered to have invented the compound microscope, which contained an eye-piece and another lens near the object to be seen called an objective, in the Netherlands around 1590.

Robert Hooke (1635–1703) described how to use microscopes in his 1665 book, *Micrographia.* Antoni von Leeuwenhoek (1632–1723) is the most famous early microscopist; this Dutch textile trader perused bacteria, blood cells, protozoa, and sperm cells. He made small microscopes consisting of a piece of metal with a hole in it that contained a hand-made lens.

In the nineteenth century, with the development of the **cell theory** and the beginnings of pathology, the microscope became a vital tool for physicians. Around 1820, achromatic microscopes, in which chromatic aberrations had been corrected, became available.

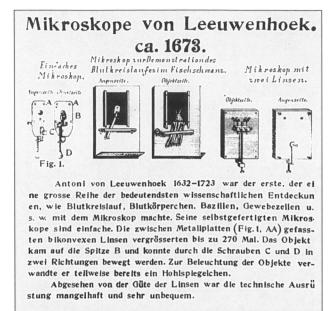

Description of the structure of von Leeuwenhoek's microscope from the Deutsches Museum, Munich, Germany, 1937. (Courtesy of Department of Historical Collections, Health Sciences Library, SUNY Health Science Center at Syracuse).

Sectioning of tissues also had to improve in order to make individual cells more clearly visible. Pieter de Riemer (1760–1831) was the first person to freeze tissues to make it easier to slice them thinly. In 1869, Edwin Klebs (1833–1913) introduced paraffin embedding (where the sample is encased in wax and then cut into very thin slices), another technique still used today. Around this time many staining techniques were developed to improve the ability to distinguish between various types of cells. These developments made **biopsy** of tissue samples an important clinical tool.

By the beginning of the twentieth century, most of the staining and sample preparation techniques used in today's microscopy were in place. In the middle of the century, **electron microscopy** and other techniques for even greater magnification became available. Operating microscopes for performing **microsurgery** became commercially available in the 1950s. Today, microscopes are used to examine **tissue** samples taken in **biopsies** to diagnose disease; to perform blood counts; and during surgery.

Additional reading: Ford, *Single Lens.*

microsurgery

Microsurgery is the surgical repair or reconstruction of near-microscopic and microscopic structures, such as blood vessels, lymph vessels, and nerves. Microsurgery has made it possible to successfully reattach severed fingers, toes, legs, and arms, as well as to repair blood vessel damage, restore fertility after surgical sterilization in both men and women, and reconstruct the breast after mastectomy.

Numerous reports of successful reattachments of parts of fingers appeared in the nineteenth century. A handful of reports of noses (bitten or sliced off in fights or amputated as punishment for a crime) being reattached appear in the 1600s and 1700s. But reattaching these appendages did not involve microsurgery, which surgeons didn't begin using until the beginning of the twentieth century, when some began attempting experimental limb reattachments in animals.

Alexis Carrel (1873–1944) won the 1912 Nobel Prize for the technique he developed to sew blood vessels together known as anastomosis. He devised several pioneering microsurgical techniques, all while practicing with animals. Operating microscopes became available commercially in 1953. Toward the end of the 1950s, fine instruments and suturing materials also became available that made microsurgery more efficient.

In 1962, Boston surgeon Ronald A. Malt (1931–) "replanted" a 12–year-old boy's right arm after it had been severed above the elbow in a train accident. Surgeons in Shanghai also reported success in replanting forearms, hands, and fingers during the early 1960s, and these operations soon became almost routine in China.

Microsurgery centers were opened worldwide in the 1970s and 1980s, and today major centers have reattachment success rates of 80 percent and better. The world's first transplant of an appendage from one human to another was performed in 1999, when an automobile accident victim's hand was attached to the arm of an Australian ex-convict by French surgeons.

Additional reading: Comroe, *Exploring the Heart,* pp. 199–202.

midwife

A midwife is a person—male or female—who cares for pregnant women and delivers babies. Some historians say that women were helping to deliver children by 6000 B.C., taking over a role that had previously belonged to the woman's husband. Midwives are mentioned several times in the Bible. Midwifery was first regulated in the fifteenth century in Ravensburg, Germany, and Henry VIII also issued legal requirements for midwives in 1512. In many parts of Europe midwives were licensed by the Church.

One of the most famous midwives in history was Louyse Bourgeois (1563–1636), who delivered six of French queen Marie de Medici's (1573–1642) children. She wrote a book that was published in 1609 called *Instruction to my Daughter* that included descriptions of how to handle several types of difficult delivery.

With the introduction of **forceps** in the seventeenth century, men began entering the baby-delivery business, sparking a tension between midwives and doctors that continues today. Doctors question whether midwives can handle difficult deliveries, while midwives question the approach doctors take. However, in the United States, women who choose to work with a midwife almost always have a physician attend the delivery as well.

For the first 150 years after the United States was settled, women received care during pregnancy and labor from friends, family, and midwives. In some colonies, midwives were required to have licenses. Some were paid and housed by the local government.

A program for experienced midwives was launched at New York's Bellevue Hospital in 1911. Nurse midwives, who are registered nurses with additional training in caring for pregnant women and in assisting during delivery, arrived in the United States in 1925 with the founding of the Frontier Nursing Service in rural Kentucky. The service was established to provide care for poor women in rural and urban areas. The first training program for nurse-midwives in the United States, the Maternity Center Association, was formed in New York City in 1931. In their early days, both programs depended on nurse-midwives who had been trained in England.

With the natural childbirth movement that began in the 1970s in the United States, more and more women began turning to midwives for assistance. In 1995, according to the National Center for Health Statistics, 207,370 births were attended by midwives, as compared with 98,000 in 1989. The 1995 figure still represents less than 6 percent of all births.

Additional reading: O'Dowd and Philipp, *The History of Obstetrics and Gynaecology*, pp. 167–90.

migraine

A migraine is an excruciating headache caused by the dilatation of cerebral blood vessels.

An "aura" marked by visual disturbances precedes the classic migraine. Then blood flow diminishes, but can increase during the painful phase. Vomiting often accompanies migraine, which may be felt on only one side of the head and behind the eye. About 8 million Americans are thought to suffer from migraines.

The first mention of migraine appears in the Ebers papyrus of about 3,500 years ago: a courtesan in the Pharoah's court suffered from a "sickness of half the head." The word "migraine" comes from the Greek word hemicrania, and first appears in English as "mygraine" in 1398.

Hippocrates (c.460–c.377) described the aura before the migraine and the course a migraine takes. The pain mechanism of migraine was first explained by Harold Wolff (1898–1962) in the 1930s. He proposed that migraine was caused by the abnormal relaxation and increased pulsing dilation of the main arteries in the brain.

In 1961, Federico Sicuteri (1920–) reported that people excreted large amounts of a metabolite of the neurotransmitter **serotonin** during migraine attacks. This eventually led to the development of sumatriptan (sold as Imitrex), a migraine drug that works by restoring levels of this chemical, which was released in 1993.

Currently migraine is best treated by avoiding migraine triggers, which can include stress and certain foods including alcohol, foods that contain monosodium glutamate (MSG), and preserved meats with nitrates and nitrites. Also drugs can be used to prevent migraine, such as propanolol and methysergide, which is derived from ergot. During migraines, patients may be given **ergotamine** and, if this doesn't work, pain killers such as codeine and Demerol. A nasal spray made to deliver ergot derivative quickly to the brain was released by the drug company Novartis in 1997.

Additional reading: Rogers and Adler, "The New War Against Migraines"; Morrow, "Struggling to Spell Relief."

minimally invasive surgery

Minimally invasive surgery is a general term for operations performed with techniques designed to minimize trauma to the body, with the assistance of miniaturized imaging systems. **Arthroscopy** (performed on the joints) and **laparoscopy** (on the abdomen) are two types of minimally invasive surgery. Today, at least one half of all surgical procedures are performed using minimally invasive techniques.

Minimally invasive surgery has many advantages over conventional "open" surgery. Recovery time is faster, there is less scarring, and the body is generally subject to less trauma. However, some surgeons are concerned that the powerful trend toward minimally invasive surgery can be dangerous if such procedures are performed by less-skilled surgeons.

Surgical telescopes were invented in the 1960s. At around this time, fiberoptics became available as well. These flexible fibers transmit light, making it possible to view the inside of the body through a curved tube. Kurt Semm (1927–) performed the first laparoscopic **appendectomy** in 1981.

Procedures involving laparoscopy, including gynecological operations and gallbladder removal, as well as arthroscopic operations, were the first surgeries to be performed using minimally invasive techniques, in the 1970s.

Video cameras were introduced during the 1980s to provide on-screen images of the interior of the body for the surgeon. During the 1990s, the quality of these images sur-

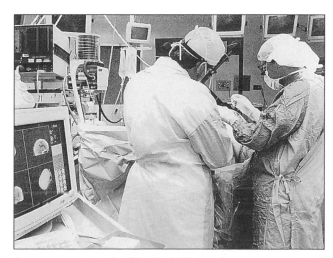

Surgeons operate at the Cleveland Clinic using computer-assisted minimally invasive surgery. The screen at the left provides three-dimensional magnetic resonance imaging scans of the brain. (Photo courtesy of Cleveland Clinic Archives.)

passed what would have been visible with the naked eye. Surgical robot assistants for laparoscopic surgery are now able, for example, to operate a video camera and to scale down the movement of a surgeon's hands.

In the 1990s, **magnetic resonance imaging (MRI)** machines were developed that are large enough for a surgeon to work inside them. These have been used only to perform **biopsies**, although surgeons believe the machines may be one day used to guide surgical procedures.

Heart surgery, such as repair of the heart valves and **bypass surgery**, has been performed using minimally invasive techniques, in which a smaller incision is made in the sternum. These surgeries were first performed in the mid-1990s. (*See also* robotic surgery)

Additional reading: Porter, *The Cambridge Illustrated History of Medicine,* pp. 350–52.

monoclonal antibodies

Monoclonal antibodies are a series of identical antibodies produced by hybrid cells.

Antibodies are very difficult to study because a single **antigen** can cause the immune system to produce thousands of different antibodies. But a hybrid cell, known as a hybridoma, can produce great quantities of a single specific **antibody**.

Georges Kohler (1946–1995), working in Cesar Milstein's (1927–) lab in Cambridge, England, created the first hybridoma. Lymphomas produce antibodies, but they are impossible to keep alive in culture. Kohler decided to try to create immortal antibody-producing cells by combining lymphomas with other types of **cancer** cells. He exposed a mouse to a specific antigen (in this case red blood cells from sheep), then removed the mouse's spleen, taking lymphoma cells out of the spleen and mixing them with a line of myeloma cells. The two cell lines mixed to form hybrids, but Kohler waited several weeks to perform the test that would determine if the hybrids in fact produced the antibody against the sheep red blood cells. When he finally performed the test, it worked.

Kohler and Milstein reported on their findings in 1975 and shared the 1984 Nobel Prize for their work.

Monoclonal antibodies are useful for diagnostic purposes, for example in counting the number of CD4 **T cells** in people with **AIDS**. Their use in medical therapy, such as the production of anti-idiotype **antibodies**, has remained largely experimental. There currently are 80 different monoclonal antibodies being tested in clinical studies (most for treating or imaging cancer). Monoclonal antibody technology also is being used to create drugs. There are currently 30 monoclonal antibody-based drugs in use, including the **breast cancer** drug **Herceptin.** One-quarter of all drugs now under development at biotechnology companies are monoclonal antibodies.

One application of monoclonal antibodies is producing passive immunity by giving a person antibodies against a disease rather than causing him or her to produce the antibodies themselves. The antibodies can be applied directly to the mucous membranes, which is where many infectious agents enter the body, protecting people against respiratory, digestive, or reproductive tract infections. Human trials are just beginning.

Other advances include the production of monoclonal antibodies by transgenic animals and plants, which should greatly lower their now-prohibitive cost.

Additional reading: Hall, *A Commotion in the Blood,* pp. 391–400; Shorter, *The Health Century,* pp. 250–56.

morphine

Morphine is an ingredient of **opium** that is used today as a painkiller. It is 10 times more powerful than opium and is used to treat severe pain, such as that experienced by **cancer** patients.

The pharmacist Friedrich Serturner (1783–1841) isolated an active alkaloid substance from opium in 1803, reporting his findings two years later. This was also the first alkaloid substance to be isolated from a plant. Alkali is a general term for substances with basic properties.

Serturner's findings did not receive widespread attention until he published an article in 1817. He named the substance morphium. The French chemist Joseph Gay-Lussac (1778–1850), who wrote an editorial accompanying the 1817 paper, suggested that this substance and all subsequent plant alkalis be given the suffix "ine," and changed the name to morphine.

By the 1830s, chemical tests to detect the presence of morphine were available and the drug was being used widely.

Physicians searched for ways to administer morphine into the blood stream so it would work quickly, for example by rubbing the drug into abraded skin and even passing a needle threaded with medicine-soaked string through the skin.

When the subcutaneous injection technique was refined in the middle of the 1800s, the door opened for more effective medical use of morphine, but it also introduced the problem of intravenous drug use that persists today.

The use and abuse of morphine spread rapidly and abuse became recognized as a problem about 20 years after the drug entered widespread use. Morphine's association with **addiction** gave it a bad reputation that has only recently been rehabilitated. Today, morphine remains a useful painkilling drug, although tight government control of its distribution and prescription have made many doctors reluctant to give it to patients who need it—even people dying of cancer. (*See also* heroin)

Additional reading: Courtwright, *Dark Paradise.*

MRI. See magnetic resonance imaging

multiple sclerosis (MS)

Multiple sclerosis (MS) is a progressive degenerative disease of the brain or spinal cord in which the myelin sheath that protects the nerves breaks down, causing the nerves to malfunction.

People with MS suffer numbness and lose motor control, and may lose vision during an attack. The disease usually first strikes between the ages of 20 and 40, and is most common in Canada, northern Europe, and the northern United States.

Although the cause of MS is unclear, the disease is known to be an autoimmune condition in which the body attacks itself. There is evidence for a genetic basis to the disease; some researchers suggest that MS is triggered by a viral infection in genetically vulnerable individuals.

Parisian anatomist Jean Cruveilhier (1791–1874) described the symptoms of multiple sclerosis in 1842, along with certain pathological characteristics. In 1883, the neurologist Jean-Marie Charcot (1825–1893) provided a more detailed description and distinguished multiple sclerosis from other paralytic diseases. He also developed criteria for diagnosing multiple sclerosis and correlated the symptoms with pathological changes found after autopsy. Charcot also suggested that the disease might be caused by the demyelination of nerves.

Toward the end of the nineteenth century, researchers began to gather evidence that MS may be a hereditary or genetic disease.

There remains no cure for multiple sclerosis, although physical therapy can help somewhat and therapy with high doses of **interferon** also can be beneficial in slowing the progression of disease.

Some people with the condition experience long remissions and can led relatively normal lives for decades, while for others the disease strikes more quickly and leads to rapid deterioration and death within months. About 5 to 10 percent of people with MS experience the steadily progressing form of the disease, while the rest have intermittent symptoms. About a quarter of people with MS are working full-time 15 years after the diagnosis, and the average life span after diagnosis is 25 years.

Additional reading: Kiple, *The Cambridge World History of Human Disease,* pp. 883–87.

mumps

Mumps is a viral infection that causes painful swelling in the salivary glands. In children, mumps is usually mild, but in males who have passed puberty mumps can cause painful swelling of the testicles that can, although rarely, produce sterility.

Hippocrates (c.460–c.377 B.C.) is believed to have described mumps. In 1755, Richard Russell (1700–1771) described mumps and said that it was communicable.

Ernest W. Goodpasture (1886–1969) and his colleagues proved that mumps was caused by a **virus** in 1934.

Maurice Hilleman (1942–) and his colleagues began working on a live **vaccine** for mumps in the early 1960s, and the first vaccine—named after his daughter Jerilynn, whose cells it was made from—was licensed in 1967.

Today the mumps vaccine usually is given as part of the measles-mumps-rubella **immunization.**

Additional reading: Kiple, *The Cambridge World History of Human Disease,* pp. 887–89.

myelography

Myelography is a technique for imaging the spine in which radio-opaque agents are injected into the fluid surrounding the spinal cord and **X-rays** are taken. Early myelography was performed by injecting air into the spinal column, which was extremely painful for the patient.

Walter Dandy (1886–1946) introduced ventriculography, for viewing the cavities at the center of the brain, in 1918 and pneumoencephalography the following year. In pneumoencephalography, air is injected into the brain to make imaging of the brain easier. He published results of using this technique to diagnose spinal tumors in 1925. He had tried a number of liquids in animals, but results were always fatal.

In 1922, Jean Athenase Sicard (1873–1929) accidentally introduced iodized poppyseed oil (Lipiodol) into the cerebrospinal fluid of a patient and found the oil's high iodine content made it possible to visualize the spine with X-rays and detect tumors. But the liquid irritated the tissue of the spine and tended to form globules in the spinal fluid, which limited its use.

When William Jason Mixter (1880–1958) reported on herniated discs as a source of low back pain in 1934, the demand for myelography become more widespread despite its problems. Researchers in Rochester began using a substance called Pantopaque in 1940 and reported on it in 1944. This thinner substance didn't dissolve in cerebrospinal fluid, didn't irritate the spine, and didn't form globules.

A number of different agents have been introduced since then, all with their own drawbacks and benefits. The most popular today are iohexol and iopamidol.

Additional reading: Kevles, *Naked to the Bone,* pp. 103–04.

N

National Institutes of Health (NIH)

The National Institutes of Health constitute the major federal agency supporting medical research in the United States.

Located in Bethesda, Maryland, the institutes also fund training of medical researchers and provide health information to the public. The institutes' requested budget for 1999 was roughly $14.7 billion.

The **U.S. Public Health Service's** Hygiene Laboratory, which began as a one-room facility on Staten Island, New York, was renamed the National Institutes of Health by the Ransdell Act of 1930, which included a grant of $750,000 for building new facilities. The buildings that the NIH now occupy were built on a donated 45-acre site in Bethesda. The first buildings opened in 1938.

In 1937, Congress unanimously passed the National **Cancer** Act, which established the National Cancer Institute, the first institute to be founded. The most recently established institute is the National Human Genome Research Institute, formed in 1989. There are currently 18 different institutes focusing on various areas of health and medical research.

Additional reading: Harden, *Inventing the NIH*.

needle exchange programs

Needle exchange programs are intended to prevent the spread of disease among intravenous (IV) drug users by providing free, clean needles in exchange for used ones. Some programs also provide bleach to IV drug users to allow them to clean their "works" themselves, and also offer counseling on drug use and safe sex to participants.

The impetus for these programs began with the rise of **AIDS** in the 1980s, a viral disease that can be transmitted from person to person by contaminated hypodermic needles. About one-third of cases of AIDS in the United States are related to IV drug use, and most of all new cases of HIV infection are thought to be IV-drug related. There are believed to be between 1.1 and 1.9 million IV drug users in the United States.

In 1984, a needle exchange was set up in Amsterdam, the Netherlands by the city's municipal health service, at the behest of a group of drug users. Several European nations and Australia followed with similar programs. Needle-exchange programs have been slow to develop in the United States, however, largely because of some **public health** and government officials' fear that by providing addicts with clean needles they will appear to condone illegal drug use.

Since the early 1980s, volunteer groups have set up unofficial, and in some cases illegal, distribution centers for clean needles. The first legal needle-exchange programs in the United States were established in New York City (1988) and Washington, D.C. (1992). There are currently approximately 75 needle exchange programs in 55 U.S. cities. Since 1988, Congress has banned the use of federal funds to help pay for these programs.

In a 1995 report, a federal panel assembled by the National Research Council and the Institute of Medicine concluded that needle exchange and bleach distribution alone would not be effective in stopping the spread of HIV and other blood-borne diseases. However, many **addiction** experts disagree with the panel's findings.

Additional reading: Stolberg, "President Decides Against Financing Needle Programs."

neurons

Neurons are the cells that make up the nervous system.

Czech pathologist Christian Gottfried Ehrenburg (1795–1896) first described neurons in 1836. One year later, Ehrenburg and physiologist Johannes Evangelista Purkinje (1787–1867) identified neurons in the central nervous system. These cells, which he found in the cerebellum and called "flask-shaped ganglion bodies," came to be called Purkinje cells. One of Ehrenburg's pupils, Gabriel Gustav Valentin (1810–1883), described the cell nucleus and capsule of the neuron in 1843.

In 1838, one of the originators of the **cell theory**, Theodore Schwann (1810–1882), described the myelin sheath that surrounds and protects neurons.

Otto Friedrich Karl Dieters (1834–1863) described the dendrites and axons of the nerve cells in 1865, while Camillo Golgi (1843–1926) provided the world's first full and accurate description of the whole nerve cell in 1873, working in his home kitchen with a silver stain he developed.

Two theories of nervous system structure, the reticular theory and the neuron doctrine, competed with one another in the nineteenth century. Adherents of the reticular theory believed that the nervous system was made up of a continuous net of dendrites. The other theory, set forth largely by Wilhelm His (1863–1934) and August Forel (1848–1931), was that individual cells were the basis of the nervous system. Heinrich Wilhelm Gottfried Waldeyer (1837–1921) coined the word "neuron" and claimed correctly in 1891 that the nervous system consisted of cells with an axon that "sent" impulses and dendrites that "received" impulses.

Santiago Ramon y Cajal (1852–1934) confirmed the neuron theory in several studies published from 1892 to 1907. Cajal and Golgi shared the 1906 Nobel Prize for physiology and medicine.

The discovery of the structure and function of these cells has made a number of advances possible, from neurological surgery to local **anesthesia**.

Additional reading: McHenry and Garrison, *Garrison's History of Neurology,* pp. 139–79.

NIH. *See* National Institutes of Health.

911

Throughout the United States, people can dial "911" for emergency assistance.

The idea for a national emergency telephone number dates back to pre-World War II Britain. In London during the war, a call to "999" prompted a flashing light at the switchboard telephone exchange, which would cue the operator to answer the call quickly and route it to the appropriate place. Belgium, Denmark, and Sweden established similar systems in the 1960s.

The impetus for establishing a national emergency number system in the United States came from the National Association of Fire Chiefs. The group recommended a single number for fire reporting in 1958. In 1967, a presidential commission suggested implementing such a number for reporting other emergencies as well as fires. The Federal Communications Commission (FCC) and the American Telephone and Telegraph company (AT&T) met that year to investigate the feasibility of a national emergency number. In 1968, AT&T announced that the number would be "911." Congress backed the proposal, and the first 911 call was made soon afterwards by an Alabama senator. AT&T began developing a pilot 911 program with selective call routing in Alameda County, California, and the state sponsored the first statewide 911 legislation in 1978.

In 1973, the White House established a Federal Information Center to help localities develop their own 911 systems. In 1979, nine states had enacted 911 legislation and about a quarter of the U.S. population had 911 service.

Currently, nearly 93 percent of the U.S. Population has access to 911 service. Systems are funded in various ways, from the tax base, from directory assistance calls, from surcharges on long distance calls, and by other methods.

Additional reading: The National Emergency Number Association's World Wide Web site at http://www.nena9–1–1.org.

nitrogen mustards

Nitrogen mustards were the first nonhormonal chemicals demonstrated to have anticancer activity.

Researchers from New Haven, Salt Lake City, Boston, and Portland tried a type of nitrogen mustard known as mechlorathamine on 67 patients with lymphosarcoma, **Hodgkin's disease**, and **leukemia** in the early 1940s. In a paper published in 1946, the team reported that nitrogen mustard brought on remission in several patients. Previously, the only treatment for these **cancers** had been **radiation therapy**.

Scientists hit on nitrogen mustard as a possible treatment for leukemias because its chemical cousin, sulfur mustard (the mustard gas used in chemical warfare during World War I) was known to cause the spleen and lymph nodes to shrink and the number of white blood cells to drop. In leukemia, white blood cells proliferate and the spleen and lymph nodes swell, so scientists surmised that the mustard compounds could be an effective treatment for the disease.

Nitrogen mustard was the first of a class of chemicals called the **alkylating agents**, which are palliatives for cancer treatment, meaning that they do not cure the disease but they can induce remission. Nitrogen mustards such as cyclophosphamide and melphalan are still used in cancer treatment today.

Additional reading: Weisse, *Medical Odysseys,* pp. 127–33.

nitroglycerin

Nitroglycerin is a chemical used to ease **angina pectoris**, the chest pain that occurs when the heart muscle doesn't get enough oxygen due to blockage of the blood vessels. Nitroglycerin is also an explosive, but is used medically in amounts too small to set off an explosion. The chemical was first synthesized in 1847.

The **homeopathic** physician Constantine Hering (1800–1880) was the first person to propose that nitroglycerin might have therapeutic use. He tested thousands of substances on healthy people to see if they had potential as medicine, a process called "proving." The homeopathic credo that "like is cured by like" suggests that if a medicine produces an effect in a healthy person, it can be used to treat a person with that symptom. When Hering and his provers found that a taste of nitroglycerin brought on a powerful headache, they deduced that it might be a good headache treatment. Hering named his nitroglycerin preparation "Glonione," and prescribed it for treating pain along the nerves (known as neuralgia) and other painful conditions

Meanwhile, **amyl nitrate**—related to nitroglycerin because it is also nitrite-based—was being used to treat angina pectoris. In 1879, William Murrell (1853–1912) proposed using nitroglycerin to treat angina pectoris as well, after trying it on himself and noticing its powerful effects. Murrell tested the substance in 35 people and treated his first angina patient with nitroglycerin in 1878, using a sphygmograph to record the man's pulse. The patient responded well. Today, nitroglycerin, which is now known to work by dilating the blood vessels in the heart, is a mainstay of angina treatment.

Additional reading: Sneader, *Drug Discovery,* pp. 140–43.

nitrous oxide

Nitrous oxide, or "laughing gas," was one of the first agents to be used in **anesthesia,** and is still commonly used in dental procedures today.

Joseph Priestley (1733–1804) discovered nitrous oxide in 1772. Although he didn't propose using the gas as an anesthetic, he did investigate the use of inhaled gases for medical purposes, a discipline known as "pneumatic medicine." Humphrey Davy (1778–1829), a superintendent at Priestley's Pneumatic Medicine Institute in Bristol, did a considerable amount of research on nitrous oxide; he coined the term "laughing gas" and invented a nitrous oxide inhaler. In his 1800 book, *Researches Chemical and Philosophical, Chiefly Concerning Nitrous Oxide and Dephlogisticated Nitrous Air and its Respiration,* Davy reported his experience of easing the pain of a wisdom tooth with periodic inhalations of the gas, and suggested it be used for surgery.

This did not happen, however, until 1844. The dentist Horace Wells (1815–1848) attended a nitrous oxide party given by his colleague Gardner Q. Colton (1814–1898), a doctor. Wells noticed that one guest bruised his leg and felt no pain. Suffering from a painful tooth, he asked Colton to anesthetize him with nitrous oxide while another dentist removed the tooth.

With his former student William Morton (1819–1868), Wells attempted to demonstrate nitrous oxide anesthesia at an amphitheater at Massachusetts General Hospital in 1845. The demonstration failed when his patient screamed, the audience booed, and Wells was physically ejected. Wells continued to use nitrous oxide in his practice, however.

Morton would go on to participate in a much more effective demonstration of **ether** anesthesia in 1846.

Although nitrous oxide did not turn out to be effective for general anesthesia, it is still used today for minor surgeries, such as dental procedures.

Additional reading: Friedman and Friedland, *Medicine's 10 Greatest Discoveries,* pp. 94–114.

nonsteroidal anti-inflammatory drugs (NSAIDS)

NSAIDS relieve pain, fight inflammation, and lower fever. **Aspirin**, discovered in 1898, was the first NSAID marketed commercially; it is derived from salicin, a substance found

in willow bark reported by Reverend Edmond Stone (unknown–1768) in 1763 to be "efficacious in curing aguish [feverish] and intermittent disorders."

There are three classes of NSAIDs: carboxylic acids (which includes the salicylates, acetic acids, propionic acids, and fenamates); the pyrazoles; and the oxicams. **Ibuprofen** and naproxen, both propionic acids, are widely used.

The mechanism by which aspirin and other salicylics act wasn't explained until 1971, when Sir John Vane (1927–), winner of the 1982 Nobel Prize, found that these drugs prevented inflammation by interrupting the synthesis of **prostaglandin**. He later observed that nearly all NSAIDs have this effect.

During the 1990s, researchers have learned that NSAIDs may also disrupt inflammation by preventing the activation of cells that promote inflammation in its early stages. Some NSAIDs have other healthful effects; aspirin's effectiveness in preventing stroke and heart attack is widely known, and NSAIDs may also prevent colon **cancer**. Aspirin's vascular effects come from its inhibition of prostaglandin, which influences blood clotting, but the mechanism by which NSAIDs protect the colon remains unknown.

Unfortunately, NSAIDs also can cause ulcers and bleeding in the gastrointestinal system; this is related to their effects on prostaglandin synthesis. New drugs known as **COX-2 inhibitors** may provide the beneficial effects of NSAIDs without their drawbacks.

Additional reading: Sneader, *Drug Discovery,* pp. 91–95.

norepinephrine

Norepinephrine, also known as noradrenaline, is a substance produced by the adrenal gland that is the chief substance involved in transmitting impulses in the sympathetic nervous system. It is a precursor to the neurotransmitter **epinephrine.**

Thomas Elliott (1877–1961) at Cambridge University had first suggested that norepinephrine was the main substance involved in sympathetic nerve transmission.

Swedish physician Ulf von Euler (1905–1983) isolated norepinephrine and identified it as a neurotransmitter, publishing his findings in 1946. Researchers at the Sterling Winthrop Research Institute in Rensselaer, New York, introduced an artificial form of norepinephrine as a treatment for **shock**.

Von Euler shared the 1970 Nobel Prize for his work, which helped in subsequent research on nerve activity and the development of treatments for nerve disease.

Additional reading: Ziegler and Lake, eds., *Norepinephrine.*

Nuremburg Code

The Nuremburg Code is a set of 10 ethical principles for medical research. Three U.S. judges devised the code in 1947, at the outset of the trial of Nazi physicians who had conducted barbaric experiments on prisoners in concentration camps. The code was the first set of ethical guidelines protecting human research subjects.

The code requires that subjects give uncoerced, **informed consent** to any experiment they participate in, and that they be able to withdraw from an experiment at any time. Also, the code demands that researchers protect subjects' rights.

Experts now believe that code writers intended the principles not just as a basis for punishing Nazi doctors but as an ethical framework for all investigators conducting research on human subjects, although the Code docs not specifically say this.

Unfortunately, the code has never been officially adopted by medical association researchers—including those in the United States or any government. The notorious Tuskeegee study, in which treatment for **syphilis** was withheld from a group of black men without their knowledge or consent, began after World War II. During the Cold War, radiation experiments were conducted on unknowing subjects, and U.S. soldiers were given experimental drugs during the Gulf War without their consent.

Although the Code itself has not been adopted by any nation or medical association, federal laws, as well as many international guidelines on medical research, are based on the principles. In 1964, the World Medical Association (a physicians' group founded during World War II), made the Helsinki Declaration, which implicitly acknowledges the Nuremburg Code. In 1966, the United Nations adopted the Code's central tenet, informed consent, in its International Covenant on Civil and Political Rights. The **World Health Organization (WHO)** also based its 1993 International Ethical Guidelines for Biomedical Research Involving Human Subjects on the definition of informed consent as presented in the Code. Finally, U.S. federal guidelines on medical research are modeled on the Code.

Additional reading: Annas and Groden, *The Nazi Doctors and the Nuremberg Code.*

oncogenes

Oncogenes are **genes** that promote the growth of **cancer**. Proto-oncogenes, the normal versions of these genes, manage cell growth, differentiation, and proliferation, while the defective versions, oncogenes, promote cancer growth by allowing unsuppressed, abnormal growth. Scientists now know that a series of molecular "mistakes" can lead to cancer, and oncogenes are one contributing factor.

In 1976, Harold Varmus (1939–) and J. Michael Bishop (1936–) of the University of California, San Francisco, reported that normal cells carry genes that can cause cancer when they malfunction. Varmus and Bishop won the 1989 Nobel Prize for their discovery.

Scientists had begun searching for genetic mutations that might be responsible for cancer growth in the 1970s. The first was found in a virus that had been discovered in 1911 and was known to cause tumors in chickens. The dangerous version contained an extra gene, which was dubbed "src," short for sarcoma.

In 1975, Bishop and Varmus found src's normal counterpart in chickens, and in virtually every other animal from fish to humans. They theorized that this gene, which was active in normal cells, was important in normal cell activity. Somehow the virus had picked up the normal gene long ago; it was then mutated into a form that promoted tumor growth.

Researchers at MIT, Cold Spring Harbor, and the National Cancer Institute isolated the first human oncogene, ras, in 1980–81. A mutation of one of the 6,600 nucleotides in the ras proto-oncogene is enough to make it **carcinogenic**. To date, more than 60 oncogenes have been isolated, including the breast cancer genes **BRCA1, 2**.

The presence of certain oncogenes can be a valuable tool to determine a cancer patient's prognosis as well as the type of treatment his or her tumor will respond to best.

Additional reading: Lyon and Gorner, *Altered Fates,* pp. 324–28; Fujimura, *Crafting Science.*

opiate antagonists

Opiate antagonists are drugs that block the activity of opiates by attaching themselves to opiate receptors in the brain without producing a euphoric effect.

These drugs are useful in the treatment of some addictions, as well as for speeding withdrawal from opiates. However, they are useful only for individuals who are highly motivated to kick their **addiction**. They were initially investigated for their potential as nonaddicting painkillers, but the fact that they tended to produce **depression** limited their usefulness.

The first useful member of this drug class was nalorphine, developed in 1942 by Elton Leeman McCawley (1915–) of Yale School of Medicine with the support of the drug company Merck. Unfortunately, these opiate antagonists also tended to produce depression, and their effects were not long-lasting.

The first opiate antagonist that was useful for treating opiate addiction was naloxone, synthesized in 1960 by Harold Blumbert (1909–) and his colleagues at Endo Labs in Richmond Hill, New York. The drug was an improvement because, unlike nalorphine, it did not produce physical dependence. However, because naloxone's effects only last for a day, it wasn't practical.

Naltrexone, a drug made by the drug company Dupont-Merck that was approved by the **Food and Drug Administration (FDA)** in 1984, acts longer (it can be given in weekly doses) with fewer side effects, and is now used to treat **heroin** addicts as well as alcoholics. It is believed to ease craving for the drug. (*See also* alcoholism)

Additional reading: Winslow, "Heroin Remedy to be Marketed for Alcoholism;" Stine and Kosten, eds., *New Treatments for Opiate Dependence.*

opium

Opium is an ancient drug that comes from the sap of *Papaver somniferum*, a type of poppy. It is the precursor of all opiate drugs such as **heroin, morphine**, and codeine.

Opium is mentioned in ancient texts as a medicine and poison, but not as a drug of abuse. Greek and Roman authors wrote about opium as a painkiller. The drug was likely not widely abused for centuries because the supply was controlled by priests and physicians.

Opium abuse was first mentioned in Arab literature in about 1000 A.D. Opium spread to the Far East, where it was used regularly as a recreational drug as well as a folk medicine. Smoking of opium is believed to have begun in the Dutch East Indies and spread to Formosa and China from there.

Opium smoking began to cause social problems in China in the eighteenth century and in the following century the Opium Wars occurred when Chinese rulers tried to stop the British from importing the drug to their country. Opium remained a medicine in Europe until the beginning of the nineteenth century, when people began using it for recreation as well as to treat pain, digestive problems, and melancholy. Babies and children were also regularly given opium to quiet them. Physicians freely prescribed opium for a constellation of conditions, and the drug was also available as a home remedy. Artists and writers, such as Thomas De Quincey (1785–1859) and Charles Baudelaire (1821–1867), wrote about the painful effects of opium **addiction** as well as its pleasures.

During the 1800s, chemists began isolating the components of opium, such as morphine, which came into use as painkillers but were also abused.

The United States attempted to control opium use beginning in the late 1800s with a series of laws, and limited the right to produce opium to American citizens, culminating with a ban on the importation of opium in 1909. The Harrison Act, passed in 1914 but not enforced until World War I, taxed the production of **cocaine** and opiates and also made it more difficult for physicians to prescribe the drug.

Today, morphine is used medically as a painkiller while heroin is the main opiate of abuse.

Additional reading: Booth, *Opium.*

ophthalmoscope

An ophthalmoscope is an instrument for examining the inside of the eye, especially the retina, the lining of the eye that receives images from the lens and transmits them to the optic nerve. The instrument allows a doctor to check the eye for cataracts, **glaucoma**, and other eye problems, and can also reveal the effects of underlying conditions, such as high **blood pressure** and **diabetes mellitus**, on the retinal blood vessels.

Hermann von Helmholtz (1821–1894) invented an instrument for viewing the retina that he presented to his colleagues in Berlin in 1851. Specially designed angles of reflection and illumination, consisting of a series of lenses and mirrors, allowed the user to peer through the subject's pupil to see the back of his or her eye, where the retina lies.

Over the years, several modifications have been made to improve visualization of the retina, including the first electric ophthalmoscope, invented in 1885.

Additional reading: Fisher, *Ophthalmoscopy, Retinoscopy and Refraction with a New Chapter on Orthoptics.*

oral rehydration therapy

Oral rehydration therapy is the use of a solution containing sugar, salt, and water to treat dehydration (usually caused by diarrhea), the leading killer of children in the developing world.

Intravenous rehydration treatment was introduced in the 1920s, but this expensive therapy had to be given in the hospital and was basically unavailable to most people in the developing world. Children given intravenous therapy were also not given food because of the mistaken belief that the digestive system needed to rest, so they often had to stay in the hospital for weeks to recover.

Doctors experimented with a number of oral therapies, from dehydrated bananas to carrot soup, but these worked much less reliably than intravenous treatment. Research on electrolytes at Yale University led investigators to advocate solutions that contained potassium, sodium, and glucose. Meanwhile, physiologists working in the 1950s discovered the mechanism by which sodium was transported through the intestine, which required the presence of glucose, providing more evidence for the wisdom of combining sodium and glucose.

Captain Robert A. Phillips (1906–) first tried an oral glucose-sodium solution in **cholera** patients in the Philippines in 1961 with great success. Phillips used a concentration that was too high in his subsequent clinical trial of the therapy, and several patients died.

Public health researchers working in Pakistan and India in the early 1960s developed oral rehydration therapy to treat diarrhea caused by cholera. The treatment was not introduced worldwide until the 1970s. Even though the therapy became widely used in the developing world in the early 1970s, the U.S. medical establishment has been slow to accept it—possibly because intravenous therapy brings higher reimbursement from insurance companies.

The **World Health Organization (WHO)** formulated a standard oral rehydration solution that was introduced in 1971. In the early 1980s, workers in Asia developed new solutions based on local foods such as rice, corn, wheat, and potato. Today, this therapy saves the lives of more than 1 million people every year. These complex carbohydrate-based solutions are more effective than glucose-based ones for treating diarrhea. However, both types of solutions are used today. Controversy continues about the ideal composition of oral rehydration therapy solutions.

Additional reading: Dahlburg, "Simple Oral Therapy Helps Third World in Fight Against Diarrhea."

orthodontia

Orthodontia is the dental specialty of using braces, retainers, and other appliances to align the teeth properly, for health reasons as well as for cosmetic purposes.

A Roman author at around the time of the birth of Christ wrote that pushing a tooth "with the finger, day by day, toward the place that was occupied by the one extracted" was an effective method for replacing a permanent tooth that had grown in too early and had to be removed.

During the Middle Ages, orthodontia basically consisted of pulling the offending teeth. A German author in the 1500s also wrote about giving the teeth a daily push toward their proper place. French dentist Pierre Fauchard (1678–1781) designed what was likely the first dental appliance, the "bandolet," in the 1700s. The device pushed apart the upper teeth, forming the palate into an "ideal arch." American and French dentists in the 1700s and 1800s used ligatures, plates, bands, wedges, and arches to pull or push teeth into proper alignment.

The specialty of orthodontia began to emerge around the turn of the nineteenth century. Edward H. Angle (1855–1930) established the first school of orthodontia in 1900 for postgraduates in dentistry. The manufacture of standardized orthodontic appliances also began during this time. In the next decade, appliance makers began to use stainless steel, rather than gold and silver.

During the 1950s, **health insurance** plans made orthodontia available to many more working families, and braces became a common sight in the mouths of American children.

Attachment of wires to brackets glued to the teeth, rather than to metal bands surrounding the teeth, was pioneered by several U.S. orthodontists in the mid-1950s. Plastic resin was used to attach the brackets of the teeth, which were often etched with acid so that the attachment remained secure. However, the brackets were not widely accepted until the late 1970s.

Recent advances in orthodontia include the use of alloys containing nickel, titanium, copper, and cobalt for brace wires. The newer materials make it possible to use smaller wires, and some exert continuous steady pressure on the teeth so that they are straightened more quickly. (*See also* dentistry)

Additional reading: Ring, *Dentistry.*

osmosis

Osmosis is the passage of a dissolved material through a semipermeable membrane from a region of higher concentration to a region of lower concentration, eventually resulting in equal concentration on either side of the membrane.

This phenomenon plays a central role in the distribution and filtering of material throughout the body, for example in the capillary system and in the kidneys.

The French physiologist and physicist Henri Dutrochet (1776–1847) discovered osmosis after observing the action of water in snail sperm sacs. He named this action "endosmose," and presented his findings to the Academy of Sciences in Paris in 1826. Dutrochet believed, correctly although simplistically, that "endosmose" accounted for the movement of sap in plants and water in animals.

Additional reading: Pickstone, "Discovering the Movement of Life."

osteopathy

Osteopathy is a school of medicine based on the ideas of Hippocrates (c.460–c.377 B.C.). The original osteopaths believed that manipulating the joints would promote better circulation throughout the body and thus improve health.

Andrew Taylor Still (1828–1917) founded the American School of Osteopathy in 1894 in Kirkville, Missouri. After his three children died of spinal meningitis, he began to experiment with manipulation of the muscles and bones as a healing technique. Before founding his school, he advertised himself as a "lightning bonesetter" and a "magnetic healer." Osteopathy is somewhat similar to **chiropractic**, but its main focus is on increasing the range of motion and treating muscle spasm, while chiropractic focuses on moving bones to ease pressure on the nerves.

Osteopathic schools soon began to offer conventional medical courses, although Still objected. The walls between osteopathic and conventional medicine in the United States began to break down in the 1950s. Today, doctors of osteopathy often enter medical residencies and internships, and their training is basically equivalent to that of medical doctors.

Additional reading: Gevitz, *The D.O.s.*

osteoporosis

In osteoporosis, the bones lose mass and become weaker and more susceptible to fracture. This "brittle bone disease" is common in post-menopausal women and may also strike men. Smoking, low calcium and **vitamin D** consumption, a sedentary lifestyle, and long-term use of corticosteroids and certain other drugs all can contribute to osteoporosis.

During a person's lifetime, new bone is continually added to the skeleton and old bone is reabsorbed. Osteoporosis occurs when resorption outpaces new bone growth, and is more likely to strike people who failed to build up enough bone mass during childhood and early adulthood.

The "shrinkage" in height that occurs with age is due to osteoporosis, which causes the vertebrae to fracture and collapse into one another. Approximately 1.5 million fractures sustained in the United States annually are due to osteoporosis.

Fuller Albright (1900–1969) and his colleagues first identified osteoporosis as a disease in 1941, but evidence of age-related bone loss has been found in skeletons more than 4,000 years old.

Today women are urged to prevent osteoporosis by consuming enough calcium, getting enough weight-bearing exercise, and quitting smoking. Hormone replacement therapy after menopause can help to slow bone loss.

During the 1990s, some drugs became available to maintain bone density and, in some cases, add bone mass. These include biphosphonates, such as alendronate (released in 1997), which increases bone density; selective estrogen receptor modulators (SERMs) or "designer" estrogens such as raloxifene, which prevent bone loss; and the hormone calcitonin, which halts bone loss and may increase bone density. Other treatments being investigated include new biphosphonates and SERMs, sodium fluoride, parathyroid hormone, and drugs derived from vitamin D.

Additional reading: Gaby, *Preventing and Reversing Osteoporosis.*

otoscope

An otoscope is a device for examining the inside of the ear. Anton von Troltsch (1829–1890) invented the otoscope in 1860. Adam Politzer (1835–1920), an otoscopy expert, took the first photograph of the tympanic membrane, or eardrum, five years later.

Today, the otoscope is an important tool for physical exams. Doctors use it to look for inflammation in the ear that could be a symptom of ear infection.

Additional reading: Moser, *Ears; Coping with Ear Infections; How to Use an Otoscope.*

ovariotomy

Ovariotomy is the surgical removal of an ovary, or the removal of a tumor from the ovary.

The first ovariotomy was the removal of a 22-pound tumor from the ovary of Jane Todd Crawford by Dr. Ephraim McDowell (1771–1830) in 1809, before the days of **antisepsis** or **anesthesia**. McDowell was Danville, Kentucky's only surgeon.

Crawford rode 60 miles on horseback to have the operation. According to her grandson, she read the Psalms during the 25-minute surgery. McDowell probably used hot water as an antiseptic.

The patient was up and about within 5 days, and she returned home on horseback 20 days later. She went on to live for 33 more years.

McDowell is believed to have performed at least 12 operations on the ovaries. His surgery on Crawford was not only the first ovariotomy; it was also the first successful abdominal surgery. Today, ovariotomy is used to treat ovarian **cancer**.

Additional reading: Ellis, *Famous Operations*, pp. 3–12.

P

pacemaker

A pacemaker is a device used to regulate the heartbeat of a person suffering from cardiac arrhythmias, which can be life-threatening. The pacemaker issues electrical impulses that pace the heart.

In 1952, Paul Zoll (1911–1999) of Boston kept a patient with heart arrhythmia alive for several weeks using electrical impulses delivered externally. The first internal pacemaker, developed by the Swedish doctor Rune Elmqvist, was implanted in a patient in 1958. Although the patient only lived for a few hours, the device did work.

Subsequent researchers have developed pacemakers that help the heart beat in a more normal rhythm, treat various types of arrythmias, and respond to variations in activity level and chemical changes within the heart.

In the 1980s, lithium batteries extended the life of pacemakers and advances in microelectronics and microprocessing made external reprogramming of pacemakers possible. Today, pacemaker batteries last from six to ten years.

Additional reading: Weisse, *Medical Odysseys,* p. 139–50.

Pap smear (Papanicolaou test)

A Pap smear is a screening exam for **cancer** in which shed cells are analyzed. The most common type of Pap test is the Pap smear for **cervical cancer**, in which cells from the vagina and uterus are sampled and analyzed for precancerous changes. The test is named for George Papanicolaou (1883–1962), the Greek scientist who invented it.

While working as a research fellow at Columbia University, Papanicolaou had noticed that vaginal discharge from guinea pigs contained many cells from the reproductive system. That evening he tried the first "Pap smear" on his wife Andromache, and subsequently observed that cell patterns could be correlated to ovarian cycles, hormonal shifts, and changes in the uterus. He published the results of his work with guinea pigs in 1917.

A number of other researchers using his technique made major discoveries, including the 1923 discovery of **estrogen**.

Papanicolaou began examining cells from women volunteers in 1925, and found that the Pap smear could detect **cancer** cells, too. He reported this finding three years later.

His colleagues took little notice of this finding until 1939, when Papanicolaou began a **clinical trial**. Starting that year, every woman admitted for gynecological care to New York Hospital had a Pap smear. By studying these samples, Papanicolaou learned that the vaginal smears could reveal early, precancerous changes in the cervix long before symptoms developed. He published his findings in 1941.

The American Cancer Society endorsed the Pap smear for cervical cancer prevention in 1945. Papanicolaou published an exhaustive book of his observations, the 1954 *Atlas of Exfoliative Cytology.*

Today the Pap smear has made **cervical cancer** much less threatening, because it allows this disease to be detected at an early, treatable stage. Cervical cancer is now the fourteenth most common cancer in the United States; it had previously been the second. Before the Pap smear, 32,000 U.S. women died of cervical cancer each year. In 1997, 4,900 women died of cervical cancer. In most developing nations, where Pap smears are unavailable, cervical cancer remains the leading killer of women.

In the 1990s, efforts began to improve the accuracy of Pap smears by using computer technology to analyze samples.

Additional reading: Speert, *Obstetric & Gynecologic Milestones Illustrated,* pp. 256–61.

parathyroid

The parathyroid glands are a set of four small glands located near the **thyroid gland** at the base of the neck that secrete hormones regulating calcium and phosphorus metabolism. Because the proper regulation of these minerals in the body is essential to life, loss of or damage to the parathyroids can be fatal. It can also produce muscle cramps and spasms because mineral metabolism is vital to normal nerve and muscle function. Hypoparathyroidism, a condition in which the gland fails to secrete these **hormones,** can be caused by **autoimmune disease** or injury during surgery.

Sir Richard Owen (1804–1892) first reported the existence of the gland, in a rhinoceros, in 1852. Ivar Victor Sandstrom (1852–1889) first described the parathyroid, in 1880, and was the first to show that removing this gland was fatal. During the following decade, the thyroid and parathyroid were proved to be distinct organs. Researchers also found that removing the parathyroid led to muscle spasms.

In 1909, William George MacCallum (1874–1944) showed that a decrease in blood calcium accompanied these muscle spasms. Two years later, removing the parathyroid was shown to cause the body to excrete more phosphate.

In the 1920s, James Collip (1892–1965) and his colleagues produced active extracts of parathyroid hormone, making it possible to treat hypoparathyroidism with hormone supplementation. (*See also* thyroid gland)

Additional reading: *McGraw-Hill Encyclopedia of Science and Technology, Vol. 13,* pp. 109–15.

Parkinson's disease

Parkinson's disease is a neurological condition in which a person develops tremors, weakness, and muscle stiffness. People with the disease eventually lose the ability to control their movements. There is no cure. The disease usually first strikes a person in late middle age. The cause is unknown.

The set of symptoms represented by Parkinson's disease is called "Parkinsonism"; a person may develop Parkinsonism after infection with **syphilis** or encephalitis, exposure to certain toxic chemicals, or from taking certain drugs. Ex-boxers may also develop Parkinsonism after suffering hundreds of blows to the head.

The disease was first described by James Parkinson (1755–1824) in his 1817 "An Essay on the Shaking Palsy," in which he described six cases of "paralysis agitans."

In the late 1950s, researchers determined that people with Parkinsonism had a deficiency of the neurotransmitter dopamine in a section of the brain called the neostriatum. In the early 1960s, trials of L-dopa, a substance that the body converts into dopamine, had varied success, although some patients' symptoms did significantly improve.

L-dopa, or levodopa, was the first drug found to reverse the symptoms of Parkinson's disease, and is still the main treatment for this illness.

Researchers tried higher dosages, which worked better but also produced more serious side effects. Changes in dosage of L-dopa and combinations with other drugs have since improved the effectiveness of the drug and reduced side effects.

In 1998, reports began coming in on a new treatment for treating Parkinson's: implanting brain cells from fetal pigs and humans in dopamine-deficient parts of patients' brains. These cells, from parts of the developing brain that produce dopamine, are intended to restore production of

the neurotransmitter in the brain. The results of the first clinical trial of fetal cell implants for Parkinson's disease, released in 1999 by researchers at Columbia-Presbyterian Medical Center in New York and the University of Colorado at Denver, found that the transplants helped some, but not all, patients.

Additional reading: Koller, *Handbook of Parkinson's Disease.*

pasteurization

Pasteurization is the heating of milk, wine, fruit juice, and other foodstuffs to a certain temperature to kill bacteria and prevent spoilage and fermentation. The technique is named for its inventor, Louis Pasteur (1822–1895).

The French scientist went against established thought—from Aristotle to Newton—and the Church by proposing that rot did not develop spontaneously and fermentation did not happen on its own. Instead, Pasteur said, tiny organisms contaminated the substance and used its sugars as food, producing byproducts such as alcohol in fermentation and vinegars when fermentation went on for too long. He described the best conditions for fermentation, including pH and temperature.

In the 1860s, Pasteur suggested that French wine producers could prevent spoilage by heating wine 55 to 60 degrees centigrade, which he believed would kill microorganisms without damaging the wine's flavor. The subsequent year, he proposed a heating method to protect the products of German beer makers. Pasteur went on to suggest that the organisms that caused fermentation were analogous to those that caused disease in humans, the beginnings of the **germ theory.**

Additional reading: Geison, *The Private Science of Louis Pasteur,* pp. 90–95.

PCR. *See* polymerase chain reaction.

pellagra

Pellagra is a disease caused by a deficiency of nicotinic acid (also known as niacin) that tends to strike people who eat diets based on corn or maize.

The Spanish physician Gaspar Casal (1679–1759) first described pellagra in 1730 in writings published in 1762. He called the disease *mal de la rosa* because one of the symptoms was redness of the face. Other symptoms include atrophy of the mucous membranes, diarrhea, and nervous system damage. The name pellagra comes from the Italian word for dry skin.

Proposed causes for pellagra included a toxic substance in corn, an infectious agent, or protein deficiency. Oversensitivity to sunlight was considered another possible cause.

Joseph Goldberger (1874–1929), a Hungarian-born American **public health** worker, began investigating pellagra in 1914 in response to an apparent epidemic of the disease in the southern United States. He noticed that although pellagra was considered contagious, hospital personnel who worked with pellagra patients did not become infected. He noted that children in orphanages who didn't eat meat or drink milk often developed pellagra, and he investigated whether the hospital diet, consisting of cornmeal, pork, and molasses, might be responsible. He sought and obtained extra funds to provide meat and milk to patients, which cleared up the disease. Goldberger and his colleagues thus attributed pellagra to overconsumption of corn.

Goldberger's claims weren't widely accepted. In 1917, a government commission concluded that pellagra was spread by the stable fly.

Another public health worker, Carl Voegtlin (1879–1960), learned in 1920 that yeast—known at that time to be rich in **vitamin B**—could cure pellagra. When it became clear that vitamin B1 and B2 did nothing to cure the disease, researchers began searching for the next B complex vitamin. Goldberger found liver was an excellent source of the "pellagra-preventing" factor. T.N. Spencer's previous discovery that a disease called black tongue in dogs was analogous to pellagra in humans made the search for the responsible factor much easier.

Goldberger and his colleagues began to narrow down the deficiency responsible for pellagra, finding in the 1920s that protein-free extracts of animal organ meats or yeast could prevent the condition.

Conrad A. Elvehejm (1901–1962) at the University of Wisconsin in Madison isolated the pellagra-preventive factor from liver in 1937, and found that it was a known substance called nicotinamide. He showed that this substance and the similar chemical nicotinic acid treated and prevented black tongue. Nicotinic acid had been synthesized 40 years before Elvehejm's discovery that it prevented pellagra.

Researchers later found that nicotinic acid in corn is in a form that cannot be absorbed nutritionally unless the vegetable is made alkaline, for example through the process of making corn tortillas, which are first soaked in lime water.

When southern farmers began to diversify crops from cotton and produce vegetables and fruits, pellagra gradually disappeared.

Additional reading: Etheridge, *The Butterfly Caste;* Kiple, *The Cambridge World History of Human Disease,* pp. 918–24; McCollum, *A History of Nutrition,* pp. 302–18.

penicillin

Penicillin, a substance produced by mold that can kill certain bacteria, was the first **antibiotic** to be discovered.

Alexander Fleming (1881–1955), a Scottish doctor and **syphilis** expert, discovered penicillin, basically by accident, in 1928 in his London laboratory. While he was growing cultures of staphylococci in Petri dishes, unbeknownst to him a colleague was culturing the mold species *Penicillium notatum.* When Fleming returned from a two-week vacation, he observed that the *Penicillium* mold had contaminated his staphylococci culture. The area around the mold contained no staphylococci, so the mold had apparently killed or repelled the bacteria.

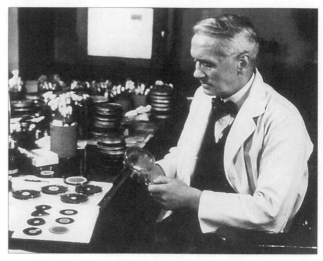

Sir Alexander Fleming in his laboratory. (Courtesy of The Wellcome Trust Medical Photographic Library, London.)

In 1929, Fleming published the results of his further research, which showed that the mold killed several different types of bacteria in culture and was nontoxic in small human and animal experiments. He did not, however, test the mold in infected animals or humans. Fleming thought the mold would be useful as a topical antibacterial agent, but he did not consider it as a drug to be taken internally. He soon abandoned his studies of penicillin for investigations of a substance he called "lysozyme," which he had found in his own nose and believed to have antibacterial properties.

A young doctor named C.G. Paine used the broth from a penicillin culture to treat eye infections in four babies, with dramatic results. He described his findings to pathologist Howard Florey (1898–1968).

In 1938, Gerhard Domagk (1895–1964) discovered the drug **prontosil,** which could cure streptococcal infections. This encouraged others to study penicillin because it proved that a drug given internally could indeed cure bacterial infections.

Meanwhile, at Oxford University in London, Ernst Chain (1906–1979), who was working under Florey, happened to have a culture of Fleming's *penicillium mold.* After he had read Fleming's paper, Chain ran into Florey's predecessor's assistant in the hall while she was carrying some of the culture, and obtained some for further experiments.

Florey and Chain found that the substance cured infections in animals, reporting their results in 1940. The Oxford team had managed to isolate penicillin, but found it difficult to produce in quantities sufficient to treat more than a handful of people. Their earliest test patients were often children or small adults, so less penicillin could be used.

A kind of "cottage industry" of small-scale penicillin producers sprang up in Great Britain, with the assistance of government aid, to supply the drug to British soldiers and civilians.

Working with Chain and Florey, U.S. scientists helped to devise methods to boost penicillin production. Kenneth B. Raper (1908–), a mold specialist working for the U.S. Department of Agriculture in Peoria, Illinois, isolated a high-producing *Penicillium chrysogenum* from a cantaloupe. Researchers at the Carnegie Institute in Cold Spring Harbor, New York, produced mutations in this mold using **X-rays** that resulted in an organism 10 times more productive than the original.

With the help of the Rockefeller Foundation and the drug companies Merck, Squibb, and Pfizer, large-scale production of penicillin in the United States began and by 1944, there was enough penicillin available to treat World War II casualties as well as civilians with serious infections. The following year, Florey, Chain, and Fleming shared the Nobel Prize for their work on penicillin and commercial sales of penicillin began.

From 1945 on, deaths from **influenza**, pneumonia, **syphilis**, and **diphtheria** fell dramatically thanks to penicillin. Penicillin also was the most effective treatment to date for **puerperal fever** and **gonorrhea.**

Today penicillin is commonly used to treat several types of bacterial infection.

Additional reading: Weisse, *Medical Odysseys,* p. 69–86; Friedman and Friedland, *Medicine's 10 Greatest Discoveries,* pp.168–91.

percussion

In percussion, a physician thumps a patient's chest and back with curved fingers and listens to the sound to check the condition of the heart and lungs.

Leopold Auenbrugger (1722–1809), an Austrian physician, first wrote about the technique in 1761. As a child, he had struck wine casks in his father's inn and noticed that the sound changed depending on how much wine was in the cask. When he later became a doctor, he began employing this technique in diagnosis.

Using percussion, physicians can tell if an area is solid or hollow or contains fluid. Percussion is especially useful for diagnosing an enlarged heart, lungs consolidated from pneumonia, or fluid in the heart and lungs.

Auenbrugger's contemporaries largely ignored his work, but Jean Nicholas Corvisart (1755–1821) translated his work into French in 1808 and practiced and taught the technique. Physicians use Auenbrugger's method today while giving patients physical exams.

Additional reading: Bynum, *Science and the Practice of Medicine in the Nineteenth Century,* pp. 35–37.

pernicious anemia

Pernicious **anemia** occurs when the stomach does not secrete enough of a substance known as intrinsic factor that allows the small intestine to absorb **vitamin** B12. This condition is usually caused by atrophy of the stomach glands. It results in a dramatic decrease in the number of blood cells, muscular weakness, and nerve dysfunction, and is fatal if left untreated.

The disease was first described in 1822, while in 1860 Austin Flint (1812–1886) suggested that some type of gastric juice deficiency caused it.

The Boston doctors George R. Minot (1885–1950) and William P. Murphy (1892–1987) were the first to develop a successful treatment for pernicious anemia. They prescribed an iron- and purine-rich diet containing liver or kidneys, muscle meat, fruit and vegetables, and little additional animal fat, publishing their results in 1926.

Minot and Murphy shared the 1930 Nobel Prize with another anemia researcher, George Whipple (1878–1976), and the three were the first Americans to be thus honored. Although they had found a treatment for pernicious anemia, they had not yet discovered the cause of the disease.

In 1928, the American doctor William Bosworth Castle (1897–1990) and his colleagues performed an experiment in which he ate hamburger, recovered a meat-and-gastric juice combination from his own stomach an hour later, and gave this substance to people with pernicious anemia, whose red blood cell count subsequently rose. Castle described the responsible substance in a 1936 article as "intrinsic factor" and argued that it must interact with an "extrinsic factor" from the meat to produce some substance that boosts the growth of red blood cells. Scientists at the drug company Merck isolated the extrinsic factor from liver in 1948. The gastritis that leads to pernicious anemia is now understood to be an **autoimmune disease,** thanks to research that began in the late 1950s and ultimately identified the specific **antigen** responsible in the late 1980s.

Treatment today consists of a special diet along with supplementation with vitamin B12 injection and iron.

Additional reading: Weisse, *Medical Odysseys,* pp. 112–24.

pertussis

Pertussis, or whooping cough, is an infectious disease of childhood that has now been largely wiped out in the developed world by **immunization**.

Pertussis was first recognized in the Middle Ages, and was called "the kink" (from a Scottish word meaning "fit") or the "kindhoest," from a Germanic word for child's cough.

The first recorded epidemic of pertussis occurred in Paris in 1578, and Guillaume de Baillou (1536–1616) gave the first detailed description of the disease in his account of the epidemic.

Jules Bordet (1870–1961) isolated the *Bordetella pertussis bacterium* responsible for the disease in 1906, and soon began attempting to make a vaccine from cultures of the bacteria. Effective vaccines were developed in the 1930s, and were routinely given to children by the mid-1940s, sometimes in conjunction with immunization for **tetanus** and **diphtheria** in the DPT vaccine.

Before immunization, pertussis was the leading killer of babies worldwide. Now there are about 600,000 deaths from pertussis each year.

Additional reading: Kiple, *The Cambridge World History of Human Disease,* pp. 1094–96.

PET scanning (positron emission tomography)

PET scanning is a technique for imaging metabolic activity in the body. It is particularly useful for following brain activity by measuring glucose consumption or blood flow in brain **tissues**.

PET scanning developed shortly after Godfrey Hounsfield (1919–) introduced **X-ray**-computed tomography, or **CAT scanning**. In CAT scanning, several X-ray images of the brain or body are taken and then combined and analyzed by a computer to create a cross-section image.

PET scanning works by the same principle, but it measures positron emission from the body after radioactive material has been introduced. PET scanning follows metabolic activity, rather than providing images alone. Hungarian physicist Georg von Hevesy (1885–1966) invented the radioactive tracers used in PET, winning the 1943 Nobel Prize for chemistry for this research.

Prototypes for PET scanning were the scintiscanner invented in 1951 at UCLA and the photoscan, invented three years later by David Kuhl (1929–), a medical student at the University of Pennsylvania. Kuhl's series of scanners were inspired by the work of his teachers Louis Sokoloff (1921–) and Seymour Kety (1915–), who were developing techniques in the 1950s to measure cerebral blood flow in live animals using radioactive isotopes. The researchers introduced positron-emitting radionuclides into the body and followed their location and concentration. The technique

was first used in humans in 1965. PET scanning involves using these techniques to make a more detailed image by combining information from multiple scans.

The first machine to provide a three-dimensional image of positron emission was the Single Photon Emission Computed Tomography (SPECT) machine, built in 1968 and based on Kuhl's system for mapping positron emission within the body.

In Michel Ter-Pogossian's (1825–1996) laboratory at Washington University in St. Louis, Michael Phelps (1939–) devised a system that measured emission rather than transmission, and featured CAT scan–like computer processing to produce a clear reconstruction of an image. His team reported the results of the new process, which they called positron emission transaxial tomography, in 1975.

The development of PET was, from the 1950s onward, subsidized by the United States Department of Energy, so it was better-funded than other developing imaging technologies such as CAT scanning and **MRI.** But PET scanning is also significantly more complex than these technologies, so it remains an expensive research tool rather than a clinical option in most cases.

Working with psychologists beginning in the 1980s, neurologists have used PET to study brain activity and have learned a great deal about cognitive function, such as the effects of psychoactive drugs on the brain, changes in brain activity and structure that accompany **addiction**, the functions of neurotransmitters, and much more. Today's PET scanners can complete scans in seconds.

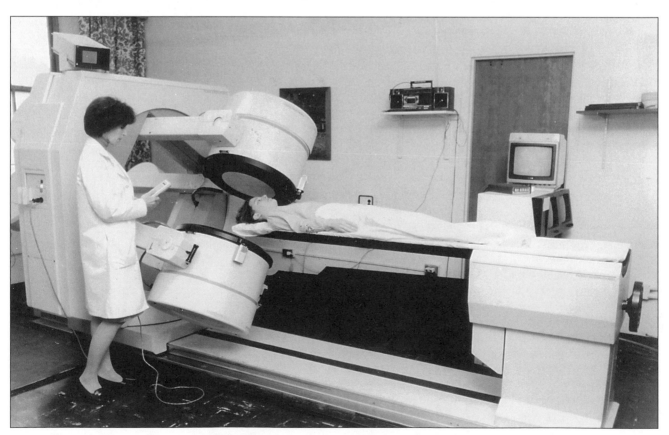

A patient receives a PET scan. (Courtesy of Archives and Special Collections, Columbia University Health Sciences Division.)

PET scanning can also reveal areas of brain dysfunction in **epilepsy**. Beginning in the 1980s, neurosurgeons began using PET scans to guide epilepsy surgery. Whole-body PET scanners were introduced in the early 1990s. These machines are used to detect and track **cancers** and follow the effectiveness of **chemotherapy**.

The clinical use of PET scanning is currently limited to diagnosing epilepsy and other brain disorders.

Additional reading: Kevles, *Naked to the Bone*, pp. 201–27.

PGD. See pre-implantation genetic diagnosis.

phagocytosis

Phagocytosis is the process by which white blood cells, called macrophages, engulf, consume, and destroy infectious agents within the body.

In 1884, Elie Metchnikoff (1845–1916) was the first person to observe and describe this process when he saw water fleas and starfish engulf foreign substances. He named the engulfment "phagocytosis." He also had seen white blood cells consuming germs, and theorized that these cells were like an army that fought infection in the body. Some other leading scientists concerned with the nascent science of immunology, including Paul Koch (1843–1910), disputed the importance of phagocytosis in the immune system, arguing that the serum of the blood and not the cells were responsible for fighting infection. It is now understood that both phagocytosis and other white blood cell actions, as well as the "humoral immunity" afforded by **antibodies** in the blood serum, make up the human immune system. Metchnikoff shared the 1908 Nobel Prize for his discovery.

Additional reading: Bynum, *Science and the Practice of Medicine in the Nineteenth Century*, pp. 159–60.

phototherapy

Phototherapy is the use of light—from sunshine to **lasers**—to treat disease. Light therapy was known to the Greeks as heliotherapy, and involved lying nude in the sun. In India, China, and Egypt light therapy was also used for skin diseases and even **mental illness**. Psoralen, a substance found in some plants that sensitizes the skin to sunlight, may be used in phototherapy, and was employed in India as early as 1400 B.C. People with vitiligo, a condition in which the skin is covered with white spots, applied pigments from seeds to the spots before lying in the sun.

In the 1800s, sunlight was used to treat **tuberculosis** of the skin and bones and to prevent **rickets**, a disease in which bones don't form properly because of the lack of **Vitamin D**.

The first person to use phototherapy in a modern sense was Niels Finsen (1860–1904), a Danish physician who treated lupus vulgaris (tuberculosis of the skin) with light from a carbon arc lamp. Finsen won the 1903 Nobel Prize in medicine for his work.

Photodynamic therapy is a version of therapy in which light is used to trigger the effect of certain medications. For **cancer**, a light-sensitive dye may be injected that goes directly to a tumor, where it is activated by laser. The first human trials of photodynamic therapy for cancer treatment were in 1978. Porphyrins are used today to specifically locate tumors, and dozens of studies of photodynamic therapy to treat various types of cancer are underway. Phototherapy is also used regularly to treat skin conditions such as psoriasis, and also to treat jaundice in newborns. It is also helpful for treating seasonal affective disorder (SAD), a condition in which people become depressed in the winter due to the lessening of sunlight.

Additional reading: Galton, *Med Tech*, pp. 307–10.

PHS. See U.S. Public Health Service.

physostigmine

Physostigmine is a cholinergic drug, meaning it intensifies the action of **acetylcholine** by inhibiting cholinesterase, a drug that breaks down this neurotransmitter. It improves muscle tone and strength, boosts the digestive system's peristaltic action, and constricts the pupils. Physostigmine is used as an antidote to strychnine poisoning and to treat **tetanus** and the muscle disease myasthenia gravis.

The drug is an extract of the Calabar bean, *Physostigma venenosum*. In the 1880s, explorers observed the use of this extract by people in West Africa in the Trial by Ordeal, in which a person accused of a crime would be given some extract. If he or she lived, innocence was proved, while death indicated guilt. A missionary living in Calabar reported on the effects of physostigmine in detail and sent some samples of the bean to Robert Christison (1797–1882) in Edinburgh. Christison tried a bit of bean himself, and found it made him weak. In animal studies, Christison's student Richard Frazer (1841–1920) discovered the bean's pupil-narrowing effects.

Douglas Argyll Robertson (1837–1909), an ophthalmologist looking for a vegetable extract that would reverse the pupil-dilating effects of belladonna and **atropine**, described the first clinical use of physostigmine, to constrict the pupil in people who couldn't tolerate light in 1863.

Today physostigmine is used to treat strychnine poisoning, tetanus, and a condition called myasthenia gravis that is characterized by muscular weakness and fatigue.

Additional reading: Brandt and Packer, "Opthamology's Botanical Heritage."

pineal gland

The pineal gland, a small structure shaped like a pine cone located at the center of the brain, produces the **hormone** melatonin. Its other functions are unknown.

The pineal gland was probably the first gland to be described anatomically. It has had mystical associations, and was thought to be the site of the "third eye" or the uppermost chakra in **Ayurveda**. The gland was described in the Indian Vedas of 300 to 400 B.C. Herophilus, an

Alexandrian physician of the third century B.C., is often credited with discovering the pineal gland; he believed it was a sphincter that controlled the flow of animal spirits. The Greek surgeon Claudius Galen (129–c.199) believed glands filled gaps in the body and supported large blood vessels, and had no other function. He named the pineal gland for its resemblance to a pine cone.

In the early twentieth century, researchers showed that removing the pineal gland in animals increased the size of sex organs and secondary sex characteristics.

During experiments, Yale dermatologist Alan Lerner (1920–) had noticed that extracts of the pineal gland lightened skin color, so he set out to try to identify the responsible substance. He isolated and identified the structure of melatonin, publishing his findings in 1958.

Several researchers in the 1960s found that the light/dark cycle had some effect on the pineal gland, and Wilbur Brooks Quay (1927–) showed in 1964 that melatonin production exhibits 24-hour periodicity. Although melatonin is believed to regulate sleep cycles, the precise role of the pineal gland in sexual development remains unclear.

In the 1990s, melatonin became a popular remedy for jet lag and sleep difficulties, but its true effectiveness for these purposes has not been confirmed.

Additional reading: Brezezinski, "Melatonin in Humans."

pituitary gland

The pituitary gland, located at the base of the skull, secretes and stores several different **hormones** to regulate the thyroid, adrenal cortex, ovaries, and testes. The gland has two sections, the anterior and posterior.

Efforts to determine the effect of secretions of the pituitary gland began in the late nineteenth century, when research into therapy with extracts of various glands began.

The first pituitary hormones to be isolated were vasopressin and oxytocin, in 1928 by scientists at the drug company Parke-Davis in Detroit. Both hormones are secreted by the posterior section of the pituitary. Vasopressin raises **blood pressure** and oxytocin increases uterine contractions. The two hormones were synthesized in 1953.

Vincent du Vigneaud (1901–1978) led efforts at George Washington University in Washington, D.C., to further purify the two hormones. He won the 1955 Nobel Prize for his work.

Human growth hormone, which is secreted by the anterior pituitary, was isolated in 1944 by Herbert Evans (1882–1971) and Choh Hao Li (1813–1987). A hormone that stimulated **adrenal gland** function was extracted from the gland in 1933 by James B. Collip (1892–1965) at McGill University in Montreal. This hormone, which came to be called adrenocorticotrophin, was initially used to treat arthritis when **cortisone** was scarce, but is rarely employed today.

Li isolated a follicle-stimulating hormone from the anterior pituitary in the 1950s.

Research into the role of the pituitary gland and its hormones continues today.

Additional reading: *McGraw-Hill Encyclopedia of Science and Technology,* Vol. 13, pp. 635–43.

placebo

A placebo is an inactive drug (usually a sugar pill) given to patients as part of a trial or, sometimes, to satisfy a patient's desire for a drug. "Placebo" is Latin for "I shall please."

The first mention of a placebo appears in George Motherby's *New Medical Dictionary* of 1785, which defines it as "a common place method or medicine." A later edition of the same dictionary, published in 1795, says placebos are "calculated to amuse for a time, rather than for any other purpose." As used here, "amuse" probably means to deceive or fool.

Thomas Jefferson (1743–1826) wrote that a placebo was a "pious fraud" intended to please the patient as well as the doctor.

During the 1940s, several placebo pills with names designed to produce an effect were distributed by doctors. These "fake drugs" were found in the 1970s to have some real physiological as well as psychological benefits, a phenomenon known as the placebo effect. Various studies have found that placebos are from 30 to 60 percent as effective as proven therapies.

Placebos are used in **clinical trials** to ensure adequate measurement of the effect of active drugs in the "double-blind" test, so named because neither doctor nor patient knows whether the patient is taking the real drug or a dummy pill.

Awareness of the powerful placebo effect is growing. Placebo or sham surgeries are increasingly being done during clinical trials, because studies have shown that the act of having an operation itself—regardless of what is done during the procedure—may help make patients better.

Additional reading: Harrington, ed., *The Placebo Effect.*

plastic surgery

Plastic surgery is performed to reconstruct body or facial structures after illness or injury or to reshape them for cosmetic reasons.

Surgery to correct facial imperfections began in the late nineteenth and early twentieth century. One pioneer was Dr. Charles C. Miller (1880–1950), who published several articles on plastic surgery and eventually his own journal. It is unclear, however, how many surgeries he actually performed and what his results were.

Modern plastic surgery was developed during World War I, after combat injuries made it necessary for surgeons to learn how to reconstruct the face and body. Trench warfare, steel helmets, and airplanes all contributed to devastating and numerous facial injuries among soldiers. Queens Hospital in Kent was a famous wartime center for reconstructive surgery. The hospital's director, Harold Delf Gillies (1882–1960), an otolaryngologist from New Zealand, invented a tubed pedicle, a surgical technique that made it possible to transfer skin from one area to another in stages without interrupting the blood supply.

The success of reconstructive surgeons during the war made what would become known as plastic surgery more respectable. Before the war, some "beauty surgeons" such as Miller performed cosmetic procedures, but mainstream physicians considered these practitioners to be unscrupulous. The reputation of surgery for cosmetic purposes alone—and the surgeons who performed these operations—improved somewhat after the war, but a faint aura of corruption persisted, according to historians of the specialty.

A group of reconstructive surgeons met in Chicago to organize a professional group in 1921, which became the American Association of Plastic Surgeons. The American Society of Plastic and Reconstructive Surgeons was founded in 1931 by Jacques W. Malniak (1889–1976). In 1937, Vilray P. Blair (1871–1955) organized the American Board of Plastic Surgery.

Plastic surgeons of the 1920s and 1930s who advertised their services were generally looked down upon by their colleagues. But plastic surgery for cosmetic purposes became increasingly acceptable to American women in the years after World War II, and enthusiastic articles in the popular press contributed to this acceptance. Cosmetic surgery began to be seen as psychologically healthy and even economically necessary. Men began seeking plastic surgery such as facelifts to restore youthful appearance in the 1960s.

Techniques to reshape the body, such as liposuction (introduced in the United States from France in 1981) and silicone implants to increase the size of breasts, calves, and even penises are now widely available and popular. Health risks of liposuction can include embolism, discolored skin, and death. (*See also* rhinoplasty)

Additional reading: Haiken, *Venus Envy*.

podophyllotoxin

Podophyllotoxin is a substance found in the mayapple or mandrake plant, *Podophyllum peltatum*, from which effective drugs for cancer **chemotherapy** have been derived. The drugs made from this substance work by breaking **DNA** strands in tumor cells. Podophyllum derivatives are also used to treat warts.

The mandrake has long been used in folk medicine. The extract of this North American plant was included in the first edition of the *United States Pharmacopoeia* in 1820, and widely used as a purgative.

Scientists at the Swiss pharmaceutical company Sandoz developed two podophyllin-related compounds in the mid-1950s that became the anticancer drugs etoposide and teniposide.

Clinical trials of etoposide began in 1971, and it was approved by the **Food and Drug Administration (FDA)** for treating testicular **cancer** in 1983. Marketing in some countries of teniposide, although not in the United States, began in the mid 1970s. In 1978, Sandoz handed over the development of its podophyllotoxin-related drugs to the pharmaceutical company Bristol-Myers.

Additional reading: Lednicer, ed., *Chronicles of Drug Discovery, Vol. III*, pp. 349–80.

poison control center

A poison control center is a facility for treating patients who have been poisoned, or for providing reference information on poisoning.

Edward Press (1913–), an Illinois pediatrician, opened the first Poison Information Center in 1953, three years after a survey found many children were injured or killed by accidental poisoning. After Press opened the center and wrote a reference guide to the toxicity of chemicals contained in household substances, other Poison Information Centers began opening around the United States.

Today the American Association of Poison Control Centers provides guidelines on how these centers, which are open 24 hours, should be run and staffed. The **Food and Drug Administration (FDA)** also helps to coordinate the efforts of poison control centers. There are more than 400 centers offering information or treatment in the United States.

Additional reading: Epstein, "Poison Control."

poliomyelitis (polio)

Poliomyelitis is the infection of the motor **neurons** with a poliovirus. Polio can lead to fever, infection of the meninges of the brain, and temporary or permanent paralysis. If the muscles of the respiratory system are paralyzed, a person will die unless he or she receives assistance in breathing.

The disease was known by several names until the 1870s, when it was called acute anterior poliomyelitis, a name later shortened to polio. There are several different strains of poliovirus and three major types, which vary in their ability to cause paralysis. The disease is spread by

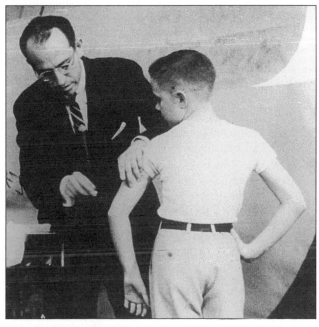

A boy receives a polio shot from Dr. Jonas Salk, one of the inventors of a vaccine for this disease, in 1955. (Photo courtesy of New York University Medical Center Archives.)

water or food contaminated with infected fecal matter, and may occasionally be contracted by drinking contaminated milk.

Epidemics of virulent polio began on the Mediterranean island of Malta in 1919. During that year an epidemic of polio struck New York City as well, affecting children under five almost exclusively. Polio infection reached a peak of 40,000 cases a year in the United States from 1951 to 1955.

Attempts to vaccinate against polio began in 1935, but resulted in paralysis and death for some who were vaccinated. Thomas Weller (1915–), John Enders (1897–1985), and Frederick Robbins (1916–) succeeded in growing the **virus** in human skin and intestine cells, and invented a dye that would indicate when the virus was growing by 1950. This made it possible to develop a safe polio **vaccine**. The three shared the 1954 Nobel Prize for their achievement.

Hilary Koprowski (1916–) tested a weakened strain of the virus as an oral vaccine in 20 adults in 1951. Two years later, Jonas Salk (1914–1995) gave a vaccine containing completely inactivated virus to more than 100 children. The following year, several hundred thousand children received the vaccine in field tests, which were successful. Tragedy resulted when some lots of the vaccine that contained live virus, which was being manufactured by several different companies, caused 250 cases of polio infection in 1955.

During the 1950s, Albert Sabin (1906–1993) produced an oral vaccine for polio. The vaccine is inexpensive and can transmit immunity to nonvaccinated individuals, but it must be given in several doses. This vaccine also is difficult to use in tropical countries, because it is not heat-stable.

Decades after the polio outbreaks of the 1950s, physicians began to observe that some patients' symptoms returned. This condition is called "post-polio syndrome." It generally occurs 20 to 30 years after a person was first infected with the virus. From one-quarter to two-thirds of people who contracted polio may be affected; estimates vary because the definition of what constitutes the syndrome varies. Generally, symptoms are considered to be a slow, progressive weakening of the muscles. The cause of the syndrome is unknown, and there is no treatment for it.

Today there are about 10 cases of polio a year in the United States. In many parts of the world polio is now rare, but because of low rates of vaccination in Central Africa and India, the disease is still relatively common in those nations. (*See also* Drinker respirator [iron lung])

Additional reading: Paul, *A History of Poliomyelitis;* Shorter, *The Health Century,* pp. 60–70, 199–203.

polymerase chain reaction (PCR)

Polymerase chain reaction is a process for multiplying **DNA** fragments that has revolutionized molecular biology.

Kary Mullis (1944–) discovered PCR, sharing the 1993 Nobel Prize in chemistry for his achievement. Cetus Corporation researchers developed the technology and commercialized it in 1988.

Using PCR, a researcher can make ten billion copies of a selected DNA fragment in three hours. The targeted section is heated so the double strand of DNA splits apart. Then huge amounts of single nucleotides are introduced to the solution, connecting to their mates on either half. The mixture is then heated again and the splitting and assembly process repeated, rapidly multiplying the number of pieces of genetic material.

This makes it possible to analyze DNA from tiny samples.

Archeology, forensics, genetics, and **AIDS** research are among the disciplines that have benefited from PCR. The test has spawned diagnostic tools, made **DNA fingerprinting** possible, and greatly accelerated the process of mapping the genome. (*See also* gene mapping)

Additional reading: Rabinow, *Making PCR.*

positron emission tomography. See PET scanning.

Prausnitz-Kustner reaction

The Prausnitz-Kustner reaction was an experiment proving that the agent responsible for causing allergic reactions circulates in the blood. It is named for Carl Prausnitz (1896–1963) and Heinz Kustner (1897–1963), who devised the experiment and reported it in 1921.

Kustner was allergic to fish, while Prausnitz was not. Nothing happened when Prausnitz received an injection of cooked fish extract. But when he first received an injection of serum (blood with cells removed) from Kustner and a day later received the fish injection, he had the same allergic reaction to fish that Kustner did, and remained sensitive to the fish injections for weeks.

This test became a standard method for screening people for certain **allergies**, but is no longer used because of the danger of transmitting **AIDS, hepatitis**, and other infections with an injection of another person's serum.

To judge whether a person is allergic to a specific substance, skin endpoint titration, in which a small amount of the allergen is injected under the skin, is commonly used today. Different types of skin tests have commonly been used to diagnose allergies since 1910, when they were first popularized by Leonard Noon. Laboratory tests may also be used.

Additional reading: Clark, *At War Within,* pp. 88–90.

pregnancy test

Pregnancy tests are used to determine whether a woman is pregnant, and today can be completed in minutes using urine analysis kits available in drugstores.

The ancient Egyptians used a pregnancy test in which the woman was to urinate on two bags, one containing wheat and one containing barley. If either germinated, she was pregnant. Barley foretold a male child; wheat, a female. Other ancient pregnancy tests relied on urine as well; during the Middle Ages in England, the "piss prophets" used urine to diagnose pregnancy as well as a multitude of other ailments.

The first truly reliable pregnancy test was devised by Bernhard Zondek (1891–1966) and Selmar Ascheim (1878–1965) in 1928. The "A Z test" involved injecting immature mice with a woman's urine and looking for changes in the ovaries and uterus of the mice after five days. Maurice Freedman (1903–1991) reported on a similar test in rabbits one year later. By 1931, he was able to recommend the test as a "simple, rapid" procedure for identifying pregnancy in its early stages. The "rabbit test" soon became the most popular pregnancy test in the United States.

Subsequently less expensive and faster tests were introduced; today it is possible to buy disposable, nearly instant pregnancy tests in any drugstore. However, these tests are not 100 percent accurate, and must be confirmed by laboratory pregnancy tests.

Additional reading: Speert, *Obstetric & Gynecologic Milestones Illustrated,* pp. 222–27.

pre-implantation genetic diagnosis (PGD)

Pre-implantation genetic diagnosis is a technique for evaluating the **genes** of an embryo that has undergone **in vitro fertilization** before it is implanted in the uterus. PGD is generally used for women who have had frequent miscarriages due to genetic problems, to give them a better chance of carrying a child to term. It may also be used for couples at high risk of bearing a child with a genetic abnormality.

The diagnosis is accomplished by either removing a polar body—an extra cell produced during egg development—from an unfertilized egg, or removing a cell from an embryo in the early stages of development. This generally is performed when the embryo is about three days old and has reached the six- to ten-cell stage.

This procedure was first performed by Alan H. Handyside and his colleagues in 1990. The group was attempting to implant female embryos rather than male embryos because the couples involved in their study were at risk of having a child with an X **chromosome**-linked disorder. In 1992, Handyside used the procedure to prevent a child from being born with **cystic fibrosis.** By the late 1990s, a few thousand of these procedures had been performed; at a cost of $20,000 per disease screening, they are prohibitively expensive for most couples.

Scientists at the Genetics and IVF Institute in Fairfax, Virginia, recently developed a less expensive method for choosing a child's sex (to avoid sex-linked disease or for personal choice.) They were able to sort sperm by whether they carried an X or a Y chromosome, using a nontoxic, light-sensitive dye, so that the egg could be fertilized using Y- or X- bearing sperm, thus producing a boy or a girl as preferred. This test is available today for about $2,500. It raises questions about whether giving couples the ability to choose a child's sex for reasons of personal preference rather than health concerns is ethical. There currently are no clinical guidelines that prescribe when this technique should and should not be used.

Additional reading: Gosden, *Designing Babies,* pp. 108–15.

premature infant care

Premature infants are defined as those who are born before the 37th week of pregnancy or weigh less than 2,500 grams at birth (about five and a half pounds). Normal pregnancies last 40 weeks. Prematurely born infants often require special care to survive and develop normally. Approximately 7 percent of white infants and 13 percent of nonwhite infants born in the United States are premature.

Alexandre Gueniot (1832–1935) first established weight criteria for premature birth in 1872. Before this, infants were seldom weighed at birth. He suggested that infants weighing 2,500 grams or less be considered premature. The American Academy of Pediatrics did not adopt a definition of prematurity as measured by weight until 1935, and the **World Health Organization (WHO)** followed in 1950.

Although it was long clear to **midwives** and others experienced with newborn infants that premature infants needed extra help in staying warm, scientific observations of premature infants' inability to maintain body temperature on their own were first made in 1829.

French doctors were pioneers in modern care for the premature infant, designing incubators and feeding methods toward the end of the nineteenth century. This was largely because Paris was home to two hospitals at the forefront of pediatric care: the Hopital des Enfants Malades, founded in 1802 as the first hospital solely for children, and the Hopital des Enfants Trouves (foundlings), founded in 1795. Also, the French government, alarmed by low birth rates and high infant mortality rates in the 1870s, took several steps to improve maternal and infant health. The obstetrician Stephane Tarnier (1828–1897) was a leader in these efforts.

Incubators began to be used for premature infants in the 1830s. These early incubators, including a model invented by Johann Georg von Ruehl (1769–1846) and described in 1837, were basically double-walled metal tubs. The space between the walls was filled with warm water. Tarnier built the first closed incubator, which he based on a chicken-egg incubator that he saw during an 1878 visit to a zoo. The first model, built for two infants, was used two years later. Tarnier's colleague Pierre Auvard (1855–1941) designed a smaller, single-infant model. Both models were warmed with stoneware containers of boiling water, which required an attendant to constantly test the incubator to make sure the temperature remained steady. Pierre Budin (1846–1907) added an electrical device to Tarnier's design that warned of overheating by ringing an electric bell. Use of the incubators brought down premature infant mortality from about two-thirds to just over one-third. In the 1890s, several U.S. companies began making similar incubators, also heated with hot water.

Tarnier introduced gavage feeding for premature infants, in which a tube is inserted through the nose and into the infant's stomach and then filled through a funnel, in

1884. Max Rubner (1854–1932) and Otto Huebner (1843–1926) published an 1898 paper on infants' caloric needs, which subsequently made it possible to gauge exactly how much to feed a premature infant. Nearly all of the early neonatal care experts recommended mother's milk for premature children.

Gueniot stressed the importance of protecting infants from infection in 1872, shortly after the **germ theory** of disease had been put forth. Budin designed the world's first isolation ward for premature infants at his Paris hospital, in about 1895.

The first hospital station for premature infants in the United States was established in 1922 at the Sarah Morris Hospital for Children in Chicago, and directed by Julius H. Hess (1876–1955).

Oxygen for premature infants became standard practice in the 1930s and 1940s. However, in the early 1950s, high concentrations of oxygen were found to put premature infants at risk of blinding eye damage. About 10,000 U.S. children were blinded by the use of unnecessarily high oxygen concentrations.

Hospital statistics in the 1930s revealed that 80 percent of neonatal deaths were due to prematurity, leading to renewed efforts to prevent premature birth with **prenatal care**. **Syphilis,** once a leading cause of premature infant birth, declined sharply after the introduction of **penicillin** in the 1940s.

A major advance in premature infant care was the introduction of the Isolette incubator in 1947, which included a scale and portals through which the nurse and doctor could insert their gloved hands.

The first specialized center for care of premature infants was opened at the University of Colorado in Denver in 1947, and 10 other centers were built in New York City from 1948 to 1953.

In the 1960s, specialists in the care of premature infants began to realize the importance of parental involvement in care for these babies, for the health of both baby and parents. Parents were encouraged to hold their premature infants and spend time with them. Federal laws were passed requiring states to provide intensive care for premature infants in the mid-1970s, after studies proved that such units greatly reduced infant mortality.

Today, the main causes of premature birth are pregnancy among adolescents, as well as drug, cigarette, and alcohol use by mothers. Lack of prenatal care also is known to be a major risk factor for prematurity.

Although 800-gram infants survive increasingly frequently and 700-gram infants survive occasionally, premature infants still often face health problems in childhood and adulthood, including learning disabilities and neurological damage.

Additional reading: Cone, *History of the Care and Feeding of the Premature Infant.*

prenatal care

Prenatal care is health care given to women during—and often before—pregnancy to prevent birth defects and ensure that mother and baby are as healthy as possible. It includes attention to proper nutrition, monitoring of fetal health, avoiding alcohol and cigarettes, and preventing infections that could damage the fetus, such as **measles**.

Before the modern understanding of nutrition developed in the last century and a half, ideas on prenatal care were based on the thoughts of Hippocrates (c.460–c.377 B.C.) and Claudius Galen (c.129–c.199), who stressed balance in the consumption of food. Nutrition was the most important consideration for prenatal care; it was thought to help to maintain balance of the humors. Birth was thought to occur when the fetus could no longer obtain enough nourishment through the navel vein; thus if the mother didn't have rich enough blood—or enough blood at all—she risked miscarriage. On the other hand, too much food could cause the fetus to become too large and outgrow the uterus. Moderation was the key. Women of the seventeenth century, for example, might be advised to avoid spicy food and salads, which could cause constipation, diarrhea, or indigestion. Beyond this, prenatal care basically consisted of counseling women to avoid frights or certain sights that were supposed to damage the child.

By the early part of the twentieth century, doctors understood that it would be possible to prevent **eclampsia** with diet and rest; they also were able to diagnose **syphilis** in the mother and thus treat a child immediately after birth to avoid blindness from the disease.

John William Ballantyne (1861–1923) of Edinburgh is considered the father of modern prenatal care. In 1901, the first bed specifically for prenatal care was endowed at his hospital. Home visits to pregnant patients began in Boston, with America's first prenatal care clinic opening there in 1911.

The **U.S. Children's Bureau** was founded in 1912 to improve health care for women and children. The bureau found that the United States had a very high rate of infant and maternal mortality for an industrialized nation. In 1921, the bureau—helped by the votes of newly enfranchised women—succeeded in getting Congress to pass the Sheppard-Towner Act, which provided funds to states for educating women on prenatal and postnatal care and ensured that resources were available for this care. But lobbying efforts by organized medicine, led by the American Medical Association (AMA), resulted in appropriations for maternal and child health ending in 1929.

Perhaps as a result, maternal mortality rates were no better and infant mortality rates had substantially grown by the 1930s. Studies found that this was because not enough women got prenatal care, and because of overly aggressive doctors who performed unnecessary procedures to speed delivery.

In response, Title V of the 1935 **Social Security** Act provided additional funding for maternal and child care, resulting in a steady decrease in the rate of maternal and infant mortality.

Research in the late 1950s linked maternal smoking with low infant birth weight. Subsequent studies have shown that women who smoke are twice as likely as nonsmokers to have low-birthweight babies, infants who weigh less than 2,500 grams (five-and-a-half pounds). Research in the early 1970s linked alcohol consumption with retarded fetal development. Kenneth L. Jones and David W. Smith at the Washington University in St. Louis described "fetal alcohol syndrome" in 1973, a group of birth defects found in the children of alcoholic mothers.

Although adequate prenatal care is known to be the best way to prevent infant mortality, many women in the United States—especially poor women—do not receive adequate prenatal care, which is considered to be care beginning in the first trimester of pregnancy. Also, there remains a large gap in infant mortality rates between blacks and whites in the United States.

Additional reading: Enkin, *A Guide to Effective Care in Pregnancy and Childbirth.*

prescription

A prescription is a doctor's authorization of a drug for a patient, with instructions on how the drug should be taken.

During the first third of the twentieth century in the United States, only a third of the drugs that people took were prescribed by doctors. These prescriptions were basically a doctor's orders for a particular medication, and had no legal connotation. Patients could obtain any drug on their own, without a prescription, and usually went to the pharmacist themselves to buy medicine. At the same time, many doctors sold drugs themselves.

The Food, Drug, and Cosmetic Act of 1938, passed largely as an effort to make drugs safer, was the first U.S. law to distinguish between prescription and nonprescription drugs. Drugs that would be "dangerous in the hands of those unskilled in the uses of drugs," according to a **Food and Drug Administration (FDA)** report, would be prescription-only. The agency did not specify which drugs would require prescriptions, although it did state that any drug with "caution" on the label required a prescription.

Most actions taken by the agency against pharmacies to enforce this law addressed sales of barbituates or sulfa drugs without prescriptions.

The Humphrey-Durham Amendment, passed in 1951, clarified this distinction, and made provisions for prescription refills and prescriptions ordered by telephone.

Additional reading: Temin, *Taking Your Medicine*, pp. 18–57.

prion

A prion is an infectious agent, even tinier than a **virus**, made up of protein. Prions —short for "proteinacious infectious particles" — cause degenerative brain diseases called **transmissible spongiform encephalopathies**, including Creutzfeldt-Jakob disease (CJD); kuru, a rare illness among New Guineans who ate the brains of deceased relatives;

and "mad cow" disease and scrapie, which affect cattle and sheep respectively as well as other animals. It had been thought that these diseases were caused by hypothetical agents known as "slow viruses," because a person might become sick with them decades after they initially were infected.

Dr. Stanley B. Prusiner (1942–), who coined the term "prion" and won the 1997 Nobel Prize for his discovery of them, began studying degenerative brain disease as a neurology resident in 1972, after seeing a patient with CJD. In 1982, Prusiner proposed that scrapie was caused by an infectious agent that did not contain RNA or **DNA**. Many scientists dismissed this idea, because only organisms containing nucleic acid were thought to be able to infect other life forms.

Prusiner argued that the body makes the protein that constitutes prions normally, in a tightly-wound helical form. It is true that every animal has the gene that makes normal prion protein. But for some reason as yet unknown, these proteins can lose their shape, shifting into a more stable, folded form. The disease spreads when other protein particles pick up this abnormal shape.

Prusiner and his supporters believe that prions may be found to be the cause of **Alzheimer's disease** and other degenerative brain disorders, either by infection or from a genetic abnormality that causes the body to make the misshapen proteins.

Additional reading: Koprowski and Oldstone, eds., *Microbe Hunters Then and Now,* pp. 407–42; Rhodes, *Deadly Feasts.*

progesterone

Progesterone is a **hormone** released by the corpus luteum in the ovary that plays an important role in the menstrual cycle, and also is vital in helping women to maintain pregnancy.

The corpus luteum was discovered in 1903 by Ludwig Fraenkel (1870–unknown), who observed that after the ovary releases an egg, yellow material collects in the empty follicle. The French researcher Paul Albert Ancel (1873–1961) proved that this material prepared the uterus for pregnancy.

George Corner (1889–1981) and Willard Allen (1904–) of the University of Rochester in New York developed an ovarian extract capable of preventing abortion in 1930. Pregnant rabbits whose corpus lutea had been surgically removed retained their fetuses when given the extract.

The active hormone was isolated by three different teams in 1934: Allen and Oscar Wintersteiner (1898–1971) at Columbia University; Adolf Butenandt (1903–1995) and Karl Heinrich Slotta (1895–1987) at Gottingen University; and Swiss researchers led by Adolf Wettstein (1907–). It was named progesterone, and clinical use of the hormone for preventing miscarriage began soon afterwards.

Because the hormone was difficult to prepare and had to be used in large quantities, efforts began to find a synthetic version. Researchers in Zurich and Berlin developed dehydroepiandrosterone in 1937, and a Berlin team (at

Schering laboratories) synthesized a more progesterone-like chemical, ethisterone, in 1938. Soon afterwards, the Schering team developed the most effective artificial progesterone, ethinylestradiol, which is still used today in **hormone replacement therapy** for menopause.

In 1950 Gregory Pincus (1903–1967) began investigating progesterone as a contraceptive. He needed more powerful artificial progesterones than were currently available. He found the most effective compounds were norethindron, developed by the Mexican drug company Syntex S.A. and patented in 1956; and norethynodrel, developed at G.D. Searle and Company in Chicago. Clinical trials of the progesterone-like **birth control pill** began in 1956. The first oral contraceptive, manufactured by Searle, went on the market in 1960.

Additional reading: Angier, *Woman,* pp. 162–76.

prontosil

Prontosil is a sulfonamide drug, originally manufactured as dye, that Gerhard Domagk (1895–1964) discovered in the early 1930s to be effective against staphylococcal and streptococcal infections. He first gave the drug to humans, including his own daughter, in 1935.

Domagk, who at the time was a biochemist at the German company Bayer, was nominated for the Nobel Prize in 1939, but the Nazi government barred him from accepting the prize.

Prontosil was the first antibacterial "sulfa" drug. It was especially effective for treating women with **puerperal fever**, which is usually caused by a streptococcal infection. Previously, this common infection was almost always fatal.

Researchers later found that sulfanilamide was responsible for prontosil's streptococcus-fighting power, and this drug replaced prontosil.

Sulfanilamide and prontosil enter bacterial cells the same way that an essential nutrient does, but they disrupt the bacterium's function rather than providing nutrition. Sulfanilamides can also damage blood-forming tissues and change blood pigmentation, turning patients blue, so they have been largely replaced by antibacterial drugs with fewer side effects, including the sulfonamides.

Additional reading: Sneader, *Drug Discovery,* pp. 282–86.

prostaglandin

The prostaglandins are a number of different fatty acids that certain organs release to produce local effects. Prostaglandins are autocoids, meaning they work within the tissues where they are produced by passing from cell to cell, rather than by traveling through the bloodstream as **hormones** do. Their formation and release is triggered by injury or hormonal action. Prostaglandins act quickly, are broken down quickly, and are not stored in the body.

In 1935, the Swedish researcher Ulf von Euler (1905–1983) found the first prostaglandin by isolating a substance from human seminal fluid that lowered **blood pressure** in rats. He coined the word "prostaglandin" to describe the substance.

Prostaglandins influence blood flow, neurotransmission, gastrointestinal activity, blood clotting, ovarian cycles, and uterine contraction, among other body processes. The discovery of prostaglandins has contributed to the understanding of these phenomena.

The body produces prostaglandins by oxidizing arachidonic acid, a fatty acid contained in cell membranes. The body releases prostaglandins after injury, and prostaglandins play a role in the development of inflammation. **Nonsteroidal anti-inflammatory drugs**, including **aspirin**, work in part by inhibiting the formation of prostaglandin.

Additional reading: Galton, *Med Tech,* pp. 311–34.

prostate cancer

Prostate **cancer** is the most common cancer in men, and the second leading cause of cancer death in men in the United States and Canada. Approximately 184,500 American men were diagnosed with prostate cancer in 1998, and roughly 39,200 died of the disease.

There are now known to be two types of prostate cancer; a slow-growing, relatively benign type that is rarely fatal, and an aggressive type. Much medical attention has focused on how to determine which type a man's cancer is, to help decide whether to pursue radical or conservative treatment. **Prostate-specific antigen (PSA)** testing, which is used to screen for prostate enlargement and prostate cancer, can provide some help but is not completely reliable.

Hugh H. Young (1870–1945), with the assistance of his teacher William S. Halsted (1852–1922), performed the first surgical removal of the prostate gland to treat cancer in 1904. A different version of the operation, which is performed from above the pubic bone rather than through the perineum, was introduced in the 1950s and has made preserving a patient's sexual function somewhat easier.

Doctors began using radium to treat prostate cancer in the early twentieth century. Megavoltage external beam **radiation therapy**, introduced in the 1950s, was more effective because it could penetrate deeper without exposing surface **tissues** to a great deal of radiation.

Charles Huggins (1901–1997) first reported castrating a patient to treat prostate cancer that had spread to the bones in 1941. The patient was not cured, but he experienced much less pain. Huggins thus showed that hormonal treatment of prostate cancer by eliminating testosterone, which can stimulate tumor growth, was somewhat effective. He won the 1966 Nobel Prize in physiology or medicine for this achievement.

Castration for this purpose is now rarely necessary. Usually drug treatment with luteinizing hormone-releasing **hormone** agonists and anti-**androgens** will produce the same effect. This type of anti-androgen therapy does not cure the cancer or prolong life, but it does make the patient more comfortable.

The National Prostatic Cancer Project, directed by Gerald Patrick Murphy (1934–), began evaluating chemotherapeutic drugs for treating prostate cancer in the late 1970s.

Now, screening with digital rectal exams, and sometimes PSA testing, is performed regularly in men over 40 to detect prostate cancer in its early stages.

Additional reading: Loo and Betancourt, *The Prostate Cancer Sourcebook.*

prostate-specific antigen (PSA)

Men are given PSA tests to screen for prostate **cancer**. Although the PSA test is not definitive, high levels of this chemical can indicate that a man has this type of cancer.

Antigens that were specific to the prostate gland and appeared to be associated with cancer were discovered by several different research teams in the early 1970s. In 1991, researchers showed that the substance was found in men with benign prostate enlargement as well as prostate cancer.

In 1994, standardized methods for PSA testing were issued by the National Committee for Clinical Laboratory Standards. A large National Cancer Institute trial of the usefulness of PSA testing for detecting prostate cancer is now underway.

Additional reading: Loo and Betancourt, *The Prostate Cancer Sourcebook,* pp. 48–53.

prosthesis

A prosthesis is a device used to replace a missing body part.

Prosthetic noses and facial masks to cover deformities may have been made as early as 1000 B.C. The earliest documented prosthetic nose was made for a Byzantine emperor, Justinian II, who had been punished with a public nasal amputation (a common sentence in those times). Around 700 A.D., he commissioned a nose made of gold.

Early limb prostheses were made of wood. The earliest surviving prosthesis was a bronze and wood artificial leg from Etruscan times found in Capri in 1858. The prosthesis, kept in London, was destroyed during World War II.

During the 1400s and beyond, prostheses were often made by armorers out of iron, and were intended more to conceal the lack of a limb than to replace its function.

Ambrose Pare (c.1510–1590), a French military surgeon, was a pioneer in prosthetics. He designed facial prostheses made of ivory, papier mache, gold, and leather, including an artificial eye and an artificial ear. In 1529, he introduced ligatures that were stitched through the stump of the amputated limb in order to attach the prosthesis more securely. He also described an artificial leg with a working knee joint in 1564. But although Pare left clear documentation of his designs, it is unclear if they were ever actually built and used.

Peg legs and hook hands were the prostheses of the poor, while the rich had their armorers make jointed prostheses of iron. The most advanced prosthesis of its time was the Prince of Homburg's (1633–1708) "Silver Leg," which replaced his left leg, lost in battle. The leg was made of wood, with ankle and foot joints as well as a spring to hold the foot at the proper angle.

A London doctor created a wooden prosthesis with artificial tendons connecting the knee and ankle, allowing these joints to flex normally. The leg became known as the Anglesley leg, because it was made for the Marquis of Anglesley after he lost his leg at the Battle of Waterloo. This design was introduced to the United States in 1839, whereupon it became known as the American leg.

Once **anesthesia** was invented, it became possible for surgeons to more carefully amputate limbs in order to preserve an effective attachment for a prosthesis. The requirement for prostheses grew in the United States after many men were injured in the Civil War, but few innovations in the construction of artificial limbs occurred until the mid-twentieth century, after World War II.

During World War I, British surgeons and artists made temporary masks for soldiers whose faces had been damaged in trench warfare to wear before they had corrective **plastic surgery**. These masks were made from a facial mold, with the missing structures sculpted in clay. The masks were then fashioned from copper or rubber and painted to resemble natural skin color.

Prevulcanized latex and silicones were both introduced in the mid-twentieth century, and were eventually incorporated into prosthesis.

From the beginning of the nineteenth century mechanics and surgeons began attempting to develop prosthesis that employed a person's remaining muscles to move the artificial limb. Most early methods for doing this, however, were crude and unpopular.

In 1945, the National Academy of Sciences launched a research program in prosthetics at the request of the Army's Surgeon General. The Armed Services, the Department of Health, Education, and Welfare and the Veterans Administration collaborated on this research, which yielded many important inventions in prosthetic joints and alignment, better methods for making upper-arm amputee prostheses, and an emphasis on saving the knee.

In 1952, a series of six-week courses in prosthetics were taught at the University of California in Berkeley and at New York University. Now there are eight educational programs in orthotics and prosthetics in the United States.

The thalidomide debacle of 1959 and 1960, in which a number of children were born with severe **birth defects** generally involving missing limbs after their mothers had taken the drug, spurred research into prosthetics in Europe.

In the United States, there is now a certification board for prosthetists and orthotists (founded in 1970) and there are 800 facilities where artificial limbs are built and fitted. The International Society of Prosthetists was established in Copenhagen in 1992.

A network of U.S. federal and state government agencies help provide prostheses to people who need them and train them in their use. These agencies include Maternal and Child Health Services, the Veterans Administration, the **U.S. Public Health Service**, the Rehabilitation Services Administration, and **Medicare.**

There currently are approximately 370,000 American amputees, with lower-limb amputees far outnumbering upper-limb amputees. As prosthetics technology has advanced, many people who have lost limbs to accident or disease (usually a vascular disorder, cancer, or infection) are able to function well and even participate in sports.

The number of amputees internationally is growing rapidly. There are currently 110 million active landmines remaining in 64 countries, according to the American **Red Cross**. These landmines are relics of wartime. People returning to war-stricken areas, such as Cambodia and Bosnia-Herzegovina, may stumble on the hidden landmines and lose a limb, or their life. In Angola, according to the United Nations, there are 70,000 amputees, or one for every 154 people. International relief agencies are struggling to provide these amputees with prostheses, while the international community attempts to clear the mines so they pose no further danger.

Additional reading: Wilson, *Limb Prosthetics.*

protease inhibitors

Protease inhibitors are a class of drugs that have been highly successful in reducing the level of the HIV **virus** in **AIDS** patients' blood, especially when used in conjunction with **AZT** and other nucleoside analogs. This combination of drugs is known as highly active anti-retroviral therapy, or HAART.

The **Food and Drug Administration (FDA)** approved four protease inhibitors, saquinavir, ritonavir, idinavir, and nelfinavir, in December 1995. These drugs interfere with the action of an enzyme essential to the HIV replication cycle. In 1996, a large study found that combining a protease inhibitor with two nucleoside analogs reduced HIV RNA to undetectable levels in 90 percent of patients in 24 weeks, and strengthened the patients' immune systems.

Protease inhibitors work so well that researchers thought it might be possible to cure AIDS with them, if treatment began early enough; unfortunately the virus is hidden in other parts of the body even when it remains undetectable in the blood, so they are most likely not a cure. Also, these drugs have serious long-term side effects including changes in body-fat distribution and increases in blood cholesterol levels. Taking HAART is difficult as well, because it requires a complicated system of taking drugs at several different times, in different combinations, some with food and some without, and the regimen must be strictly adhered to in order for it to work.

Protease inhibitors are extremely expensive, making them basically unavailable to people in the poor areas hardest hit by AIDS, such as sub-Saharan Africa.

A new protease inhibitor, aprenavir, was synthesized at the Cambridge, Massachusetts company Vertex Pharmaceuticals in 1993. The drug is now undergoing **clinical trials**. One promising aspect of the new medication is that patients need only take it twice a day.

Additional reading: Waldman, "When You Want to Live, But Can't Afford It"; Altman, "With AIDS Advance, More Disappointment."

Prozac. *See* antidepressant drugs.

psychoanalysis

Psychoanalysis is a method of **psychotherapy** in which a detailed account of a person's past and present is obtained in order to eliminate unconscious conflicts that are thought to be the source of mental and emotional problems. Psychoanalysts must first go through analysis themselves as part of their training.

Psychotherapy focuses on treating the milder forms of mental illness. Psychiatrists now generally agree that it is not useful for treating severe **mental illness**, such as **schizophrenia** or manic depressive illness.

Sigmund Freud (1856–1939) is considered the father of psychoanalysis. He was the first person to develop the idea of an unconscious, and to suggest that emotional problems were caused by the repression of past traumatic events. Repression of these events would lead to their surfacing in neurotic symptoms, a theory that is known as the psychodynamic model of mental illness.

Freud wrote several books outlining his theories, including *Three Essays on the Theory of Sexuality, Ego and the Id,* and *Civilization and its Discontents.* His seminal work, *The Interpretation of Dreams,* was published in 1901.

Among Freud's most familiar theories are that people's problems often arise from childhood sexual desire for the parent of the opposite sex (the Oedipal complex), and that humans have a death instinct—Thanatos—as well as the impulse to life, or Eros.

Freud's ideas on psychology and society have had great influence on twentieth century thinking, and on the treatment of mental illness.

Carl Jung (1875–1961), Alfred Adler (1870–1939), and others developed their own schools of psychoanalytic thought.

Jung developed the theories of extroverted and introverted personality, as well as the idea that people's dreams and fantasies express a collective unconsciousness shared by all humans. In his *Psychological Types,* published in 1921, he set forth his concepts of the four mental functions: thinking, feeling, sensation, and intuition. He was the first person to advocate psychoanalysis for the middle aged and elderly, and also focused on the link between psychology and religion. Part of analysis for patients, in Jung's school, was the development of his or her personal "mythology" as expressed in dream and imagination.

Adler based much of his work on the "inferiority feeling" (later incorrectly popularized as the "inferiority complex"), and focused his school of psychotherapy on helping people disabled by feelings of inferiority. He established Vienna's first child guidance clinic in 1921, and until his death strongly advocated the importance of educating children. Both Jung and Adler disagreed with Freud on his insistence that neurosis was based on sexual factors.

Psychoanalytic therapy requires a person to attend several sessions each week, usually indefinitely; for this reason this type of therapy is usually limited to people who can afford to pay for these therapeutic sessions themselves, as health insurance companies have begun to sharply limit reimbursement for psychiatric therapy.

Although psychoanalysis and psychodynamic theory held sway for much of the twentieth century, recent discoveries on the biochemical and genetic roots of mental illness, along with the discovery of effective drugs for treating mental illness, has led to the gradual phasing out of psychoanalysis as the dominant psychiatric discipline. However, Freud's theories of personality and civilization have been a major influence on society.

Additional reading: Porter, ed., *Medicine*, pp. 161–62.

psychotherapy

Psychotherapy is the treatment of mental illness with counseling.

Hypnotherapy, discovered in the nineteenth century, is thought by some to be the earliest form of psychotherapy. The French psychiatrist Hippolyte Bernheim (1840–1919) claimed that the power of suggestion in hypnosis could be used to cure patients with minor **mental illness** and also physical ailments. While practicing and advocating this technique, he learned that for some patients who resisted hypnosis, suggestion without hypnosis worked well also. In the 1880s, he began recommending nonhypnotic suggestion to his colleagues.

In 1887, Frederik Willem von Eeden (1860–1932) opened an outpatient hypnotherapy clinic in Amsterdam called the "Clinic for Psychotherapeutic Suggestion," which was the first use of the term psychotherapy.

Psychotherapy, with or without hypnosis, spread throughout Europe by the mid-1890s. Two Paris neurologists, Pierre Janet (1859–1947) and Jules-Joseph Dejerine (1849–1917), were leaders in the French school of psychotherapy. Dejerine's technique was basically to listen attentively and sympathetically to patients. By the beginning of the twentieth century, many neurologists—including Sigmund Freud (1856–1939), the inventor of **psychoanalysis**—were opening private psychotherapeutic practices in their offices.

Psychotherapy soon became popular in the United States as well, again with neurologists leading the charge. For much of the twentieth century psychoanalysis was the most influential form of psychotherapy, but other schools of thought such as **behaviorism,** along with a growing understanding of the biological and genetic roots of mental illness, challenged Freudian theory.

Today in the United States psychotherapy can be provided by psychiatrists (who have medical degrees), psychologists, and social workers. It remains an important part of treatment for mental illness.

Additional reading: Bromberg, *Man above Humanity.*

public health

Public health is the science of protecting the health of individuals through community efforts, such as sanitation and **prenatal care**.

Early public health efforts of the Middle Ages included isolating people with **leprosy** and placing travelers under **quarantine** from **bubonic plague**-ridden areas.

The "sanitary science" movement, which arose in the early nineteenth century, could be considered a forerunner to modern public health. Sanitary science recommended ventilation, isolation of sick people, and disinfection. Disease was thought to be spread by dirt, sewage vapors, and other types of "filth," and extreme cleanliness was considered the best way to prevent disease. Sanitation had become a kind of fad among upper-class Americans by the end of the nineteenth century.

The sanitary science movement led to sophisticated public health measures, such as sewage systems, land drainage, and clean drinking water. These measures were needed more than ever because of the overcrowding of cities that developed during this century and the corresponding rise in infant mortality and death from infectious disease.

The Shattuck report of 1850 by the Massachusetts Sanitary Commission reviewed poor health conditions, and recommended that public health organizations be established. New York City created the first such organization in 1866. By the end of the nineteenth century, most large U.S. cities had a safe drinking water supply. The **U.S. Public Health Service** was founded in 1912.

The "golden age" of American public health is generally thought of as the time from 1890 to 1930, after the acceptance of the **germ theory** of disease, when scientists conveyed to the public the fact that germs caused disease and that sick people spread disease by coughing, spitting, and sneezing.

Today public health efforts in the United States focus on vaccination, healthy diet, exercise, smoking cessation, and disease-prevention measures, such as safe sex to prevent HIV infection.

Additional reading: Rosen, *A History of Public Health.*

puerperal fever

Puerperal fever is a pelvic infection that was once a common killer of women after childbirth.

Early nineteenth-century treatment involved bleeding, purging, blistering, and hot douches. Alexander Gordon (1752–1799), a Scottish physician, was the first to suggest that puerperal fever might be transmitted by the doctor or **midwife** attending the birth; he implicated himself, as well as some midwives, in 28 cases between 1789 and 1792,

In Boston, Dr. Oliver Wendell Holmes (1809–1894) published a careful and logical explanation of the contagiousness of puerperal fever in 1843.

Many in the medical establishment rejected the idea, however; they may not have wanted to claim responsibility for this devastating, common illness. Also, the idea that germs spread disease would not become widely accepted until later in the century.

Ignaz Semmelweis (1818–1865), a Hungarian-born doctor working in a Vienna obstetrical clinic in the 1840s, observed that the mortality rate in the division of the clinic where medical students delivered babies was much higher than in the division that employed midwives. Medical students performed **autopsies**, while midwives trained on models, and Semmelweis believed that something from the corpses was responsible for spreading disease. Once he got his colleagues to begin washing their hands with chlorinated lime before attending births, the mortality rate dropped. Unfortunately, his colleagues resented his tough stance and his hospital appointment was not renewed.

Once disease-causing microbes were discovered in the 1870s, it became clear that Semmelweis and Gordon were right.

When **antisepsis** had finally became common practice around the early 1900s, puerperal fever was less common, but there was still no effective way to treat infections that did occur. **Prontosil**, the first of the sulfa drugs, became available in the 1930s and was found to produce rapid improvement in puerperal fever. **Penicillin**, introduced in the 1940s, also was an effective treatment. Today, infection after delivery is much less common and can usually be treated effectively.

Additional reading: Speert, *Obstetric & Gynecologic Milestones Illustrated*, pp. 370–88.

pulse watch

A pulse watch is an instrument used to measure the pulse.

Sir John Floyer (1649–1734) is considered to be the inventor of the pulse watch. He wrote a 1707 book, *The Physician's Pulse Watch*, and the instrument he designed was commercially available at that time.

Measuring the pulse with a watch became possible when the minute hand was invented in 1670. Floyer's watch, made by Samuel Watson (c.1674–1709), included a second hand. The watch also had a button to stop the watch. Floyer used the watch to record pulse and respiration rates, and tabulated these rates in an early form of a bedside chart.

Keeping track of the pulse made it possible to begin studying its rate scientifically and use the pulse as a diagnostic tool.

Additional reading: Floyer, *The Physician's Pulse-Watch*.

purgatives

Purgatives are drugs used to cause vomiting and diarrhea, and thus purge harmful substances from the body. Examples of purgatives include **ipecac**, senna, and castor oil.

Medicine from ancient times to the present has employed purgatives, often to harmful effect. Much medical theory was based on the idea that getting bad substances out of the body by bleeding or purging would restore health. Unfortunately, purging tended to dehydrate patients and often caused fatal irritation of their digestive systems. Ancient Egyptians were particularly devoted to purging, as they saw intestinal decay as the source of disease. Ancient Greek physicians also extolled purging, along with starving and bleeding of the patient, as a cure for all ills.

Up until the nineteenth century—and even today, with the current fad for high-colonic enemas—purging remains a popular if rarely useful method for restoring health.

Additional reading: "Laxatives—and Alternatives," *Consumer Reports on Health*.

quarantine

Quarantine is the isolation of people, animals, or plants that may be infected with a disease to prevent the spread of the disease. The word comes from the Italian phrase for "40 days," which is about how long the first quarantines lasted.

In 1371, the council of the Italian town of Ragusa established history's first quarantine when it voted to require travelers from Black Plague areas, along with their luggage, to be isolated temporarily before entering the city. Visitors would have to spend a month on a nearby island, and could come to Ragusa once it was clear they didn't have the plague.

In 1397, the town converted a monastery on the island into a quarantine hospital. Unlike many towns of the time, Ragusa had a democratic legislature and a **public health** service. The service consisted of a physician, two surgeons, and an apothecary.

Other ports followed with their own quarantines: Marseilles in 1383, Venice in 1403, Pisa in 1464, and Genoa in 1467. The first quarantine in the Western Hemisphere was established at the island of Hispaniola (now Haiti and the Dominican Republic) in 1519, and London introduced a quarantine in 1626.

Quarantine hospitals were named lazarets after Saint-Lazar, a plague hospital in Rome. Some cities also introduced continental quarantines and military "cordons sanitaires" to protect cities or countries during larger epidemics. The largest cordon sanitaire ever established was along the border between Austria and Turkey to prevent the **bubonic plague** from entering Europe. Set up in 1728, it was 200 miles long, and lasted until 1872. The plague managed to break the cordon only once.

During the nineteenth century, better understanding of contagion as well as greatly increased travel made the old quarantine system obsolete. Nations began to confer and organize international plans for preventing the spread of disease. In 1881, the conferees decided to establish an international office for information on infectious disease, and in 1903 they signed the International Sanitary Agreement to prevent the spread of **yellow fever, cholera**, and plague. Under the agreement, ships were classified as infected, sus-

pect, or clean, and infected or suspect ships were held for five days.

Today, the **World Health Organization (WHO)** is in charge of directing quarantines, while countries—and even states within countries—can enact their own quarantines.

Additional reading: Rosen, *A History of Public Health*, pp. 43–45.

quinine

Quinine is a drug used to prevent and treat **malaria** and is also used to reduce the frequency and severity of muscle cramps.

Derived from the bark of the cinchona tree, a plant native to South America, quinine reached Europe in the 1600s. The first description of the material appears in a book by a monk who lived in Peru, Father Antonio de la Calancha, who reported that a type of bark could cure malaria. The tree grew in the part of the continent now known as Ecuador.

Because malaria was a common disease in Europe, demand quickly grew for the bark. It was called "Jesuit bark" because Jesuit priests controlled its distribution. The use of cinchona became widespread, and it was employed to treat any type of fever as well as malaria.

In 1819, German chemist Friedlieb Runge (1794–1867) isolated a substance from cinchona bark that he called "China base." Joseph Bienaime Caventou (1795–1877) and Pierre-Joseph Pelletier (1788–1842), French pharmacists, isolated a substance they called quinine (which turned out to be the same as China base) and reported their findings in 1820. It had the advantage of being more palatable than powdered cinchona bark. Quinine was listed in Francois Magendie's (1733–1855) *Formulaire*, a list of medicinal chemicals, in the following year.

Pelletier soon began large-scale processing of quinine, and others followed because the French chemists had freely released the details of how to prepare the chemical from cinchona bark.

Additional reading: McGrew, *Encyclopedia of Medical History*, pp. 298–99.

173

R

rabies

Rabies is a viral infection of the nervous system that strikes warm-blooded animals, especially carnivores, and leads to paralysis and death. The disease usually is spread by the bite of an infected animal.

Treatment is effective if the disease is still in its incubation period, the 2 to 16 weeks it takes for the **virus** to travel from the bite to the brain. After the wound site is thoroughly washed, the person is given several injections of human immune globulin and then a series of **vaccine** injections.

Rabies is also known as hydrophobia, or fear of water, because people and animals with the disease may be extremely thirsty but suffer throat spasms when they try to drink.

The earliest certain mention of rabies appears in a Chinese text of around 600 B.C. Early treatments included washing and performing **cauterization** on the wound and **bloodletting**. Ambrose Pare (c.1510–1590) observed that rabies appeared to involve the central nervous system.

The British doctor John Hunter (1728–1793) suggested inoculating animals with the saliva of rabid creatures to see if this was how the disease spread. Experiments followed that proved rabies was indeed spread by saliva. Knowledge that rabies was a contagious disease and not a mental disorder contributed nothing to treatment, however, which ranged from **electroconvulsive therapy** to ocean immersion.

Louis Pasteur (1822–1895) developed the first rabies vaccine, which he made from rabbit spinal-cord tissue, and gave it to a human for the first time in 1885. The patient, a boy of nine who had been bitten by a rabid dog two days before, was given progressively stronger preparations of the vaccine. He lived, as did all but one of the hundreds of people who received the vaccine in subsequent months.

Adelchi Negri (1876–1912) observed dark spots in the nerve cells of dogs with rabies in 1903, which came to be known as Negri bodies and were used for years as a method for detecting rabies. The virus itself was first observed in 1962, and Negri bodies were shown by an electron **microscope** to be clumps of virus three years later.

A vaccine for rabies based on human cells was developed in the late 1970s, and an improved version was released in the United States in 1988.

Rabies vaccines for pet dogs, invented in the 1920s, have kept the disease in check in much of the developed world. There now are rabies shots for cats, sheep, cattle, horses, and ferrets.

There have been one or two cases of rabies in humans in the United States each year since 1965, and 20,000 to 30,000 people in the United States receive rabies treatment annually.

Additional reading: Kiple, *The Cambridge World History of Human Disease,* pp. 962–67; Flieger, "Mad Dogs and Friendly Skunks."

radiation therapy

Radiation therapy is the use of ionizing radiation to destroy cancerous cells while damaging healthy **tissue** as little as possible. It may involve directing beams of radiation at abnormal tissue or implanting radioactive material inside the tumor or in a nearby body cavity. Radiation may also be used as palliative treatment in situations where the **cancer** cannot be cured; for example, it might be used to reduce the size of a tumor in the esophagus to allow a patient to swallow comfortably or to destroy painful bone metastases.

At present, more than half of cancer patients in the United States will receive radiation therapy as part of their treatment. Roughly half of these patients are given radiation with intent to cure, and half of them are cured. Radiation therapy is believed to work by damaging the **DNA** of cancer cells.

Attempts to treat cancer and other diseases with radiation began soon after Wihelm Konrad Roentgen (1845–1923) discovered **X-rays** in 1895. Three weeks after Roentgen announced his discovery in 1896, the Chicago vacuum tube manufacturer Emil H. Grubbe (1875–1960) reportedly used radiation to treat cancer for the first time. Rose Lee, who had **breast cancer**, received daily one-hour treatments over 18 days. Her diseased breast was placed against a

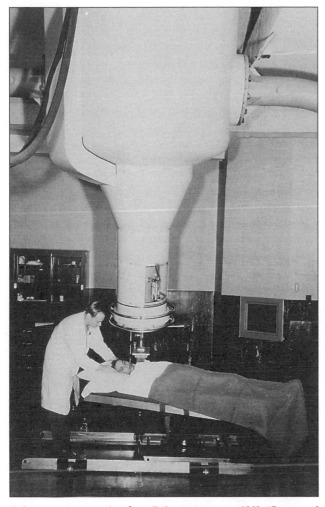

A doctor prepares a patient for radiation treatment, ca. 1960. (Courtesy of Archives and Special Collections, Columbia University Health Sciences Division.)

vacuum tube while the surrounding skin was shielded with lead foil. Treatment was stopped because of skin damage, and Lee died about one month later. Several attempts to treat cancer and skin disorders were also reported in 1896.

Radiation therapy was used, with some success, to treat many types of skin disorders such as lupus, acne, and excess hair. It is no longer used today to treat benign disease, although light therapy is frequently used for these purposes.

In 1900, Tage Sjogren (1859–1939) in Stockholm reported the first cancer cures using radiation therapy, of two patients with skin cancer. From Roentgen's discovery until the early 1920s, radiation therapy of other types of cancer was given most often via localized doses of radium, which could deliver gamma rays relatively deep into tissue, because X-ray machines of the time couldn't penetrate much beyond the skin.

Robert Abbe (1851–1928) was the first to treat a tumor by directly inserting radium into the abnormal tissue, reporting his results in 1904. Radium did not become widely and inexpensively available in the United States until the mid-1910s, when a radium recovery plant was established in Denver. The Memorial Hospital in New York became a leading center for radium implantation treatment of cancers.

William D. Coolidge (1873–1975) invented the hot-cathode tube, capable of generating up to 140 kilovolts, in 1913. He developed another tube that could generate 200 kilovolts that became available in 1922. Such machines were known as X-ray cannons because of their appearance, and described technically as "deep" or orthovoltage machines. These made it possible to use X-rays, rather than radium, to treat tumors lying deep in the body.

The roentgen, the first dosage unit of radiation to be developed, was adopted in 1928 at the Second International Congress of Radiology in Stockholm. The unit now used to measure the amount of absorbed radiation, the rad, was adopted in 1956.

Claude Regaud (1870–1940) introduced the concept of fractionation in 1919, when he reported the results of his experiments in using radiation to sterilize a ram. A single large dose of radiation did not sterilize the animal and extensively damaged the skin of the testes; however, several daily doses sterilized the animal without skin damage. Regaud suggested that the testis, with its rapidly dividing sperm cells, made a good model for researching cancer. He also proposed that distributing the dosage of radiation made it possible to reach all of the cells at their most vulnerable stage of division. Destruction of cancer without destroying healthy cells soon became the goal of treating cancer with radiotherapy.

In 1922, Regaud and Henri Coutard (1876–1950) reported on the apparent cure of six patients with advanced laryngeal cancer using such multiple small doses of radiation. Coutard, who went on to have dramatic success in treating patients with cancer of the larynx and tonsil with radiation, stressed the importance of making daily observations of the patient and his or her cancer.

The 1920s also saw the first systematic attempts at radiation therapy treatment planning, and the appointment of hospital physicists to oversee this planning.

Although curative radiotherapy became possible for some patients at this time, its applications were limited because the "deep" X-ray machines didn't go deep enough. In the early 1930s, several groups worked on developing more powerful treatment machines that offered one megavolt of energy and more. The first megavoltage therapy was given at California Institute of Technology in 1933.

Robert J. Van de Graaf (1901–1967) developed a generator capable of producing more than a million volts using very little power in the early 1930s, but an X-ray tube capable of handling that voltage had not yet been developed. The first Van de Graaf generator was built at Huntington Hospital in Boston and was first used to treat patients in 1937. These machines became the standard through the 1940s.

Ralston Paterson (1897–1981), working in Manchester, England, at the Holt Radium Institute, declared in 1936 that X ray therapy had to be given in the maximum tolerable dose. Paterson and his colleagues also developed standardized techniques for arranging the radioactive field around a patient, as well as a standardized dosage system.

The first linear accelerator machine for delivering radiation therapy was built by the company Metropolitan Vickers and installed at the Hammersmith Hospital in London, where the first patient was treated in 1953.

Cobalt 60 machines, also developed around this time, became more popular than linear accelerators for several decades because they were relatively easy to maintain. In the late 1960s, linear accelerators became more reliable and became the radiation therapy machines of choice, remaining so today.

A technique called radiosurgery, in which a single high dose of radiation is delivered to a site precisely located within the body, was envisioned in 1951 by the Swedish neurosurgeon Lars Lekskell (1907–1986). Lekskell invented the **gamma knife,** a tool for radiosurgery, and used it in patients for the first time in 1968. Today, about 14,000 patients are treated with the gamma knife each year. The treatment is effective for small tumors that can be precisely targeted, especially in the brain and nervous systems.

In order for radiosurgery to develop, the idea of stereotaxis—locating a point within the body by placing it at the intersection of three axes—had to be developed, so that the surgical site inside the brain could be pinpointed. Several researchers, including Lekskell, invented **stereotactic surgery** techniques and instruments in the late 1940s.

A major advance in radiation therapy occurred in the 1970s with the development of three-dimensional medical imaging. Techniques such as **CAT scanning** and **magnetic resonance imaging (MRI)** have made it possible to identify the size and shape of tumors precisely and thus deliver radiation to the tumors more accurately. During the 1970s, investigators at the Harvard Medical School in Boston and London's Royal Free Hospital began using computer-controlled radiation therapy to treat patients. A number of teams carried out National Cancer Institute-funded work on developing three-dimensional radiation delivery systems through the 1980s and 1990s, including the University of Pennsylvania School of Medicine, Massachusetts General Hospital, Memorial-Sloan Kettering Cancer Center, and Washington University in St. Louis.

Another development in radiation therapy, which followed the refinement of three-dimensional delivery of radiation treatment, has been the technique of 3–D conformal radiation therapy, in which a dosage of radiation is "wrapped" around the tumor to maximize the amount delivered to the cancerous tissue and minimize damage to normal tissue. This is done with movements of both the treatment machine and the couch on which the patient lies.

By the late 1990s, three-dimensional radiation treatment planning systems had become the standard of care.

Additional reading: Eisenberg, *Radiology*, pp. 481–526; Alexander, Loeffler, and Lunsford, eds., *Stereotactic Radiosurgery*; Steiner, ed., *Radiosurgery*.

rapid opiate detoxification

In rapid opiate detoxification, an opiate-addicted person is anesthetized and given an **opiate antagonist**, thus speeding the withdrawal process. Sedation or **anesthesia** is given because the process would otherwise be extremely painful.

Normally, a person suffers withdrawal symptoms including muscle aches, pains, and flu-like symptoms for five days or more after they stop taking **heroin** or any other opiate drug. With the rapid process, he or she undergoes complete detoxification in roughly six hours.

One major benefit of this process is that it is less painful, although a person may still suffer discomfort after waking up from anesthesia. The other is that most people who try to "detox" on their own are unsuccessful, returning to drug use before the last vestiges of the drug have left their bodies. However, people who go through the rapid opiate detoxification process must undergo treatment for the conditions that brought on the **addiction** afterward, and may not be successful in remaining drug-free. Some advocates of the procedure argue that people who complete it experience less craving for drugs afterward, but currently there is no scientific evidence for this claim.

Dr. Norbert Loimer first performed the procedure under anesthesia in his Vienna clinic in 1978. There are a handful of clinics in the United States performing the procedure. It costs from $5,500 to $7,000, and is rarely covered by insurance.

Additional reading: Matthews, "A Solution of Substance for Substance Abuse?"

receptors

Receptors are binding sites on molecules that "accept" or "refuse" other molecules (called ligands), which then can stimulate the receiving molecule to action, shut it down, or block it from accommodating other ligands. Receptors are found everywhere in the body and are responsible for many physiological actions, such as the functioning of the nervous system. Many drugs work on this principle, by mimicking a substance that a receptor normally accepts and thus blocking it from receiving the actual substance.

John N. Langley (1852–1925) first proposed the existence of receptors in 1878, when he wrote that specific drugs were capable of forming compounds with some type of other substance in nerve endings and gland cells. He described this phenomenon more precisely in 1905, noting that nicotine and **curare** block stimulation of nerves and thus prevent a muscle from contracting, not acting on the muscle itself but on "some accessory substance."

Around that time, Paul Ehrlich (1854–1915) proposed that drugs could be designed that would fit with the molecular structure of a parasite but not with normal **tissues**, thus blocking infection. In 1913, he dubbed the receiving molecule area the "receptor."

Additional reading: Silverstein, "Paul Ehrlich's Passion."

recombinant DNA

In **DNA** recombination, genetic material from different species are combined for various purposes.

Herbert Boyer (1936–) and Stanley Cohen (1922–) were the first to recombine DNA in 1973, when they spliced DNA from an African clawed toad with genetic material from bacteria by using **restriction enzymes**.

Recombination is used in agriculture to give certain desirable traits—such as insect resistance—to crops. The major role of DNA recombination in human health has been to facilitate the production of huge amounts of a particular protein by engineering the gene that expresses that protein into an organism that reproduces rapidly, such as bacteria. For example, human **insulin** is now produced by recombination.

Recombination technology has given rise to fears that genetically altered animals or plants will "breed" with other living things and thus give rise to dangerous life forms, but thanks largely to tight regulation by the Recombinant DNA Advisory Committee, formed by the **National Institutes of Health** in 1974, there have been no such disasters to date.

Additional reading: Grace, *Biotechnology Unzipped*, pp. 31–44.

red blood cells

Red blood cells are cells in the blood that are responsible for transporting hemoglobin and oxygen through the body.

During the 1600s, both Dutch microscopist Antoni van Leeuwenhoek (1632–1723) and Italian anatomist Marcello Malpighi (1628–1694) observed and described red blood cells.

Leeuwenhoek wrote about the cells in a letter to a colleague in 1674, calling them "red globules" and describing how they deformed themselves in order to pass through tiny vessels (later found to be **capillaries**). Malpighi made most of his observations in the course of performing dissections. In 1661, he wrote to a colleague that the red part of the blood—which he said contained particles—mixed with the white part of the blood in a frog's lungs rather than in its liver, and he described capillary circulation in the organ. In 1666, he described a clot he found in the heart of a corpse that contained "some very small red particles" that "can roll and turn helter-skelter in the little spaces." He also observed that red blood cells were depleted from the blood after the blood returned from the "nutrition of the parts."

However, Leeuwenhoek, perhaps because he promoted his own primacy assiduously, is generally thought of as the discoverer of red blood cells.

Additional reading: Harris, *The Birth of the Cell*, pp. 15–22.

Red Cross

The International Red Cross, based in Geneva, is a politically neutral organization devoted to providing medical care during wartime, while the 122 national Red Cross and 24 Red Crescent organizations provide emergency relief, first aid training, and other **public health** services locally.

The founder of the International Red Cross was Henri Dunant (1828–1910), a Swiss aristocrat. Dunant saw the aftermath of a battle at Solferino in 1859 and wrote a pamphlet, "A Memory of Solferino," that was published three years later. He called for a neutral organization that would provide medical care to war casualties. At this point, about 60 percent of people wounded in battle died from lack of medical care.

The International Committee of the Red Cross was established in 1863, and the following year 12 European countries signed the Geneva Convention and agreed to abide by rules for humane treatment of prisoners of war as well as of the sick and wounded.

The United States did not sign the Geneva Convention until 1882, after a campaign in which Clara Barton (1821–1912) played a major role. Barton founded the American Red Cross and directed the organization for 23 years.

Several additions to the Geneva Convention have been made, including rules addressing soldiers injured in battles at sea (1907), requiring humane treatment of prisoners of war (1929), and protecting civilians during wartime (1949).

The U.S. Red Cross provides first-aid training; blood collection, banking, and transfusions; and relief services during national disasters.

Additional reading: Hutchinson, *Champions of Charity*.

reflex

A reflex is an action performed without conscious thought, triggered by an impulse that travels from the sensory nerve to the spinal cord back to the motor nerve and to the muscle. This path is known as the reflex arc. Reflex actions can include pulling one's hand away from a hot stove or the response of the pupil to changes in light levels. The mind does not become aware of the movement, if it does at all, until after it has happened.

Rene Descartes (1596–1650) provided the first description of reflex action, calling what would become known as the nervous impulse the "animal spirits," which acted without "the intervention of the soul." Thomas Willis (1621–1675) further enunciated the idea, writing that sensation caused animal spirits to rebound from within and produce "local movement."

Robert Whytt (1714–1766) established, using decapitated frogs, that an intact spinal cord is necessary in order for reflex action to take place. Marshall Hall (1790–1857) described reflex action as distinct from volition, instead being "aimless" and even "frequently opposed to his [the individual's] volition." He wrote that the reflex was carried from the irritated nerve to the spinal marrow to the nerve passing from the marrow, and suggested that these structures must be related or connected. Hall was the first to demonstrate that the spine was not an appendage to the brain, but in fact an independent organ, in experiments on decapitated snakes. He coined the terms reflex arc and reflex action.

John Hughlings Jackson (1835–1911) refined the idea of reflex by describing the effect of nervous system injury such as a **stroke** on reflexes, noting that the least automatic movements were impaired first and took the longest to be regained.

Checking a person's reflexes is now a standard part of neurological examinations. Flaws in reflex response can reveal brain or nerve damage.

Additional reading: Spillane, *The Doctrine of the Nerves,* pp. 84–89.

refractive surgery

In refractive surgery, the cornea is reshaped in order to correct nearsightedness or farsightedness. These surgeries were first performed with tiny scalpels, but are now generally done with excimer lasers (*see* **laser surgery**).

In radial keratotomy, the first type of refractory surgery to be developed, a series of incisions are made on the cornea in a spoke-like pattern. The incisions allow the cornea to flatten, thus correcting nearsightedness. Surgeons began attempting this surgery in the nineteenth century. Japanese surgeons began using surgery to correct keratoconus, a malformation of the cornea, in the 1930s. They found the surgery worked for nearsightedness as well, but their patients suffered subsequent eye damage. Soviet surgeons began testing the procedure on rabbits and began operating on humans two years later. The procedure was first performed in the United States in 1978.

The excimer laser, which became commercially available in 1979, made it possible to perform these procedures with more precision. **Food and Drug Administration** trials of refractive surgery with excimer lasers began in 1987. The following year, Marguerite B. McDonald (1950–) at the Louisiana State University Eye Center achieved the first successful result with photorefractive keratectomy in nearsighted person after extensive experiments in rabbits and

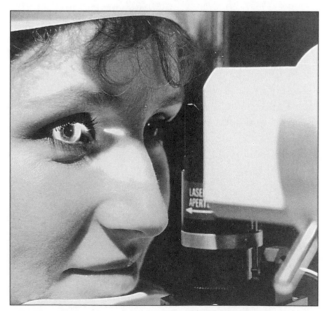

A patient receives laser surgery to correct nearsightedness in 1989. (Courtesy of Archives and Special Collections, Columbia University Health Sciences Division.)

primates. The "photo" refers to the fact that a laser is used to perform the procedure.

The FDA approved lasers made by the U.S. companies Summit and VISX for certain procedures in 1995. Refractive surgery centers soon sprang up around the United States to offer people the chance to throw away their glasses forever. The procedure still remains somewhat controversial; critics say it weakens the eye and makes it more susceptible to damage.

Additional reading: Galton, *Med Tech,* pp. 264–66.

relaxation response

The relaxation response is a mental state attained by meditation, prayer, yoga, or other techniques in which oxygen consumption drops, heart and breathing rates slow, and muscles relax.

The relaxation response has been known for centuries in both Western Christian and Jewish traditions and in Eastern religions, such as Buddhism.

Harvard psychiatrist Herbert Benson (1935–) and his colleagues described the relaxation response in a 1974 article, reporting that this state could be obtained by transcendental meditation, yoga, and prayer. Benson proposed that the relaxation response is the opposite of the fight-or-flight response, and results in decreased sympathetic nervous system activity and increased parasympathetic nervous system activity. (The sympathetic nerves generally stimulate the organs to work harder, while the parasympathetic nerves have the opposite effect.)

Regular practice of the relaxation response (twice a day for 15 minutes is the usual recommendation) has been shown to have positive effects on many stress-related physical and mental problems, such as **hypertension** and anxiety.

Additional reading: Benson, *The Relaxation Response;* "East Meets West," "How to Find Help," Consumer Reports.

REM

Rapid eye movement is a stage of sleep that is associated with dreaming. During REM, the eyes move back and forth quickly under the eyelids. REM alternates with non-REM sleep in about four or five cycles during a single sleeping period. Eugene Aserinsky (1921–1998) and Nathaniel Kleitman (1895–1999) discovered rapid eye movements during sleep and published their observations in 1953.

The significance of REM sleep remains unclear, although it is thought to be essential to health. Experiments have shown that depriving people of this sleep cycle is psychologically harmful.

Additional reading: Jouvet, *The Paradox of Sleep.*

renin-angiotensin system

The renin-angiotensin system is the body's mechanism for maintaining **blood pressure** at the optimal level, which, when it malfunctions, may contribute to **hypertension** and heart disease.

The **adrenal gland** releases renin in response to low amounts of sodium in the blood, or low blood pressure. Renin is converted into angiotensin and then into angiotensin II. These substances raise blood pressure by constricting blood vessels and affecting the heart in other ways.

Robert Tigerstedt (1853–1923) and his colleagues in Finland were the first to propose the existence of such a system, when they showed in an 1898 paper that kidney extracts raised blood pressure. They named the responsible substance "renin." About 40 years later, scientists confirmed this, but suggested that renin itself didn't raise blood pressure but instead formed another pressure-raising substance. They named this substance angiotensin. In 1956, others delineated the products of renin as angiotensin I, angiotensin II, and angiotensin-converting-enzyme (ACE). Angiotensin II was synthesized in 1956, but the actual structure of renin wasn't described until the early 1970s.

Today, the renin-angiotensin system is known to be active in all of the body's tissues. Also, we know that this affects the heart directly, not just through blood pressure, and that by inhibiting the action of the system with drugs called **ACE inhibitors** it is possible to bring down blood pressure and even reverse the harmful effects of heart disease to a certain extent.

Additional reading: Comroe, *Exploring the Heart*, pp. 310–13.

reserpine

Reserpine is a blood pressure-lowering and sedative drug derived from the plant *Rauwolfia serpentina*, which is named after the German botanist Leonhard Rauwolf (1535–1596), who described the plant in 1582.

The first record of the plant's medical uses appears in an Indian medical treatise written in about 600 B.C. called the *Charaka Samhita*. The drug was used to treat snakebite.

Scientific investigation of the plant began with the efforts of several Indian researchers. In 1931, Calcutta doctors reported that extracts of the plant lowered **blood pressure** and also had a sedative effect. Researchers at the School of Tropical Medicine in Calcutta investigated the plant and its extracts for more than a decade, and proved that it did indeed lower blood pressure and produce sedation. Rauwolfia became an accepted blood-pressure treatment in India, and it is estimated that one million citizens received it for this purpose during the 1940s.

News of the drug spread beyond India when the *British Heart Journal* published a paper by an Indian doctor on his trials of the drug in patients at a Bombay hospital. Robert Wilkins (1906–), head of the hypertension clinic at Massachusetts General Hospital, tested the drug for five years in his patients, reporting his results in 1952. That year, Nathan Kline (1916–1983) tried using the drug to treat psychotic patients.

The active alkaloid of Rauwolfia, reserpine, was isolated from the plant in 1951. The drug company Ciba began selling the drug two years later. Robert Woodward (1917–1979) of Harvard University synthesized reserpine in 1956.

The drug was used for many years to treat high blood pressure and also as a sedative, but became less popular once more powerful tranquilizing drugs (such as chlorpromazine, used as an **antipsychotic**) became available. Also, reserpine's effects on blood pressure were relatively modest and the drug also could bring on severe **depression** in some people.

The drug is now used less frequently because of its side effects. But recent research has found interesting links between the drug and certain dopamine **receptors** in the brain, which may point the way toward other therapeutic uses.

Additional reading: Curzon, "How Reserpine and Chloropromazine Act."

restriction enzyme

A restriction enzyme is a chemical that "snips" a specific point on a **DNA** molecule, cued by the sequence of nucleotides.

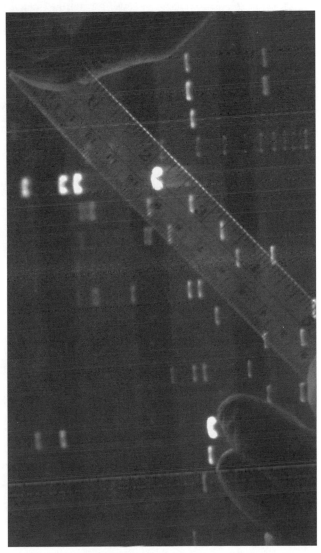

DNA fragments, cut apart using restriction enzymes, are displayed on an electrophoresis gel. (Courtesy of National Institute for Human Genome Research.)

There are more than 800 known restriction enzymes, each of which cuts DNA at a different point. Restriction enzymes cut the two sides of DNA unevenly, leaving a "sticky end" that allows DNA particles to attach to others that have been cut by the same enzyme, no matter what species they are from. This has made it possible to combine different types of DNA in a process known as recombination. Restriction enzymes are also used in **DNA fingerprinting.** (See also recombinant DNA)

Additional reading: Grace, *Biotechnology Unzipped,* pp. 35–41.

retroviruses

Retroviruses are viruses made of RNA that put their host's **DNA** to work, instructing it to make more of the **virus.** Some of these viruses may cause **cancer.**

Retroviruses consist of a single strand of RNA. Once they enter a cell, retroviruses collect nucleotides and assemble themselves as a double strand of DNA, which splices itself into the host's genetic material. Other RNA viruses exist, but they are not capable of incorporating themselves directly into the host's DNA. Because retroviruses can do this, they are more difficult for the immune system to recognize and fight. Furthermore, when a cell divides it carries the instruction for making more copies of the virus with it.

David Baltimore (1938–) at the Massachusetts Institute of Technology and Howard Temin (1934–) at the University of Washington discovered retroviruses, and shared the 1975 Nobel Prize for their achievement.

Temin had first hypothesized the existence of retroviruses in the 1960s, but this idea was met with skepticism in the scientific community. He and Baltimore then put together a case for how such a virus might function. They showed that retroviruses carry an enzyme called reverse transcriptase with them when they enter a cell in order to facilitate the process of forming their own DNA. The presence of this enzyme in a cell indicates retroviral infection.

The first retrovirus attacking humans was discovered in 1979 by Dr. Robert Gallo (1937–) at the National Cancer Institute in Bethesda, Maryland, in the white blood cells of a man with lymphoma. Gallo called the virus human **T cell** lymphoma virus, or HTLV.

HIV, the virus that causes **AIDS,** was the second human retrovirus to be discovered. Gallo and Luc Montagnier (1932–), at the Pasteur Institute in France, both claimed to have been the first discoverers of HIV in the early 1980s. The international scientific community agreed to give credit to both.

Retroviruses have been put to therapeutic use; the first human **gene therapy** employed a retrovirus to insert correct genetic information into a patient's T cells, with some success.

Additional reading: Garrett, *The Coming Plague,* pp. 226–33.

Rh factor

Rh factor is an **antibody** that coats the surface of most people's **red blood cells.** A person may be Rh positive, meaning they have the antibody, or negative, meaning they don't. About 85 percent of humans are Rh positive.

A fetal condition known as erythroblastosis fetalis can occur if an Rh-negative mother is pregnant with an Rh-positive fetus. An Rh-negative mother who has given birth to an Rh-positive child may, in a subsequent pregnancy with an Rh-positive child, produce antibodies that cross the placenta and attack the fetus's red blood cells, resulting in **anemia,** enlargement of the spleen and liver, and possibly death.

Giving a woman Rh immune globulin, which contains Rh antibodies, shortly before delivery will suppress her immune response and prevent erythroblastosis fetalis in subsequent pregnancies.

Louis K. Diamond first named and described erythroblastosis fetalis in 1932. A few years later, Philip Levine (1900–1987) observed a severe transfusion reaction, resulting in destruction of red blood cells, in a woman who had delivered a stillborn infant. He reported that this was due to a previously unknown blood type.

Karl Landsteiner (1863–1943), the discoverer of ABO blood groups, named this human blood factor "Rh," after rhesus monkeys, because his experiments using animal serum found a similar proportion of red blood cells positive and negative for a factor in rhesus monkey blood: 85 percent and 15 percent, respectively. The human and rhesus blood factors were later found not to be identical, but the name has remained.

Diamond initially tried treating erythroblastosis fetalis with transfusions of Rh negative blood to newborns via the umbilical vein in 1946. In the early days of treatment, about half the children survived; this proportion grew to more than 95 percent. In 1960, Dr. A. William Liley (unknown–1983) of New Zealand developed a method for measuring the severity of fetal anemia. Three years later, he began transfusing fetuses in utero. The first such successful transfusion, in 1963, after three unsuccessful attempts, was also the first successful **fetal surgery.**

In 1960, a method for preventing erythroblastosis fetalis by giving an Rh-negative mother Rh antibodies after the birth of her first Rh-positive child was developed by Levine and his colleagues, and became widely available later in the decade. The antibodies were gathered from other Rh-positive mothers of Rh-negative children who had high concentrations of these proteins in their blood. This antibody is known as the "Big D" antibody.

Additional reading: Speert, *Obstetric & Gynecologic Milestones Illustrated,* pp. 436–46

rheumatoid arthritis

Rheumatoid arthritis is an **autoimmune disease** that causes painful inflammation of the joints. Osteoarthritis, or degenerative arthritis, is a separate disease related to aging and exacerbated by injury.

Early treatment of rheumatoid arthritis involved sending people to spas where they could bathe in warm water to ease joint pain. Salicylates, drugs related to **aspirin,** were also found to be helpful in the nineteenth century. In the 1920s and 1930s, surgeries to repair arthritic joints were performed with some success. In the 1930s, gold salts were found to ease inflammation. It was at this time that physicians began treating rheumatoid arthritis as a separate disease from osteoarthritis. In the early 1950s, antimalarial drugs and immunosuppressive agents began being used to treat mild arthritis.

Cortisones, medications based on **hormones** produced by the adrenal cortex that were introduced in the 1950s, are extremely effective for treating rheumatoid arthritis. But their benefits decrease with extended use and long-term use also produces serious side effects.

Penicillamine, introduced in 1963, was found to have effects similar to gold salts, but the drug also had some severe side effects.

Methotrexate, an immune-suppressing drug introduced in 1990, and other immunosuppressants such as cyclophosphamide and azathioprine, also are used to treat rheumatoid arthritis. Anti-**tumor necrosis factor,** developed in the late 1990s, is very effective but remains extremely expensive. The first drug of this class is etanercept, which was approved for release by the **Food and Drug Administration (FDA)** in late 1998. During that same year, the FDA approved the first in another new class of drugs for rheumatoid arthritis, the **COX-2 inhibitor** Celebrex. This is preferable to **nonsteroidal anti-inflammatory drugs (NSAIDs),** because continued use of these medications can lead to damage of the intestinal tract. (*See also* immunosuppression)

Additional reading: Kiple, *The Cambridge World History of Human Disease,* pp. 599–602.

rhinoplasty

Rhinoplasty is surgery to reconstruct or reshape the nose.

The first mention of reconstructive rhinoplasty appears in the writings of the Indian surgeon Susruta, who around 600 B.C. described using a flap of skin from the cheek to create a new nose. A technique for using skin from the forehead may have been used by Indian surgeons as early as 1000 A.D.

In the late nineteenth century, U.S. surgeons began attempting surgery to decrease the size of the nose and to reshape "saddle" or sunken noses that were often caused by syphilitic infection. Paraffin injections were used at first to rebuild depressed noses, but the material migrated, sometimes caused tumor growth, and was difficult to remove.

Today, rhinoplasty is a generally safe and routine part of **plastic surgery** practice.

Additional reading: Gilman, *Making the Body Beautiful,* pp. 43–118.

rhodopsin

Rhodopsin is a pigment, also known as visual purple, that is found in the rods of the retina and helps the eye adapt to darkness. The discovery of the significance of rhodopsin in vision paved the way for the understanding of the role of **vitamin A** in preserving sight, because the visual pigment is a derivative of the nutrient.

Franz Christian Boll (1849–1879) discovered rhodopsin in a frog's retina in 1876. He noted that the pigment turned yellow when held to the light, and named it "sehpurpur," or visual purple.

Willy Kuhne (1837–1900) and Carl Anton Ewald (1845–1915) confirmed that rhodopsin is found in the human retina in the late 1870s by dissecting the eye of a criminal who had been executed in the dark. Kuhne also discovered visual violet, or porphyropsin. The study of the eyes of recently killed animals and humans became a popular scientific pursuit; because light bleached the purple and violet out of the retina, with specific preparation the retina produced an "optogram" showing light and dark that represented the dead person or animal's last sight.

Pigments of the light-viewing cells, the cones, were not discovered until much later. They were called throlabe, chromolabe, and cyanolabe, for red-, green-, and blue-catching, respectively.

Additional reading: Brown, "Chemical Found to Absorb Radar"; "How Humans Learn to See in Red, Green and Blue," *The Economist.*

rickets

Rickets is a disease in which the limbs fail to grow straight and strong because sufficient minerals are not deposited in newly forming bone and cartilage. This disease is caused by a lack of **vitamin D**, and was among the first deficiency diseases described. It has been common among poor children, particularly in cities. When rickets is left untreated, it can affect the brain and spine, and may be fatal.

The first descriptions of rickets appear before the tenth century. Francis Glisson (c.1597–1677), an English physician, wrote the definitive text on rickets, *De Rachitide,* published in 1650. He suggested, incorrectly, that the disease was caused by poor hygiene and an unwholesome home environment.

Researchers working during the late 1890s and early 1900s found that 80 percent or more of infants in several large European and U.S. cities showed signs of rickets. Lack of sunlight was suspected as a cause, but the reason for why this might be was not understood for decades.

Animals raised in London's Zoological Gardens were plagued by rickets and other bone disorders. In 1889, Sir John Bland-Sutton (1855–1936) suggested giving lion cubs cod liver oil and crushed bones along with their regular meat diet, with excellent results.

Edward Mellanby (1884–1955), after extensive research using puppies, concluded in 1919 that rickets was caused by dietary deficiency and could be prevented and cured with cod-liver oil. However, two years later he proposed incorrectly that **vitamin A** prevented rickets. The following year, Elmer V. McCollum (1879–1967) and colleagues discovered a second fat-soluble vitamin, D, that was essential for normal bone formation.

Researchers discovered by the 1920s that the body itself produced vitamin D when exposed to sunlight, and that foods exposed to ultraviolet light would be enriched with the **vitamin**. Thanks to supplementation of bread and dairy products with vitamin D in the United States, the disease is now rare in this county.

Additional reading: McCollum, *A History of Nutrition*, pp. 266–90.

Ritalin. *See* attention-deficit hyperactivity disorder.

robotic surgery

Surgeons are increasingly using robots, which can allow the surgeon to operate on the interior of the body through tiny holes, to assist them in performing operations. There are surgical robots that can be directed by voice commands, and others that "translate" the movement of the surgeon's hands into much finer and steadier motions. Robots may also be used to guide a camera during **minimally invasive surgery**, while the surgeon performs the operation him or herself.

Surgeons are using robot technology in relatively uncomplicated bypass surgeries—for example, operations in which only one vessel must be bypassed. They sit at a console across the room from a patient. The first United States **clinical trial** of robot-assisted endoscopic coronary artery **bypass surgery**, conducted at the Milton S. Hershey Medical Center in Hershey, Pennsylvania, found in early 2000 that the technique was safe and feasible.

The Goleta, California company Computer Motion, Inc., is a leader in the production of surgical robots.

Advocates of robotic surgery believe the uses of this technology will increase, and that it may one day make it possible for a surgeon to operate on a patient from a location miles away.

Additional reading: Kolata, Gina. "Next Up: Surgery by Remote Control." *The New York Times*.

rubber gloves

Gloves made with rubber and other waterproof, protective materials are used in a variety of medical procedures to prevent the spread of infection. They were invented at about the same time that **germ theory**, the idea that microbes spread disease, became generally accepted.

Willam S. Halsted (1852–1922), a legendary surgeon who worked at Johns Hopkins Hospital in Baltimore, is generally agreed to have introduced the surgical use of rubber gloves. He wrote in 1913 that one of his operating nurses suffered from dermatitis on her arms and hands from exposure to the corrosive **antiseptic** solution used in surgery. In or around 1889, Halsted asked the Goodyear Rubber Company to make two pairs of thin rubber gloves with wrist-protecting extensions called gauntlets. Gradually, surgeons themselves began using the gloves. The first surgeon to wear them, according to Halsted, was Joseph C. Bloodgood (1866–1935) of Johns Hopkins in an 1893 operation.

As the use of rubber gloves spread, some surgeons objected to them, arguing that the gloves interfered with their surgical technique. But their use soon became standard practice.

Additional reading: Miller, "William Stewart Halsted and the Use of Rubber Gloves"; "The Pre-Halstedian and Post-Halstedian History of the Surgical Rubber Glove," *Surgery, Gynecology, and Obstetrics.*

rubella

Rubella is an infectious viral disease. In childhood, rubella infection is mild, and once a person has had rubella he or she is immune to infection. But rubella infection during pregnancy can cause serious **birth defects**.

Rubella had long been thought to be the same thing as **scarlet fever** and **measles**, but was officially recognized as a separate disease in 1881 by the International Congress of Medicine in London.

Japanese scientists in 1938 showed that a **virus** caused rubella. Australian ophthalmologist Norman McAlister Gregg (1892–1966) observed in 1941 that children of mothers who had been infected with rubella early in pregnancy were born with defects, including cataracts and other eye problems, low birthweight, heart malformations, skin problems, deafness, and retardation. These children also had a higher-than-normal death rate. Gregg's findings were not confirmed or widely known until the end of the 1940s.

Paul D. Parkman (1932–) at the Walter Reed Army Hospital in Washington, D.C., and Thomas Weller (1915–) and Franklin Neva (1922–) at the Harvard School of Public Health, working separately, isolated the rubella virus in 1962.

Parkman and his colleagues produced a weakened form of the rubella virus in 1966, making it possible to develop **vaccines** against rubella. An **antibody** test, which determines whether a person is immune to rubella, was developed in 1967. Widespread rubella vaccination for children began in the early 1970s.

Today, many U.S. states require women to have been vaccinated for rubella, or have proven their immunity to rubella infection, before granting them a marriage license.

Additional reading: Williams, *Virus Hunters,* pp. 396–400.

S

Salvarsan

Salvarsan is an arsenical drug that targets the spirochetes that cause **syphilis**. Despite its drawbacks, the drug helped revolutionize the treatment of venereal disease when it was introduced in 1910. It was better than the syphilis treatment previously available, which consisted chiefly of mercury-based drugs that tended to be quite toxic.

Paul Ehrlich (1854–1915) announced that he had discovered an effective syphilis drug in 1910, the 606th compound that he evaluated for this purpose. Hoechst began manufacturing the drug later that year and called it Salvarsan. The drug had to be given intravenously, which in those times involved a surgical procedure.

Salvarsan was difficult and painful to administer and had serious side effects, such as kidney damage. But the success of the drug in eliminating contagious symptoms prompted the opening of venereal disease clinics, as well as the admission of syphilis patients to general hospitals.

By 1918, the **U.S. Public Health Service** had created a Venereal Diseases Division. When a shortage of Salvarsan threatened as World War I loomed, U.S. laboratories were licensed to make the drug under the name "arsphenamine."

Penicillin, the first **antibiotic**, revolutionized the treatment of syphilis in 1944 and made salvarsan obsolete.

Additional reading: Weatherall, *In Search of a Cure,* pp. 58–63.

scarlet fever

Scarlet fever, or scarletina, is an infectious disease whose symptoms include fever, sore throat, rash, and rapid pulse. People with the infection also develop a "strawberry tongue," in which the papilla of the tongue project like strawberry seeds and the tongue itself is bright red. Scarlet fever is rarely fatal, but can be dangerous if complications such as meningitis (infection of the membranes surrounding the brain) develop. It is treated with **penicillin**.

The disease is caused by certain types of streptococcal bacteria that produce a toxin, and appears in both mild and virulent forms.

Scarlet fever was first described in Europe in the sixteenth and seventeenth centuries. Thomas Sydenham (1624–1689) distinguished scarlet fever from **measles** in 1683.

Edward Klein (1844–1925), a Yugoslavian doctor working at St. Bartholomew's Hospital in London, isolated streptococci from scarlet fever patients' blood in 1887, but he was unable to prove that the germ caused the disease. George (1881–1967) and Gladys Dick (1881–1963) showed in the early 1920s that scarlet fever was caused by an infection of the throat with type A hemolytic streptococci. They developed the Dick test, which gauges a person's susceptibility to scarlet fever.

Scarlet fever is common in an extremely mild form in the United States, Canada, and Europe. In the nineteenth century, however, a virulent strain was prevalent in Europe, persisting in certain parts of the continent until the early twentieth century.

Additional reading: Kiple, *The Cambridge World History of Human Disease,* pp. 990–92.

schistosomiasis

Schistosomiasis is a disease caused by infection of the blood with flukes that live in the body of a certain type of snail. People catch the disease by wading in water that contains these snails. The flukes are called cercariae. The disease is endemic to Asia, Africa, and tropical regions of the Americas. It is rarely fatal, but can lead to chronic ill health.

There are different types of the disease in different regions: *Schistosoma mansoni* in Africa, South America, and the Caribbean; *S. japonicum,* in China and Southeast Asia; and *S. haematobium* of Africa and the Middle East. *S. mansoni* and *S. japonicum* are associated with liver disease, while *S. haematobium* causes urinary tract disease and bladder **cancer**.

The German physician Theodor Bilharz (1825–1862) discovered the cause of the disease in 1851, finding a long worm in the bloodstream of a person undergoing an **autopsy** at a hospital in Cairo. The disease is sometimes called bilharzia in honor of his discovery.

In the chronic form of the disease the liver and spleen are enlarged. The infected person also suffers from fatigue and gastrointestinal problems. Symptoms occur because the parasite's eggs clog the liver; the immune system's reaction to the parasite also produces some symptoms. However, some people can be infected with the parasite and remain relatively healthy.

The first drug discovered to be effective against schistosomiasis was tartar emetic, introduced in Africa in 1916. This drug has become obsolete, as it is extremely toxic. New more helpful **antiparasitic** drugs introduced in the 1980s include praziquantel (sold as Biltricide), which can also be used to prevent the infection.

Additional reading: Kiple, *The Cambridge World History of Human Disease*, pp. 992–97.

schizophrenia

Schizophrenia is a group of **mental illnesses** characterized by delusions, hallucinations, and a loss of identity. People with schizophrenia also tend to have paranoid delusions, disordered thought processes (for example, they may speak in a "word salad" of unrelated terms), disorganized behavior, and abnormal affect (meaning they are not able to respond emotionally in an appropriate fashion).

Schizophrenia is treated with **psychotherapy** and **antipsychotic drugs**. It usually strikes people in their 20s or 30s, and about one-third of patients recover or get somewhat better within 25 to 30 years of their diagnosis. The cause of the disease is unknown. About one in 100 people in the United States suffers from schizophrenia.

Philipe Pinel (1745–1826) described schizophrenia for the first time in 1809. The disease was called *dementia praecox,* or premature dementia. Eugen Bleuler (1857–1939) coined the word "schizophrenia"—German for "divided mind"—in 1908. He saw the disease as a split in psychic function due to unknown causes.

In the early twentieth century, attempts were made to treat schizophrenia with a wide variety of approaches, ranging from adrenaline injections to vasectomy, with no success. The first successful treatment for psychosis was coma therapy, followed by **convulsive therapy** and **electroconvulsive therapy**. The first antipsychotic drugs became available in the 1950s, and were effective in relieving psychotic symptoms for many patients but also had severe neurological side effects. More tolerable and more effective antipsychotic drugs became available in the 1990s.

Some historians believe schizophrenia is a relatively new disease, caused by a virus or by the stresses of modern life, while others believe it has been with us since prehistoric times.

Studies of twins, beginning in 1928, gradually established a genetic basis for schizophrenia, although the disease does not follow a classic pattern of inheritance. The best of these studies were done in Denmark, thanks to the extensive hospital and adoption records kept in that country. The identical twin of a person with schizophrenia has a 50 percent chance of developing the disease, while a fraternal or nonidentical twin has a 15 percent chance.

Epidemiological studies have also found that people born in urban areas and in the spring and winter months are more likely to develop schizophrenia. However, doctors are not certain why this occurs. Studies of the brain using **CAT scanning** and **magnetic resonance imaging** have revealed that people with schizophrenia tend to have less brain tissue that people without the disease, as well as less activity in the frontal lobes.

As evidence accumulates, more and more researchers believe that there are a number of causes that work together to cause schizophrenia, rather than a single source. Most see schizophrenia as caused by errors in brain development, particularly in connections among the neurons that make up the brain. Basically, people with schizophrenia have abnormalities that lead to errors in information processing. The theory that schizophrenia was caused by "schizophrenogenic mothers" has been proved to be totally false.

Although there are now effective medications for treating schizophrenia, not all patients respond to them. Also, these drugs must be taken for the rest of a person's life and they tend to have troubling side effects. Schizophrenics often stop taking their medication because of these side effects. Other treatments that are important for helping a person—and his or her family—cope with schizophrenia include family therapy, **behavioral therapy**, and skills treatment. A recent study found that fewer than one half of schizophrenics in the United States receive adequate treatment. (*See also* mental hospitals)

Additional reading: Keefe and Harvey, *Understanding Schizophrenia.*

scoliosis treatment

Scoliosis is a condition in which the spine is curved laterally in a C- or S-shape. This disorder ranges from mild to disabling, and is seven times more common in women than in men. It may be caused by **tuberculosis** or **poliomyelitis**, although it usually has no apparent cause.

Early attempts to treat scoliosis, beginning with Hippocrates (c.460–c.377 B.C.) , consisted of traction—pulling the spine into the proper shape—or suspending a person by the head and armpits, or even the feet, to straighten the spine.

Ambrose Pare (c.1510–1590) thought scoliosis was caused by bad posture, and he devised a girdle made of thin, perforated iron sheets to treat spinal curvature. Nicholas Andry (1658–1717) blamed scoliosis on uneven muscular contraction, and used rest, suspension, and padded corsets, along with care in the design of furniture, to promote proper posture.

Beginning in the early 1800s, extension chairs were developed to hold a person upright. Some included instruments for traction. Exercise also was attempted beginning about this time. Jean-Andre Venel (1740–1791) developed a traction bed that the patient could use at night and while resting during the day. In 1850, Max Langenbeck (1818–1877) invented a device in which the person was bound to a post with a padded board. The board was thrust forward by a screw to push against the convexity of the spine. Around this time, braces were introduced that exerted lateral as well as vertical pressure on the spine, and attempts were made to correct scoliosis surgically, with varying success.

Lewis Sayre (1820–1900) invented a plaster jacket that was used while suspending the patient by his or her head and armpits.

Russell Hibbs (1869–1932) performed the first spinal fusion in 1911, for back deformity caused by tuberculosis infection. He used the operation to treat scoliosis in 1914. A more effective brace, the Risser plaster jacket, was introduced in the late 1920s.

Some problems with plaster casts were that they compressed the lungs, caused pressure sores, and could not be used to control spinal rotation. Robert Ray (1914–) and his colleagues developed an effective brace consisting of a halo around the head and a hoop around the spine, reporting on their research in 1970. The brace was attached by bone screws to the skull and pelvis.

Today, a person with scoliosis usually receives treatment during adolescence, and this treatment may consist of exercises, bracing, traction, or surgery (or a combination of these) depending on the severity of the spinal curvature.

Additional reading: LeVay, *History of Orthopaedics,* pp. 529–46.

scurvy

Scurvy is a serious illness caused by deficiency in the nutrient **vitamin C.** Humans cannot synthesize this nutrient themselves, but must consume it in food. The disease is treated with vitamin C suplementation.

The word "scurvy" comes from northern European words meaning "to itch." Scurvy became well known in the late 1400s, when the crews of long sea voyages began to develop the illness. Symptoms include bleeding gums and weak and swollen limbs. If a person is deprived of vitamin C for long enough, old wounds will reopen and he or she will eventually die.

There were scattered accounts of using preparations of leaves and citrus fruit or juice to prevent scurvy in the fifteenth, sixteenth, and seventeenth centuries. During French explorer Jacques Cartier's (1491–1557) voyage to North America, in 1536, a Native American reportedly showed the ship's captain how to treat the disease with evergreen tree leaves.

James Lind (1716–1794), a Scottish naval surgeon, conducted the first ever **clinical trial** in 1747 to investigate how to best treat scurvy. On the ship Salisbury, Lind divided 12 sailors with scurvy into 6 pairs and fed each pair a different diet. He found that those who ate oranges and lemons healed the fastest. The British Navy waited until 1795 to include lime or lemon juice in sailors' diets. Cap-

tain James Cook (1728–1779) stocked fresh fruit and vegetables as well as lemon juice on his second voyage around the world. None of his crew died from scurvy.

The "antiscorbutic," or antiscurvy vitamin was not discovered until the 1930s, but Axel Holst (1861–1931) had first suggested that such a substance must exist in 1907. He and his colleague Alfred Frohlich (1871–1953) showed that scurvy was indeed a deficiency disease.

Additional reading: Gordon, *The Alarming History of Medicine,* pp. 56–64; Kiple, *The Cambridge World History of Human Disease,* pp. 1000–05.

seat belts

Seat belts are devices used to prevent injury in automobile accidents by restraining drivers and passengers.

The first U.S. automobile manufacturer to introduce seatbelts was Nash, in 1949. The seatbelts proved to be unpopular, but a report by the Cornell Aeronautical Labs in 1953 found that aircraft-style seat belts were indeed effective at preventing injury. After the report, various automobile manufacturers began testing seat belts, and the Society of Automotive Engineers formed a committee to develop criteria for their strength and performance.

With much publicity, Ford Motor Company introduced its "Lifeguard" safety package, including front and rear seatbelts, in 1956. But because General Motors cars sold better that year, many in the industry took this to mean that "safety doesn't sell." Meanwhile, Chevrolet introduced a shoulder belt in 1957 and Volvo made lap and shoulder belts standard equipment in 1959.

Legislation requiring seat belts in cars began in Wisconsin, which ruled that all cars sold in the state be equipped with safety belts beginning in 1962. Several states followed, enough so that the industry made seat belts standard by 1964. The National Traffic and Motor Vehicles Safety Act of 1966 brought automobile design and manufacture under federal regulation.

Beginning in 1973, the federal regulatory body, the National Highway Traffic Safety Administration (NHTSA), required that cars be designed so that they wouldn't start unless all safety belts were latched. Congress reversed the NHTSA's decree the following year.

The world's first law requiring seat-belt use was passed in Victoria, Australia, in 1971. The first year the law was in effect, highway fatalities dropped 21 percent. Other Australian states, along with European countries, followed with seat-belt requirements of their own, but the United States did not, arguing that the public would protest.

In 1977, however, Tennessee passed a law requiring the use of restraints for children. Other states followed.

In 1984, Transportation Secretary Elizabeth Dole (1936–) created incentives for states to pass laws requiring seat belt use. New York was the first state to require seat belt use, with a law passed in 1984, and by 1985 17 states had done so.

According to the NHTSA, seatbelts saved 9,000 lives and prevented 200,000 injuries in 1990. In 1998, the federal government launched a campaign to promote seat belt and safety seat use for children, and also provided $1.2 billion in grants to states to promote seat belt use.

Today, all states have a law requiring adults to use seatbelts, except for New Hampshire, which only requires that people younger than 18 use the devices.

Additional reading: Kent, "Report."

sensors

Sensors are devices capable of detecting and measuring chemical, biological, electrical or other physical signals that are becoming increasingly important in health care. Technology for developing these devices has advanced greatly thanks to microchip technology and molecular chemistry. Sensors will soon be used to monitor a patient's health remotely, as well as to detect bacteria in the environment and make implanted devices such as **pacemakers** "smart."

The leading applications of sensor technology at present are for instruments that measure blood glucose and blood gases. Patients with **diabetes** must continually monitor their blood sugar levels with blood glucose tests that require them to draw a small blood sample by pricking the skin. Glucose sensors were first tested in the lab in the 1960s, and in animals in the early 1970s. The main technology being investigated for use in glucose sensing uses the enzyme glucose oxidase, which is secured at a charged electrode. The enzyme oxidizes glucose, producing hydrogen peroxide, which the sensor detects electrochemically. These sensors are placed on the end of a fine wire or needle and implanted under the skin.

Researchers are also investigating tissue sampling for blood glucose monitoring, because the amount of glucose in the tissue is a relatively good indicator of blood levels and this could eliminate the need for puncturing the skin. Cygnus Inc. has developed a sensor that is worn like a watch, which brings glucose to the skin surface by applying an electric current. Other potential technologies include optical techniques such as infrared spectroscopy and tissue light scattering.

The Food and Drug Administration approved, in 1999, a device that is implanted beneath diabetes patients' skin and continually monitors and records their blood glucose levels. However, the patient must still use finger-prick tests to monitor his or her own glucose levels, because the information is only available to the physician. The next generation of these machines, currently under development, will allow a physician to read this information remotely with a hand-held device or desktop computer.

Physicians predict that patients entering the hospital may soon be implanted with sensors that will monitor the levels of various chemicals and gases in the blood, making conventional blood tests obsolete.

Sensors are also under development for detecting bacteria and poisons in the environment. Experts believe these devices will be in use within the next few years to assist in infection control in hospitals; for example, they could sample air for bacteria. Sensors can also be used to help guide **robotic surgery.**

Sensor technology is also being used to allow devices such as **pacemakers** to "read" and adapt to changes in the body. For example, the pacemaker could monitor blood oxygen levels and pressure within the heart and adjust its function accordingly. **Cochlear implants** are another type of biological sensor now in common use, and Johns Hopkins researchers have invented a biochip that senses light and can be implanted in the eye, acting as an artificial retina to restore sight to patients with diseases that damage the retina such as macular degeneration and retinitis pigmentosa. Researchers also believe that devices that will dispense medication in response to changes in the environment within the body will also become a reality within the next few years.

Additional Reading: Wilson, Charles B. "Sensors 2010." *British Medical Journal.*

serotonin

Serotonin is a naturally occurring chemical in the body that acts as a neurotransmitter and is thought to be related to many psychological factors. Serotonin is found in the platelets in the blood, the mucous membrane lining the stomach, and the mast cells of the immune system. It is a potent blood vessel constrictor.

Serotonin was first isolated and synthesized in 1948. It was found in the brain shortly afterwards, and research increasingly pointed toward a role for serotonin in the regulation of mood. As researchers began to identify several different types of serotonin **receptors** in the brain, work began to develop drugs that would either cut down or emphasize the activity of serotonin.

For example, antimigraine drugs such as sumatriptan were developed that would block serotonin receptors, while **antidepressants** were developed that slowed the brain's reabsorption of serotonin so there would be more of this neurotransmitter present in the brain. Appetite-suppressing drugs that increase serotonin levels have also been developed. Two of these drugs, fenfluramine and dexfenfluramine, have been withdrawn from the market because they may cause heart valve defects, but sibutramine (sold as Meridia) is still available. (*See also* weight-loss drugs)

Additional reading: Cowley, "A Little Help from Serotonin."

serum therapy

Serum therapy was an early method for fighting infectious disease in which patients received injections of serum (the cell-free liquid portion of blood) from animals that had been intentionally infected with the disease, producing "passive immunity."

Emil von Behring (1854–1917) and Shibasaburo Kitasato (1852–1931) learned in 1890 that blood from animals given small doses of certain toxins could neutralize these toxins in the laboratory. The first human treated with serum therapy was a child given **diphtheria** antitoxin a year later. Behring won the first Nobel Prize for Physiology and Medicine for his work in 1901.

The problem with serum therapy was that it produced "serum sickness": people would develop swelling, itching, swollen lymph nodes, fever, and even a drop in white blood cell counts after several injections. These symptoms occurred because repeated injections caused the formation of "immune complexes," large clusters of cells produced when the body's immune system massed to attack the foreign animal cells.

A report in 1905 outlined these problems, but the real death blow to serum therapy probably occurred when the child of the well-respected, popular German pathologist Paul Langerhans (1847–1888) died after receiving several injections of horse **antibodies**. Now serum treatment is used only in emergencies; for example, in treatment of poisonous snake bites.

Additional reading: Bynum, *Science and the Practice of Medicine in the Nineteenth Century,* pp. 160–64.

sexually transmitted disease (STD). *See* AIDS; gonorrhea; hepatitis; syphilis.

shock

Shock occurs when there is not enough blood flow for the heart to function properly and to deliver sufficient oxygenated blood to body **tissues**. Shock has many potential causes, including traumatic injury, heart attack, poisoning, infection, and dehydration.

Shock had long been observed but was not understood. Around the turn of the twentieth century, Dr. George Crile (1864–1943) observed that shock caused more deaths during surgery than any other factor. In experiments with dogs using blood-pressure-measuring equipment he made himself, Crile confirmed that a severe, sudden drop in **blood pressure** accompanied shock. He developed an inflatable rubber suit for shock victims that maintained blood pressure, which he used from 1902 to 1907. The suit, though cumbersome, kept shock victims alive by squeezing their bodies and maintaining their blood pressure. In 1905, Crile treated a victim of shock with a direct **blood transfusion** from the victim's brother; the donor's artery was sewn to the recipient's vein. The patient recovered. Crile also developed a combined system of local and general **anesthesia**, that brought down mortality from shock during surgery.

During World War I, doctors and nurses observed thousands of cases of shock and learned more about the process. But because blood transfusion technology was not advanced enough for battlefield use, the main treatment available to World War I medics was keeping the shock victim warm.

Medical personnel observed that when a person was in shock, his or her blood became very thick and dark and flowed sluggishly. This led to the idea of using transfused plasma—the liquid part of blood—to treat shock, which worked well because plasma lasted longer than blood in storage and did not have to be typed. The treatment was first tried in animals in 1918, and became regular treatment for humans in shock by the mid-1930s. The development of freeze-dried plasma in 1934 advanced shock treatment further, because the dried version of plasma could be stored for five years rather than two.

Edwin Joseph Cohn (1892–1953) and his colleagues at Harvard, working to develop blood products for treating soldiers wounded in World War II, found that the blood protein albumin was an effective treatment for ending shock. Albumin was used extensively by the Allies during the war.

Today, shock is treated with blood or plasma transfusion or the administration of drugs that increase blood volume, along with oxygen.

Additional reading: Saunders, "In Case of Shock."

sickle-cell anemia

In sickle-cell **anemia, red blood cells** take on an abnormal, sickle-like shape because of a structural defect in the hemoglobin molecule. Sufferers are anemic, and the malformed cells can also block **capillaries**, which leads to damage of tissues supplied by these tiny blood vessels. The disease is also very painful.

There is no cure for sickle-cell anemia, aside from **bone marrow transplant**; treatment consists of hydration, painkillers, and blood transfusion.

This disease affects 1 in 500 black people, and more rarely people from the Mediterranean nations, Saudi Arabia, and India. Sickle-cell anemia appears in these populations because people who carry the sickle cell trait but do not have the disease are protected against **malaria**; when the malaria parasite attacks red blood cells, the cells of people with the sickle-cell trait are taken up and destroyed by the spleen, and thus do not spread the infection within the body.

Researchers believe the sickle-cell trait arose independently in Senegal, Benin, and the Central African Republic. Because people with the trait lived longer, the disease persisted.

Sickle cells were first observed in human blood in 1910 by James B. Herrick (1861–1954). Five years later, scientists at Washington University in St. Louis described the disease. The disease was first called "sickle-cell anemia" in 1922. In 1935, Lemuel Diggs (1900–1995), after performing **autopsy** studies of patients with sickle cell, proposed that organ damage occurred because the abnormal cells blocked capillaries.

In 1949, Linus Pauling (1901–1997) showed with electrophoretic studies that sickle-cell anemia was caused by an abnormal hemoglobin molecule. This discovery is considered by many people to be the birth of the molecular understanding of disease.

Despite the high prevalence of sickle-cell anemia, no definitive cure has been found. The U.S. Congress passed the National Sickle Cell Anemia Control Act in 1972, establishing a sickle-cell disease branch at the **National Institutes of Health (NIH)**.

187

In 1988, a team of surgeons at the Cliniques Universitaires Saint Luc, in Brussels, Belgium, reported performing **bone marrow transplants** in five children to treat sickle cell anemia. The children were all cured. More than 100 patients with sickle cell anemia have been treated with bone marrow transplants so far, with excellent results. Researchers believe that transplants of **stem cells** will also be useful for curing sickle cell anemia. Research continues.

Additional reading: Kiple, *The Cambridge World History of Human Disease,* pp. 1006–08.

six-mercaptopurine (6-MP)

Six-mercaptopurine is a drug used to treat **cancer,** suppress the immune system, and manage ulcerative colitis. It was the first drug to be based on a **DNA** component; the drug's inventors, Gertrude Belle Elion (1919–) and George H. Hitchings (1905–), were working on making a molecule that would resemble a purine, but would not be metabolized properly, thus interrupting DNA function. It is a member of a class of drugs known as **antimetabolites.**

While working at the Wellcome Research Laboratory in North Carolina, Elion and Hitchings came up with 6–MP, which they first tested in children with acute **leukemia.** Hitchings and Elion shared the 1988 Nobel Prize for designing this and other drugs.

Around 1960, 6–MP also was found to be a useful immunosuppresant for use in **kidney transplant** by Roy Calne (1930–). Calne showed that an animal could accept a kidney from a completely unrelated donor if 6–MP was used to suppress immunity.

Although today other immunosuppresant drugs have largely replaced 6–MP for this purpose, the drug remains in use as an effective treatment for ulcerative colitis and for some cancers. (*See also* immunosuppression)

Additional reading: Sneader, *Drug Discovery,* pp. 347–48.

skin grafts

Skin grafts are patches of skin removed from one part of the body and placed on another part, usually to repair damage from burns or in other types of **plastic surgery.**

Indian physicians treated mutilated ears, noses, and lips with skin grafts from the face and the buttocks as early as 2500 B.C. There have been numerous other anecdotal reports of skin grafts, including an account of a master receiving a nose donated by his slave, but it was not until the nineteenth century that researchers rediscovered the work of the Indian physicians and began systematically attempting skin grafts.

The British surgeon Astley Cooper (1768–1843) reported grafting skin from an amputated thumb to the wound in 1817. Other European physicians performed skin grafts with varying success. In the early twentieth century, instruments called dermatomes were developed to collect skin for grafting more precisely. Dermatomes could slice off thinner layers of skin than had previously been possible.

The problem with using skin grafts is that the material is scarce, especially when one is trying to treat a badly burned person with his or her own skin, and skin from a donor—when it is available—may be rejected.

In the late 1970s, skin banks were introduced in which the skin was preserved by freezing. A better technique, in which the grafts were preserved with glycerol and the skin was subsequently better accepted by recipients, was introduced in 1984. Today, "donor banks" of cadaver skin provide skin grafts to badly burned people. Unfortunately, the issue of disease transmission from donated **tissue** has complicated matters. Researchers are now developing various types of **artificial skin** to help solve this problem.

Additional Reading: Klasen, *History of Free Skin Grafting*; Skouge, *Skin Grafting.*

sleep apnea

In sleep apnea, a person stops breathing for a period of time while he or she is asleep. This may be caused by obstruction in the upper airway (usually due to obesity), by respiratory-muscle problems, or by a combination of the two. Obstructive sleep apnea is the most common type.

Sleep apnea leads to daytime sleepiness, as well as nervous-system disturbances. About 40 percent of people with sleep apnea who do not receive treatment die within 10 years of the diagnosis from related conditions including car accidents, high **blood pressure**, heart arrhythmia, and **stroke**.

In the late 1800s, some doctors had suggested that sleepy, obese people's airways became obstructed during sleep, leading to "periodic states of suffocation." Late eighteenth-century doctors prescribed weight loss for treating sleepiness, an effective method that remains the best treatment today.

The condition that came to be known as sleep apnea was first called "Pickwickian syndrome," from Charles Dickens's *Pickwick Papers,* which describe an obese and sleepy character named Fat Joe. William Osler (1849–1919) is generally credited with coining the name in 1918.

Scientific evidence that blockage of the pharynx indeed caused breathing lapses was provided in the late 1960s. During the 1960s, some people with sleep apnea were surgically treated with **tracheotomy.** A more refined operation called uvulopalatopharyngoplasty (UPPP), originally developed in 1964 to correct snoring, eventually replaced tracheotomy. This surgery is basically a type of **plastic surgery** in which excess tissue in the soft palate, uvula, and elsewhere in the pharynx is removed.

Other treatment for sleep apnea includes trycyclic **antidepressants** and various devices that a person uses during sleep to ensure steady breathing, such as a mask that provides continuous positive pressure on the airways.

Addition reading: Strauss, "Help for the Weary."

smallpox

Smallpox is an infectious disease caused by the smallpox **virus** that has plagued humans since 10,000 B.C., but thanks to vaccination was completely wiped off the globe by 1980.

Smallpox produced high fevers and a rash, was fatal in 20 to 60 percent of cases, and left permanent scars on many of those who survived infection.

Smallpox scars have been found on mummies of 1000 to 1500 B.C. The first recorded epidemic of smallpox occurred in 1350 B.C. The Arab physician Rhazes (c. 864–c.936) provided the first clinical description of smallpox, in 910. He noted that smallpox could be transmitted from person to person, and observed that people infected once would not get it again. This is the first recorded theory of acquired immunity.

Smallpox, a disease of the Old World, also played a role in the conquest of the Americas. The disease wiped out the majority of the population of the New World soon after European explorers arrived in the fifteenth and sixteenth centuries, because the native people had absolutely no immunity to it.

Variolation, a technique for preventing people from developing smallpox by purposely exposing them to small amounts of infectious material, was an ancient and sometimes effective—though sometimes deadly—treatment. In China, powdered scabs from a person with smallpox were blown into a person's nose through a tube.

Lady Mary Wortley Montague (c.1689–1762), wife of the British ambassador to the Ottoman Empire, introduced variolation and inoculation to Europe. After observing the technique, she had her son inoculated in 1718 and her daughter three years later, and also wrote home to friends about the technique. Soon variolation became accepted in Britain, and the London Smallpox and Inoculation Hospital was founded in 1745.

European folk wisdom held that milkmaids never got smallpox. Edward Jenner (1749–1823), a British physician, theorized that this was because they were infected with cowpox, a similar disease that didn't make humans sick but did protect against smallpox. He tested his theory in 1796 by inoculating an eight-year-old boy with pus taken from a milkmaid's cowpox lesion. He wrote up his experiment and sent it to the Royal Society. The society was scandalized, but inoculation was quickly accepted because it was very effective.

Jenner coined the term "vaccination," based on the Latin word for cow, *vacca*. Harvard Medical School professor Benjamin Waterhouse (1754–1846) performed the first smallpox vaccinations in the United States when he inoculated his five-year-old son and six servants. King Charles IV of Spain (1748–1819) sent smallpox vaccine to his colonies around the world in the first global immunization effort.

People were sometimes used as "reservoirs" of infected material for long-distance vaccination efforts because the infected material was difficult to transport. Freeze-drying, invented in the 1940s, was used for vaccines produced in the 1950s.

Smallpox continued to decline until 1977, when a Somalian cook was reported to be the last person infected by smallpox. By 1980, the **World Health Organization (WHO)** declared that smallpox had been eradicated from the earth.

Today strains of the smallpox virus are stored at the **Centers for Disease Control and Prevention (CDC)** in Atlanta and the Institute for Viral Preparations in Moscow. A major fear is that stores of smallpox have fallen into the hands of other nations and could be used in biological warfare. (*See also* vaccine)

Additional reading: Kiple, *The Cambridge World History of Human Disease*, pp. 1009–113.

Social Security

Social Security, established in the United States by the Social Security Act of 1935, is a system of government programs designed to protect people at risk of poverty because of unemployment or old age. The act also made provisions for mothers, children, and some disabled people. The program that collects money from workers' paychecks and distributes it to people older than 65 is run at the federal level, while other programs are run individually by states.

The "old-age insurance" portion of the Social Security program was first amended in 1939, when benefits were extended to the families of workers who had retired or were deceased. The program was now called Old Age and Survivors Insurance. Disability benefits were added in 1956.

In 1965, a series of Social Security Amendments established "Health Insurance for the Aged," or Medicare; and "Medical Assistance," or Medicaid. Medicare pays for medical care for the elderly and disabled, while Medicaid covers care for the poor. Amendments in 1977 increased the payroll tax for old-age benefits, and the rate was increased again by Congress in 1983.

In 1984, Congress passed the Social Security Disability Benefits Reform Act. Under the new law, a person's benefits cannot be terminated unless the government supplies evidence that their medical condition has improved and that they are now able to work for pay.

In the 1970s, amendments to Social Security were passed to make unemployment insurance available to more people. Currently, about 95 percent of U.S. workers are eligible for unemployment insurance. A person on unemployment receives compensation based on their previous wages, for a limited amount of time.

Other Social Security programs provide assistance to families with dependent children, aid to permanently disabled people, and aid to blind people.

Additional reading: Richards, *Closing the Door to Destitution.*

sperm bank

Sperm banking is the technique of freezing semen so it can be used later for **artificial insemination**.

In 1776, Lazzaro Spallanzani (1729–1799) made the first scientific observations of frozen sperm. However, it was not until 1949, when scientists discovered that glycerol protects mammalian sperm from the damaging effects of freezing, that sperm banks began to be viable. Farmers soon began using frozen sperm to fertilize their livestock.

The first successful human pregnancy using frozen sperm occurred in 1953. Although it took years for sperm banking to be widely accepted, sperm banks are now commonplace. Main users of sperm banks are single women, lesbian couples, or infertile couples who want to have children. Some men may also use the banks to preserve their sperm for future use.

Additional reading: Daniels and Haimes, *Donor Insemination.*

sphygmomanometer (blood pressure cuff)

The sphygmomanometer is a device used to measure **blood pressure** that was invented by the Italian doctor Scipione Riva-Rocci (1863–1937) in 1896. The instrument he designed was small enough to use at a patient's bedside, and the cuff provided even pressure around the arm, making measurement more accurate. The instrument doctors and nurses use today is basically the same as Riva-Rocci's original.

The device was brought to the United States by the neurosurgeon Harvey Cushing (1869–1939), who had seen it being used during a 1901 visit to Italy.

Before the blood pressure cuff became available, physicians had measured blood pressure subjectively by feeling the radial pulse. Cushing and his colleagues Theodore Janeway (1872–1917) and George Crile (1864–1943) were advocates of the blood-pressure cuff, pointing out that it could be used by nurses and orderlies who would record the pulse figures for the physician's review.

Additional reading: Comroe, *Exploring the Heart,* pp. 218–28.

spinal cord injury treatment

Injury to the spinal cord, the column of nervous tissue that extends from the medulla to the second lumbar vertebra and coordinates reflex action and sensory and motor nerve impulses throughout the body, can lead to functional impairment and paralysis. However, advances in the late 20th century that continue into the 21st century have dramatically improved the prospects for people with these injuries. Strategies for rehabilitation, first developed in the mid-20th century, have also helped people with spinal-cord injuries live independent and productive lives.

According to the American Paralysis Association (APA), there are 250,000 Americans living with spinal cord injuries, and an average of 11,000 spinal cord injuries occur annually. About 55 percent of paralyzed Americans are paraplegic, meaning their lower body function and sensation is impaired, while 45 percent are quadriplegic, meaning they have lost function and sensation in both the arms and legs. Car accidents are the leading cause of spinal cord injuries, followed by violence and falls, according to the APA.

Neurons, the fundamental cell making up the nervous system, consist of a cell body where the nucleus is located,

dendrites surrounding the cell body that receives impulses and transmit them to the cell body, and axons that carry impulses from the cell body on to the dendrites of another cell. Camillo Golgi (1843–1926), an Italian physician and cytologist, provided the first complete and accurate description of the entire nerve cell in 1873.

The spinal cord consists of a bundle of axons. When the cord is injured, it is usually crushed, not severed. Much of the damage to the cord results from the body's response to injury, such as inflammation, which can lead to swelling and further damage the nerves. While the cells of the peripheral nervous system (beyond the brain and spinal cord) can regenerate, a phenomenon first observed by the German physiologist Theodor Schwann (1810-1882) in the 1830s, those within the central nervous system cannot.

Scientists are now attempting to discover why central nervous system cells don't regenerate, and whether using **growth factors** and other substances may stimulate regeneration. One extremely challenging aspect of coaxing these cells to regrow is that the regrown axons must establish a connection with the dendrites of another cell. This contact is not physical, but occurs across the synapse, a gap between the cells. Chemicals called neurotransmitters convey impulses across this gap.

Drugs given soon after the injury, as well as specialized rehabilitation, can restore a considerable amount of motor and sensory nerve function.

The first generation of neural **prostheses,** which restore motor function, entered clinical use in the mid-1990s. These prostheses can help patients move their hands and can also help restore physiological functions such as breathing. Devices for quadriplegic patients who depend on artificial respiration, which would use electrical impulses to "pace" breathing, are in clinical trials. Devices that allow patients to control urinary and bowel function using electronic stimulation, have shown promise in early tests. Experimental work in animals with injections of immature nerve stem cells in damaged spinal cords and surgical repair of severed spinal cords suggest that in the future it may be possible to reconnect a severed spinal cord.

The first, and at this point the only, drug that improves recovery from spinal cord injury is methylprednisolone, approved by the Food and Drug Administration in 1990 after clinical trials showed its benefits. Given within eight hours of injury, methylprednisolone restores an average of 20 percent of spinal cord function. Today most patients receive the drug within three hours of injury if possible. Scientists are unsure why the drug helps; one possibility is that it blocks inflammation and other immune system responses to injury. Other drugs, including GM ganglioside, are currently in clinical trials.

Sir Ludwig Guttman of the Stoke Mandeville Hospital in England established the first center for rehabilitation of spinal cord-injured patients during the early 1940s. The center became a model for others around the world, and a centralized approach is now considered the best strategy for helping these patients regain function and live independently. Rehabilitation can consist of passive exercise and stimulation of the muscles to maintain strength and improve function; patients are also instructed on how to use adaptive devices. Patients may also receive counseling to help them cope with their injury.

Hughes Barbeau at McGill University in Montreal and Anton Wernig at the University of Bonn, working independently, have developed techniques for training patients with spinal cord injuries to walk. This research is based on the discovery, made by Anders Lundberg at the University of Goteborg in Sweden in 1967, that the spinal cord contains a "generator" that causes the nerves on either side of the body to fire alternately and rhythmically to produce walking motions. Lundberg made this observation in tests with cats whose spinal cords had been severed; he found the "rhythm generator" could function independently of the brain.

Patients with spinal cord damage can take advantage of the rhythm generator and relearn how to walk on a treadmill, with a harness that supports part of their weight. Animal and human studies have shown that this training can restore near-normal function. Although patients may only be able to walk a few steps, with the help of a walker or cane, this makes a dramatic impact on their quality of life. Wernig's team reported in 1995 that 33 of 36 recently injured wheelchair-bound patients learned to walk using the technique, and 25 of 33 patients with older injuries. Only half of 24 patients treated with traditional rehabilitation techniques learned to walk again. Unfortunately, this technique is not useful for quadriplegic patients, who are unable to support their upper body weight effectively.

However, these patients could one day benefit from stem cell implants or surgery to bridge the damaged part of the spinal cord. Dennis Choi and John McDonald, working at Washington University in St. Louis, reported in 1999 that laboratory rats treated with immature nerve cells (which had been grown from embryonic stem cells) regained some motor function. At the Karolinska Institute in Stockholm, Sweden, Lars Olson, Heinrich Cheng and Yihai Cao developed a strategy, also in rats, for bridging a severed spinal cord. The team grafted nerve cells from the peripheral system onto the gap, holding them in place with a mixture of fibrin glue and fibroblast growth factor. The team reported in 1996 that the technique produced some regeneration of nerve growth in the spinal cord. Some scientists have urged caution in interpreting the results; the Swedish team continues to investigate this technique in animals today.

Wise Young, a physician and the head of New York University Medical Center's Neurosurgery Research Laboratory, developed the rodent model of human spinal cord injury that is now used in nearly all animal studies of new drugs and surgeries for these injuries. He also organized the first multi-center animal study of spinal cord injury treatment, in 1994. Centralized, large studies like this one promise to bring effective new treatments from the laboratory to the clinic more quickly.

Other advances for paralyzed patients include drugs for treating spasticity, a condition caused by contraction of the muscles that can lead to atrophy.

Christopher Reeve, the actor who played "Superman," became a leading activist for spinal cord injury research and treatment after he suffered a spinal cord injury in a fall from a horse. His foundation, the Christopher Reeve Paralysis Foundation, sponsors a consortium of scientists conducting spinal cord injury research (the first such collaborative effort), funds research, and provides grants to improve the quality of life of patients with spinal cord injuries.

Additional reading: National Library of Medicine's Medline Plus Web site on spinal cord injuries: http://www.nlm.nih.gov/medlineplus/spinalcordinjuries.html.

St. John's wort. *See* antidepressant drugs.

stem cell

A stem cell is an immature cell with the capability to mature into several different types of cells. Embryonic cells are stem cells, for example, while cells in the bone marrow and circulating in the blood are stem cells that mature into the various types of blood cells. The therapeutic potential of stem cells is just beginning to be investigated.

Transplanting blood stem cells has become an accepted method for treating blood disorders and restoring bone marrow function, since these cells can graft themselves to the recipient's bone marrow and begin forming normal blood cells. In theory, a single cell can create an entire blood-forming colony. In the case of diseases of blood cell formation such as **leukemia,** for example, stem cells are collected, existing bone marrow is destroyed with radiation or **chemotherapy**, and the stem cells are reinfused into the patient to establish new, disease-free bone marrow.

The first human trials of peripheral stem cell transplantation, in which the cells are collected from the bloodstream rather than the bone marrow, began in 1977. This therapy is sometimes more effective than **bone marrow transplantation**, because the stem cells are not contaminated with tumor cells and also tend to establish themselves in the marrow more rapidly.

In the 1980s, a number of different substances that stimulate blood cell growth, such as **erythropoietin** and interleukins, became available for clinical use and helped speed bone marrow recovery. These materials also make it possible to boost the number of stem cells in the blood—a process called "mobilization"—so that they can be collected more easily. During this decade scientists also developed methods for identifying, collecting and storing a patient's stem cells for future use.

In 1998, researchers at the University of Wisconsin in Madison and Johns Hopkins University in Baltimore reported that they had cultured embryonic stem cells in the laboratory. The Baltimore team used primordial germ cells—pre-egg and pre-sperm cells from frozen embryos—while the Wisconsin team used cells from human embryos.

The cells have many potential uses, including growing tissues for organ transplants, but the use of cells from human fetuses (aborted fetuses or in some cases embryos produced by **in-vitro fertilization** that couples do not use) has raised ethical questions that have yet to be resolved.

Additional reading: Wade, "Discovery Bolsters a Hope for Regeneration"; Westphal, "The Promise of Stem Cells."

stent

Stents are devices that prop blood vessels open. They may be used in the blood vessels of the heart after **angioplasty**, in blood vessels in the brain to treat **stroke**, and in any other part of the body where it is necessary to maintain blood flow.

Charles Dotter (1920–) first suggested the possibility of using spiral-shaped stents to keep blood vessels open in 1969.

Stents were first implanted experimentally in patients in 1986. The **Food and Drug Administration (FDA)** approved the first stent for human use in 1993. The introduction of **anticoagulant** therapy with ticlopidene and **aspirin** as well as inserting balloons into the stents after implantation to ensure that they were fully expanded helped improve the function of these devices.

Reported in 1994, European and U.S. trials comparing stents and angioplasty found that for some patients stenting was more effective.

The term "stent" is thought to come from the name of the British dentist Charles T. Stent (1807–1885) who invented a tubular mold for skin grafting.

Additional reading: Colburn, "Propping Arteries Open Lets Blood Flow."

stereotactic surgery

In stereotactic surgery, an area within the body is pinpointed by locating it along three axes, or in three dimensions, in relation to sites on the surface of the body using a special instrument.

Two teams working independently in 1947 developed a stereotactic surgery frame for humans: Ernest A. Spiegel (1895–unknown) and Henry T. Wycis (1911–1972) and Robert Hayne and Frederic Gibbs (1903–1992). Spiegel and Wycis called their instrument a stereoencephalotome. Hayne and Gibbs used their version to make recordings of electrical activity deep within the brains of **epilepsy** patients. Spiegel and Wycis used their stereoencephalotome for the first time to place therapeutic lesions, or incisions, in the brains of patients with neurological and psychiatric disorders. Their success was limited.

In 1948, Lars Lekskell (1907–1986) invented his own stereotactic surgery apparatus; he would go on to invent the **gamma knife**, which used concentrated radiation to destroy brain tumors. This technique is called radiosurgery.

In the 1950s and 1960s, several groups around the world developed their own stereotactic instruments and used them in surgery. **CAT scanning** and **magnetic resonance**

imaging, techniques that allow a "view" inside the body and brain, have made stereotactic surgical techniques much more precise. The first computer-assisted stereotactic procedure was reported in 1979, and these operations became routine by the mid-1990s. Image-guided technology, in which images are projected on a video screen to guide the surgeon's hand, is now the standard.

Stereotactic surgery and radiosurgery are now used to destroy tumors inside the brain and throughout the body with considerable success.

Additional reading: Alexander, Loeffler, and Lunsford, eds., *Stereotactic Radiosurgery.*

stethoscope

A stethoscope is an instrument for listening to the sounds of a person's heart, lungs, and other organs. One end of the device is placed against the patient's chest while a doctor holds the other end to their ear.

The French doctor Rene Laennec (1781–1826) invented the stethoscope in 1816. One of his female patients had heart problems, but propriety forbade Laennec from placing his ear against her chest, as he would to listen to a

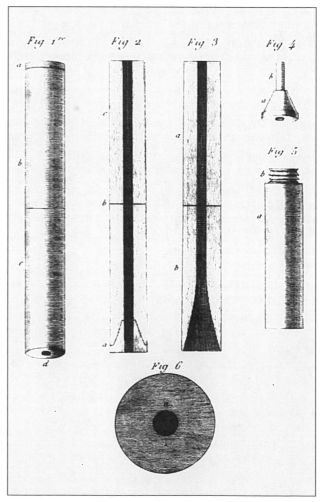

Illustration of a stethoscope from the 1819 book *L'ausculation mediate* by Rene Laennec, the stethoscope's inventor. (Courtesy of National Library of Medicine.)

male patient's heart. To sidestep this problem, Laennec placed one end of a rolled piece of paper on the patient's heart region and the other to his ear. He found this makeshift instrument allowed him to hear the heart more clearly. Laennec designed a more durable stethoscope, a wooden tube with a hole in the middle that could be taken apart and carried easily.

The American physician George P. Cammann (1804–1863) added another earpiece in 1852, to create the binaural version now in use.

Additional reading: Bynum, *Science and the Practice of Medicine in the Nineteenth Century,* pp. 37–41.

streptomycin

Streptomycin is an **antibiotic** and the first drug effective against **tuberculosis**. It comes from the fungus *Streptomyces griseus,* and works by degrading the cell membrane of bacteria and stopping the organism's synthesis of protein.

Selman Waksman (1888–1973), then a professor at Rutgers University in New Jersey, and his colleagues Albert Schatz (1920–) and Betty Bugie were studying the antibiotic properties of the fungus *S. griseus.* In 1943, Schatz began working with a culture from the throat of a sick chicken that a poultry breeder had brought to Rutgers's Agricultural Research Station. This culture was one of 10,000 the team evaluated.

Schatz found the culture from the chicken had powerful antibiotic properties. The Rutgers team named the substance streptomycin. One of the initial tests of the drug was in a girl with a tubercular infection of her meninges, the membranes surrounding the brain. Four months of daily injections with streptomycin cleared up her infection.

Clinical trials of streptomycin for tuberculosis began in 1946, and were the first randomized controlled clinical trials in history.

Waksman won the 1952 Nobel Prize for his discovery. He also coined the word "antibiotic" to describe chemicals made by microorganisms that could kill other microorganisms.

The death rate from tuberculosis worldwide began declining sharply in 1947 due to the discovery of streptomycin. Unfortunately, resistance to streptomycin and other drugs has developed in tuberculosis. Neomycin, which Waksman discovered in 1949, proved effective against streptomycin-resistant tuberculosis.

Streptomycin belongs to a class of antibiotic drugs known as aminoglycosides. Others in this class include neomycin, kanamycin (1957), gentamycin (1963), netilmicin (1976), tobramycin (1967), and amikacin (1972). Although effective, streptomycin and these drugs are all capable of causing permanent deafness and loss of balance.

Additional reading: Bottcher, *Miracle Drugs,* pp. 169–78.

stroke

A stroke occurs when blood vessels in the brain become blocked or hemorrhage, resulting in a loss of blood and oxygen flow that can lead to brain damage and death.

The **Hippocratic Corpus** refers to stroke as "apoplexy," which means "struck with violence as if by a thunderbolt" in Greek. Physicians of the time thought strokes occurred when the blood vessels of the head heated up, which attracted phlegm or black bile to the head. Aretaeus of Cappodocia (120–180) thought apoplexy was caused by congestion of blood flow. Both Hippocrates and Aretaeus noticed that apoplexy sometimes led to one-sided paralysis, and that right-sided paralysis and loss of speech tended to accompany one another.

Johann Jacob Wepfer (1620–1695) of Schaffhausen made the first connection between apoplexy and hemorrhage in the seventeenth century. He made careful studies of the blood vessels in the brains of people with apoplexy, which were published in his "Treatise on Apoplexy" in 1658. He observed that anything that impeded blood flow through the carotid arteries to the brain or back to the heart through the jugular veins could cause apoplexy. He said obese people with red faces and hands and people with irregular pulses were most prone to apoplexy. He also realized that brain tissue could not live if deprived of blood flow for even a short time, and that some people would recover from stroke.

William Heberden (1710–1801) of London described what are now known as transient ischemic attacks, ministrokes that warn of an impending major stroke.

Even though there was extensive evidence that cerebral hemorrhage caused stroke by this time, Philippe Pinel (1745–1826), a leading psychiatrist of the nineteenth century, considered apoplexy to be a form of neurosis.

John Cheyne (1777–1836) of Dublin in 1812 first put forth the idea that lack of blood flow in the brain, not vascular congestion, led to stroke. By carefully observing people who suffered from apoplexy, both before and after death (with **autopsies**), researchers gradually learned more about the specifics of stroke and developed different classifications. After studying 200 cases, Henri Duret named common sites of lesion in the brain following stroke in the 1870s.

Hans Chiari (1851–1916), a Viennese pathologist, was the first to suggest that **atherosclerosis** might be linked to stroke, in 1905, after observing atherosclerosis in the carotid arteries of people who suffered stroke.

Egas Moniz's (1874–1955) development of cerebral **angiography** in the 1930s furthered understanding of stroke by providing images of the blood vessels inside a living person's brain. Efforts at rehabilitation of people paralyzed by stroke began in the 1930s, becoming further stressed in the 1950s and 1960s. **Carotid endarterectomy**, a surgical procedure for preventing stroke by clearing out obstructions in the carotid arteries, was introduced in the 1950s and is still used frequently today.

Today it is known that high **blood pressure**, cigarette smoking, and **diabetes** are the main risk factors for stroke, and that taking **aspirin** regularly can, for some people, prevent stroke. Large studies completed in the late 1990s helped doctors to specify those at risk of stroke who will benefit from carotid endarterectomy, which is a risky operation.

Thrombolytic drugs also are useful for treating stroke caused by vessel blockage, but can worsen hemorrhagic stroke. (*See also* thrombolysis)

Additional reading: Fields, *A History of Stroke.*

sunscreen

Sunscreen protects against sunburn, aging, and **melanoma** by blocking some of the sun's ultraviolet rays from reaching the skin.

There are dozens of chemicals that block the sun to some degree. Zinc oxide, which is opaque, totally blocks the sun, and a version that is transparent but still completely blocks light became available in 1998.

Sun protection factor (SPF) is a number that indicates the strength of a sunscreen. For example, a sunscreen with SPF 10 allows a person to remain in the sun ten times longer than normal before getting a sunburn.

The first sunscreen sold commercially was developed in 1928, and contained benzyl salicylate and benzyle cinnamate. Para-aminobenzoic acid (PABA) also became available in the 1920s. Derivatives of PABA that last longer and don't stain clothing are in wide use today.

Campaigns to urge the public to begin wearing sunscreen began in 1980, after researchers in the 1970s noticed an epidemic of melanoma that they suggested was probably linked to increased sun exposure. **Public health** advocates now recommend that people wear the strongest available sunscreen year-round.

Additional reading: *Handbook of Nonprescription Drugs,* American Pharmaceutical Association, pp. 615–32.

surgical staples

Surgical staples are used to close surgical incisions. Surgical staplers became widely used in the late 1960s, but were first invented by Hungarian scientists in the 1920s.

Several studies of using staples for reattaching two openings mouth-to-mouth, a technique called anastomosis, have found that surgical stapling is quicker than hand suturing and is also less likely to produce complications such as leakage or infection. These studies and others have also shown that stapling appears to be better in general for surgery on the gastrointestinal system. This may be because stapling makes it possible to close the wounds with less manipulation of the organs.

The Soviet Union led the development of surgical staplers in the 1950s. These devices were cumbersome and difficult to sterilize, however. The United States Surgical Corporation in Connecticut produced the first Western-made staplers in 1967, which were easier to use and sterilize. Disposable, plastic staplers were made in the early 1980s.

The two main manufacturers of surgical staplers are U.S. Surgical and Ethicon.

Smaller staplers for use in **minimally invasive surgery** are now made as well.

Additional reading: Ravitch, et al., *Current Practice of Surgical Stapling.*

sutures

Sutures are stitches used to close wounds that may be made of thread, metal, or other material.

Medical historians believe that people probably used biting ants since ancient times to close wounds, based on the fact that some groups of people use the technique today. The insect is held where it can close its jaws around the wound, and then its body is snapped off, leaving the jaws embedded in the skin.

The oldest suture found on a human appears on an Egyptian mummy embalmed about 1100 B.C., but it is unclear if the Egyptians used sutures to close wounds on living people.

Hippocrates (c. 460–377 B.C.) mentioned stitching a wound using a threaded bronze needle, and there is evidence that Chinese physicians also used sutures around 200 B.C. Indian apprentice physicians practiced sutures on cloth. Celsus recommended using a woman's hair for fine stitches on the face.

Additional reading: Despain, "A Stitch in Time."

syphilis

Syphilis is a sexually transmitted disease caused by infection with the *Treponema pallidum* bacterium.

The name "syphilis" comes from a 1530 poem by Girolamo Fracastoro (c.1480–1553), but was not used widely until the late eighteenth century.

At first, infection with syphilis causes chancres (sores or lesions) in the genital area. In about one-third of cases of untreated syphilis, the tertiary stage develops, resulting in lesions throughout the body and in some cases infection of the cardiovascular and nervous systems with dementia.

Nonvenereal forms of syphilis include yaws, pinta, and bejel, all of which appear mainly in children. Venereal syphilis first appeared in Europe around 1490, and was called "morbus gallicus" or the "French Pox."

In the 1830s, Philippe Ricord (1800–1889) proposed that syphilis appeared in several stages of infection. Fritz Schaudinn (1871–1906) isolated the syphilis germ in 1905. One year later, several German scientists—including August von Wasserman (1866–1925)—developed blood tests for syphilis.

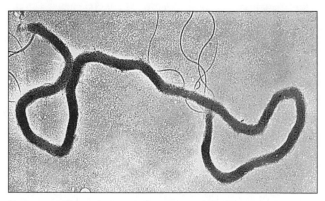

Treponema pallidum, the bacteria that causes syphilis. (Courtesy of American Society for Microbiology Archives Collection.)

Syphilis was extremely common throughout the late nineteenth century and the first half of the twentieth century. During this era, the disease was the leading cause of premature birth. Unfortunately syphilis appears to be on the rise today in certain geographic areas.

Salvarsan was the first drug found to be effective for treating syphilis; **penicillin,** which became widely available in the late 1940s, was more effective and less toxic. After penicillin became available, the disease became much less common in the United States. Penicillin remains the treatment of choice for syphilis, but some patients are being found with drug resistance.

Much of what is known about late-stage syphilis comes from the Tuskegee Study, an experiment conducted on 431 black men in the United States from 1932 to 1972. The men were purposely kept untreated (and not informed of this), even though a cure for syphilis became available during the course of the study.

Additional reading: Jones, *Bad Blood;* Karlen, *Man and Microbes,* pp. 121–28.

syringe

A syringe is a device used to inject medication under the skin or into a vein. Although instruments with a syringe-like mechanism were probably used as early as 1666, they were used to drain fluid, not to inject it.

The impetus for the development of injection syringes was the isolation of **morphine** in 1803, the most effective pain medication discovered up to that time. Some patients couldn't take the drug by mouth, and physicians reasoned that getting morphine into the bloodstream would relieve pain more quickly. Some cut the skin and rubbed medication in, others made incisions in the skin and squeezed the medication into the wound. Charles Pravaz (1791–1853) is credited with inventing the first syringe that could be used without making a previous incision in the skin; the French physician recorded his invention of a metal device with a hollow needle in 1853. Others in Europe and North America also came up with syringes. Because the danger of the spread of infection with the syringe was not yet understood, few syringes were sterilized.

All-glass and other sterilizable syringes were invented around the turn of the nineteenth century. Today, syringes or "needles" are usually made from disposable materials.

Additional reading: Boraker, "The Syringe"; McAuley, "The Hypodermic Syringe."

T

T cells

T cells are a special type of white blood cell with several different immunological duties.

In the 1940s, researchers first began to suspect that a "second arm" of the immune system, beyond **antibodies**, might exist. While studying chickens in the 1950s, Bruce Glick (1927–) made the discovery that pointed the way toward the existence of T cells. He found that chickens whose bursa of Fabricus (a small pouch off the digestive tract) was removed shortly after birth lost their ability to produce antibodies. However, he and his colleague Timothy Chang (1925–) observed that these chickens could still fight viral infection and reject skin grafts. The part of the immune system responsible for this type of immune function, the T cells, was discovered in the 1960s.

There are helper T cells that inform B cells which antibodies to make by releasing **cytokines**, and there are killer T cells that find and destroy infected or cancerous cells.

Several attempts have been made to treat **cancer** by growing quantities of a person's T cells, instructing them to kill tumors, and giving these cells back to patients with cancer, with limited success. The first **gene therapy** in humans employed genetically altered T cells to treat a rare immune deficiency disease, and this was more successful.

Additional reading: Weisse, *Medical Odysseys*, pp.186–95.

tamoxifen

Tamoxifen is a drug for treating **breast cancer** which was recently found to also prevent breast **cancer** in some women.

The drug, introduced in 1973, was one of the earliest designer **estrogens**, so called because they have some of the beneficial effects of this **hormone** without the undesirable ones. Tamoxifen protects bone and guards against fracture, a serious problem for post-menopausal women whose bones begin to thin as their estrogen levels drop. But the drug does not stimulate breast-cell growth as estrogen does, thus reducing the chance that breast cells will divide and become cancerous.

National Cancer Institute researchers started a trial of the drug for breast-cancer prevention in more than 13,000 women at high risk for the disease. They halted the trial early, in 1998, when they learned that tamoxifen cut women's chances of developing breast cancer by 45 percent.

Tamoxifen is useful for preventing breast cancer for about 15 percent of women. Its side effects, which include promoting endometrial cancer and causing blood clots in the lung and in major veins, mean it is only suitable for women at a high risk of developing breast cancer.

Additional reading: Cimons, "Should She Take Tamoxifen?"

taxol

Taxol is an anti-tumor drug derived from the bark of *Taxus brevifola*, a tree native to the Pacific Northwest. Taxol is among the most effective drugs for treating ovarian and **breast cancer.**

The laboratory of Monroe E. Wall (1916–) and Mansukh C. Wani (1925–) at Research Triangle Institute in North Carolina received samples of the tree bark along with tissue from hundreds of other plants collected in California, Washington, and Oregon in 1964. The team isolated the substance and investigated its structure, publishing their results in 1971. Taxol was first reported to halt cell division in 1978 by scientists at the National Cancer Institute. Animal testing of taxol started in the early 1980s, and trials in humans began in 1983.

Additional reading: Lednicer, ed., *Chronicles of Drug Discovery, Vol. III;* pp. 615–32.

Tay-Sachs disease

Tay-Sachs disease is a hereditary disorder of the central nervous system. Infants born with the disease develop symptoms within their first six months of life, and die within three or four years. Dr. Warren Tay (1843–1927) first described the disease in 1881, and Dr. Bernard Sachs (1858–1944) provided a fuller report in 1896.

The disease appears most commonly, although not exclusively, in people of Eastern European Jewish heritage.

A group of parents of children with Tay-Sachs formed the National Tay-Sachs and Allied Diseases Association in the 1950s. By the 1960s, researchers understood that the disease is caused by an absence of the enzymes that normally break down cellular waste, so these wastes collect and interfere with normal function. Tay-Sachs and other diseases of this type are known as "storage diseases."

John O'Brien (1934–) developed a test in 1971 that could identify people affected with Tay-Sachs, as well as healthy people who carry the Tay-Sachs gene. Soon, the National Tay-Sachs and Allied Diseases Association began promoting screening of parents to prevent the birth of children born with the disease. There is still no treatment or cure for Tay-Sachs disease.

Additional reading: Kiple, *The Cambridge World History of Human Disease*, pp. 1036–43.

TB. *See* tuberculosis.

telemedicine

Telemedicine is the use of telephone and video technology in medicine. Applications include allowing doctors to examine patients in rural areas remotely via television links, and sending images from diagnostic exams such as **X-rays** and CAT scans over the Internet (*see* **CAT scanning**).

Pilot telemedicine programs were introduced in the 1950s. Early projects included the 1950s STARPAHC, or "Space Technology Applied to Rural Papago Advanced Health Care," in which a van hooked up to **hospitals** via telephone and microwave television provided medical care at the Papago Indian Reservation in Arizona. The **U.S. Public Health Service**, NASA, and Lockheed (a technology corporation), collaborated on the project.

In 1959, the first psychiatric consultation was conducted by closed-circuit TV, and the first medical image was transmitted by coaxial cable.

In a Massachusetts General Hospital program organized in 1968, the hospital was linked by microwave television to a local airport and a Veterans Administration (VA) hospital. Dartmouth Medical School in Hanover, New Hampshire, initiated its Interact system that year as well, serving eight towns in Vermont and New Hampshire and the local VA hospital.

These early projects proved impractical because technology basically wasn't ready to support them. STARPAHC was the longest-lived, at 20 years. The only project still in place from that era is Canada's Memorial University program serving Newfoundland.

After a lull, several new telemedicine projects were launched beginning in the 1980s. Current projects include the Texas Tex HealthNet Project, serving the rural western part of the state. The Medical College of Georgia initiated a program in 1991 in which its emergency room in Augusta is connected to the Dodge County Hospital in Eastman 150 miles away. The network plans to add several stations so that ultimately any doctor in the state will be able to examine any patient in the state.

In the 1990s, telemedicine got a boost from high-speed, high-bandwidth telecommunications and medical devices that can produce digital images. Today most states have at least one telemedicine project in place.

One of the largest, most comprehensive projects is run by Boston's Partners Health Care System, which was formed by the merger of Massachusetts General and Brigham & Women's hospitals. The ongoing $100 million project includes plans for 50 locations for interactive video, and also systems for monitoring the vital signs of critically ill patients while they are at home. Doctors using the system will be able to make "virtual house calls," and radiologists are online to interpret diagnostic images.

Massachusetts General also established the first permanent international telemedicine link with Riyadh, Saudi Arabia, in 1994. Now the hospital, along with the Cleveland Clinic, Johns Hopkins, and Duke University Medical Center, is connected with several other Middle Eastern countries as part of the World Care Inc. system.

The Internet also has begun to play a major role in health care. Many patients consult their doctors via e-mail, and the World Wide Web provides a huge variety of medical information, varying greatly in quality.

Additional reading: Horvitz, "Dialing for Diagnoses."

telomere

A telomere is a region of repeating nucleotide bases at the end of a **chromosome** that shortens each time the chromosome replicates. Scientists believe telomeres, which carry no essential genetic information, limit the number of times that a given cell can divide. Once a chromosome's telomeres "run out," the chromosome begins losing parts that contain important genetic information, resulting in death of the cell or mutation. Barbara McClintock (1902–1992) first proposed the existence of telomeres and named them in the 1950s.

Telomerase is an enzyme that adds to the length of telomeres so that cell division can continue. About 85 percent of human cancers contain telomerase, making the enzyme a possible clue to early **cancer** diagnosis and also perhaps presenting a target for drug treatment of cancer.

The study of telomeres and telomerase has exploded since a simple test to detect and quantify telomerase was developed in the early 1990s.

Researchers had thought that because of its link with cancer, telomerase might be carcinogenic, but apparently this is not the case. Cancerous cells use telomerase differently than do normal cells that express it. Bone marrow cells and germ cells (egg and sperm cells) express telomerase while they are dividing actively, and also have longer telomeres, because they need to remain in a "youthful" state for a longer time.

Dr. Jerry Shay (1945–) of M.D. Anderson Cancer Center in Houston and his colleagues reported in 1998 that genetically manipulating human cells **in vitro** so they expressed telomerase extended their lifespan by at least 20 doublings and reduced certain indicators of aging, meaning that telomerase may one day prove useful for reversing the aging process.

Telomerase detection will likely be used widely for cancer diagnosis and screening within the next few years, but treatment of cancer and other degenerative diseases with telomerase is several years away.

Additional reading: Clark, *A Means to an End*, pp. 107–13.

tetanus

Tetanus, or lockjaw, is caused by a toxin produced by the bacteria *Clostridium tetani*, and can be fatal. Thanks to immunization, this disease is now extremely rare in the developed world; there were 36 cases reported in the United States in 1996 and 46 cases in 1997.

The disease occurs when the toxin enters a wound and produces muscle stiffness and spasms. Treatment for tetanus infection includes a dose of tetanus immune globulin. Mortality is 50 percent without treatment.

In 1914, the British began using equine antitoxin to immunize soldiers against tetanus during World War I. In 1933, Gaston Ramon (1886–1963) cultured the *C. tetani* bacteria, purified the toxin, and prepared a fluid toxoid for a **clinical trial**. This immunization was confirmed to be safe and effective during World War II; U.S. soldiers were given the tetanus antitoxin, and in one series of more than 2.7 million admissions for wounds and injuries, there were only 12 cases of tetanus.

Today, children receive a tetanus **vaccine** as part of their DPT (**diphtheria, pertussis,** tetanus) shot. **Public health** organizations recommend that adults receive a tetanus booster shot every five to 10 years to maintain their immunity.

Additional reading: Kiple, *The Cambridge World History of Human Disease*, pp. 1043–46.

thermometer

A thermometer is a device used, in medicine, to measure body temperature.

Although Sir Isaac Newton (1642–1727) invented a thermometer filled with linseed oil to measure human body temperature in 1700 and Daniel Fahrenheit (1686–1736) invented his mercury-filled thermometer and an accompanying temperature scale soon afterwards, physicians spent more time measuring the climatic temperature than their patients' body temperatures. Fever was not well understood, and climate was thought to have more bearing on health than body temperature. Although body warmth has been used to diagnose fever since ancient times, up until the mid-nineteenth century fever was thought of as a disease in itself, and was considered to be more closely associated with elevated pulse than with high body temperature.

The first thermometer developed specifically to test body temperature was invented by Sanctorius Sanctorius of Padua (1561–1636). The first doctor to actually use such a thermometer, in the late eighteenth century, was James Currie (1756–1805), who evaluated the body temperature of his **typhoid fever** patients who were given cold baths to reduce their temperatures.

Until 1867, when the short clinical thermometer was introduced, these devices were cumbersome. They were more than a foot long and took about 20 minutes to register a person's temperature.

German physician Karl R. A. Wunderlich (1815–1877), whose 1868 book *Medical Thermometry and Human Temperature* included observations of body temperature in more than 25,000 patients with febrile illness, is generally considered to be the father of modern thermometry. A French physician living in New York City, Dr. Edouard Seguin (1812–1880), translated Wunderlich's book and had it published in the United States in 1871.

Seguin's son Edward (1843–1898) had begun clinical studies of thermometry in 1865, designing a bedside chart for recording a patient's temperature, pulse, and respiratory rate. The younger Seguin's writing on using such charts in patients with pneumonia introduced the phrase "vital signs" into the medical literature.

The elder Seguin wrote the first of his 11 works on thermometry in 1867. He sought to popularize thermometry, so that families could use thermometers at home to determine whether it was really necessary to call a doctor. He wrote an 1873 monograph on thermometry directed at the lay public.

Today, partially due to Seguin's efforts, the thermometer is a standard feature of the American medicine cabinet.

Additional reading: McGrew, *Encyclopedia of Medical History*, pp. 73–74.

thrombolysis

Thrombolysis involves giving a patient who is having a heart attack drugs that will break up the blood clot, or thrombus, and restore blood flow to the heart.

The first thrombolytic drug was streptokinase. Researchers had found in 1933 that a streptococcus bacterium isolated from patients produced a substance that broke up fibrin. Eight years later, they discovered that a substance found in the plasma was necessary for this process to take place. L. Royal Christenson worked out the system by which the process occurred, and named the plasma factor "plasminogen" and the bacteria-produced substance "streptokinase."

In 1965, another thrombolytic substance, urokinase, was isolated from urine. **Clinical trials** of urokinase and streptokinase were conducted in the 1960s and 1970s throughout Europe and the United States. When researchers proved it was possible to safely perform contrast visualization of the heart during a heart attack, in 1980, this brought the technology forward a great deal, because researchers could actually "see" the drug working. Studies continue on what is the best thrombolytic agent to be given after a heart attack.

Additional reading: "A New Clot Buster," *Harvard Heart Letter.*

thyroid gland

The thyroid gland is located at the base of the neck. This gland was first described in 1656 by Thomas Wharton (1614–1673), who thought its purpose was to make the neck shapely.

Theodor Kocher (1841–1917) was the first person to perform thyroid surgery extensively once **anesthesia, antisepsis,** and hemostasis became available. Kocher brought his mortality rate down to 1 percent for a simple **goiter** operation, and he won the 1909 Nobel Prize for this accomplishment.

There are a number of diseases related to problems with thyroid **hormone** secretion, for example, cretinism and myxoedema (caused by too little thyroid hormone) and **Graves' disease** (caused by an excess of thyroid hormones in the body).

Myxoedema was discovered by Sir William Gull (1816–1890), a prominent doctor at London's Guy's Hospital, in 1873. He observed that some of his female patients with a series of mental and physical symptoms including drowsiness, apathy, swelling of the flesh, and low metabolism also had atrophied thyroid glands, and decided that this condition was caused by low thyroid function.

In 1888, the Committee of the Clinical Society of London established that cretinism and myxoedema were caused by low thyroid function. Cretinism is a congenital disease resulting in stunted growth and mental function.

After Charles Edouard Brown-Sequard's (1817–1894) famous experiment in 1889, in which he injected himself with an extract of animal testicles and claimed it improved his strength and intellectual function, researchers began to consider treating thyroid disease with injections from the gland. It turned out that thyroid extracts were the only glandular therapy that really worked. In 1891, George R. Murray (1865–1939) reported treating a 48–year-old myxoedemic woman with an extract from a sheep thyroid, with excellent results. The following year, several researchers found that oral thyroid preparations were as effective and could also cure infants with cretinism.

Iodine was not then used as a treatment for these thyroid diseases. Although the mineral had long been employed as a remedy for goiter, the treatment fell into disrepute in Europe after people suffered toxic effects.

Eugen Baumann (1846–1896) brought iodine back into favor in 1895 when he showed that it was a natural constituent of the thyroid gland. Other researchers soon began discovering other natural body chemicals that played various complementary and complex roles in regulating thyroid function. Edward C. Kendall (1886–1972), working at Parke-Davis in Detroit, isolated thyroxine, the active substance produced by the thyroid gland, in 1915. The first patient was treated with thyroxine in 1927, the same year that the chemical was first synthesized. Thyroid-stimulating hormone, a substance that the **pituitary gland** produces to activate the thyroid gland, was discovered two years later.

Today, thyroid disease may be treated with hormone supplementation, iodine, surgery, or radiation.

Additional reading: Alpert, "The Thyroid Gland."

tissue

A tissue is a group of similar cells in the body, along with the intracellular substance, that work together to perform a certain function. Francois-Xavier Bichat (1771–1802) was the first to describe tissues, which he called "membranes," in his 1800 work *Traite des Membraines.*

He described 21 different tissues, including connective, muscle, and nerve tissue, and said that pathological understanding of disease would come not from studying the organs but from examining the individual tissues that composed them. Tissues, he said, should be considered the functional unit of the body, not organs. Many of the individual tissues Bichat described do not stand up to our current understanding of the definition of a tissue, but his idea of this functional unit transformed pathology. Pathologists began to study the characteristics of tissues composing an organ, as well as the organ as a whole. Also, they observed that similar tissues would exhibit similar disease states, although they were located in different parts of the body.

Additional reading: Harris, *The Birth of the Cell.*

tissue culture

Tissue culture is a technique for growing living cells in the laboratory in an artificial medium.

The first person to culture **tissue** successfully was Ross Granville Harrison (1870–1959). While studying the embryonic development of nerve cells at Johns Hopkins University in Baltimore, he devised a tissue culture consisting of the medullary tube of a frog embryo immersed in frog lymph. In a 1907 article, he reported that using this technique with "reasonable aseptic precautions" made it possible to keep a tissue culture alive for a week or longer.

Harrison received little publicity for his discovery, but pioneering surgeon Alexis Carrel's (1873–1944) success in 1912 in keeping chicken-heart cells alive in a culture medium for 120 days was widely reported and recognized. After Carrel's initial experiment, however, the cells were preserved with regular additions of new chicken-heart cells, so his culture was not truly immortal. Through some inaccurate reporting, however, the legend of the immortal cells grew. In 1961, Leonard Hayflick (1928–) showed that normal human cells can in fact only divide 50 times, a figure now known as the "Hayflick limit." Late 1990s research showed that manipulation of **telomeres** allows cells to divide past this limit.

A major advance was the success of Thomas Weller (1915–), Frederick Robbins (1916–), and John F. Enders (1897–1985) in growing the **poliomyelitis virus** in tissue culture at their Harvard Medical School laboratory. This advance, reported in 1949, made development of a polio **vaccine** possible. Enders won the Nobel Prize in 1954, which he shared with his colleagues.

One drawback to cell culture for decades was the fact that normal cells—unlike **cancer cells**—did not grow well in culture. Richard Ham (1932–) at the University of Colorado developed completely synthetic and chemically controlled media for normal cell growth in the late 1970s.

Additional reading: Friedman and Friedland, *Medicine's 10 Greatest Discoveries,* pp. 131–52.

TNF. *See tumor necrosis factor.*

tonometer

A tonometer is a device used to check the pressure of the fluid within the eyeball in order to diagnose and treat **glaucoma**.

Before the invention of tonometers and after it became understood that high pressure within the eyeball was linked to glaucoma, ophthalmologists would use their fingers to check the firmness of a patient's eyeball. In 1905, Norwegian physician Hjalamar Schiotz (1850–1927) introduced an indentation tonometer, which was used for 50 years. The more precise applanation tonometer was introduced in 1955.

Noncontact tonometry, in which the changes that occur in the cornea in response to a puff of air are measured, is now used to gauge tension within the eyeball.

Additional reading: Dekking and Coster, "Dynamic Tonometry"; Pain, "Progress in Ophthalmological Instruments."

toothbrush

Toothbrushes are devices for cleaning the teeth. The earliest toothbrushes weren't brushes at all, but chewed sticks. Early dental hygiene was largely motivated by religious belief. The Talmud and the Koran, as well as the writings of Buddha, recommend using a chewing stick to clean the teeth and tongue several times a day. Sponges and cloths were also used to keep teeth clean.

The bristle toothbrush dates back at least to the 1700s; one of the fathers of **dentistry**, Pierre Fauchard (1678–1761), said horse hair toothbrushes were too hard on the teeth. Nylon bristles were introduced shortly after World War II.

Regular toothbrushing is important in dental hygiene, and helps to prevent tooth decay.

Additional reading: Ring, *Dentistry;* Wynbrandt, *The Excruciating History of Dentistry.*

tracheotomy

A tracheotomy is a surgical incision in the windpipe made so that a person with blockage in this area caused by disease or a foreign object can breathe. The surgery has been used—probably always on an emergency basis—since Roman times, with refinements in technique appearing gradually through history.

Antonia Musa Brasavola (1500–1570) reported performing a successful tracheotomy in 1546. In 1617, Italian anatomist Giralmo Fabrici (1537–1619) suggested that inserting a tube into the tracheotomy would allow for easier

breathing with a smaller incision. Sanctorius Sanctorius (1561–1636) described such an operation in 1636 but he probably did not perform it. The German surgeon Laurentius Heister (1683–1758) introduced the term tracheotomy in 1718, and performed a number of successful operations.

The operation became less necessary with the introduction and popularization of **endotracheal intubation** in the late nineteenth century.

Additional reading: Wangensteen, *The Rise of Surgery,* pp. 168–86.

transmissible spongiform encephalopathies (TSEs)

Transmissible spongiform encephalopathies are a type of degenerative brain disease that is spread when an animal comes into contact with infected nervous system matter, usually by eating it.

These diseases, which include the animal maladies scrapie and "mad cow disease" (known officially as bovine spongiform encephalopathy, or BSE), as well as the human illnesses Creutzfeldt-Jakob disease and kuru, are caused by an infectious protein particle known as a **prion**. Prions are an abnormally folded form of a naturally occurring protein; scientists believe the normal proteins in the body somehow pick up the abnormal shape from the infecting prion, thus spreading the disease. TSEs may have an incubation period of months or even years, but once the disease strikes, a person suffers rapid brain deterioration and eventual death. Prions are nearly impossible to destroy by normal sterilization methods.

Scrapie, the first TSE to be identified, was described in sheep in the eighteenth century. Infected animals rubbed themselves against posts, bit themselves, and eventually became emaciated and died. Scrapie was recognized as contagious, but it was not believed to strike humans. The disease's transmission by infected central nervous system material was confirmed in the mid-twentieth century.

Creutzfeldt-Jakob disease (CJD) was first described in the 1920s by Hans Gerhard Creutzfeldt (1855–1964) and Alfons Maria Jakob (1884–1931). In 1957, Carlton Gadjusek (1923–) described kuru, a disease that struck Papua New Guineans who had participated in ritual cannibalism. Researchers soon observed similarities between kuru and scrapie, both in the behavior of the victims of the disease and the appearance of post-mortem brain tissue samples of victims of the diseases. Gadjusek, who with Baruch S. Blumberg won the 1976 Nobel Prize for his research, proposed that these diseases were spread by some type of "slow **virus**," but he was unable to identify an infectious agent.

During the 1980s, grafts of certain types of tissue, such as corneas, and injections of **human growth hormone**, transmitted CJD to dozens of people. More careful screening of donor tissue and the introduction of recombinant growth hormone ended the spread of the disease. The disease was also spread among some residents of the Appalachian Mountains in the United States who ate the brains of TSE-infected squirrels.

Changes around 1980 in livestock feeding in Great Britain—scrapie-infected sheep carcasses began to be recycled in cattle feed—resulted in an epidemic of BSE. British officials eventually outlawed this type of cattle feeding, placed restrictions on meat processing, and ordered the destruction of millions of cows and bulls to stop the spread of the disease.

In 1996, British researchers first identified a new type of TSE they dubbed new variant CJD or Will-Ironside syndrome. The disease struck much younger people than CJD, and investigators increasingly think it is a result of eating BSE-infected beef. So far there have been about 30 cases of the new disease. It remains unclear whether these are isolated victims or the beginning of an epidemic.

Additional reading: Rhodes, *Deadly Feasts.*

transmyocardial revascularization

Transmyocardial revascularization is a surgical technique used to restore blood flow to the heart muscle to treat **angina pectoris** and prevent heart attack in patients whose coronary arteries are blocked by **atherosclerosis**. Introduced in the late 1980s, the procedure involves making several holes in the heart muscle using a carbon dioxide laser.

Researchers had shown in 1933 that there were channels between the ventricles and the coronary arteries called myocardial sinusoids that helped supply blood to the heart muscle. Bombay surgeon P.K. Sen proposed using **acupuncture** to treat blocked blood flow to the heart, and he showed in 1965 with animal studies that puncturing the left ventricle with needles prevented acute ischemia. However, these channels closed soon after they were made, so they were not a long-term solution.

Attempts to revascularize the heart muscles with **laser surgery** were first reported in 1986 by Mahmood Mirhoseini (1930–) and colleagues at the Heart and Lung Institute of Wisconsin and researchers at the Kobe University School of Medicine in Japan. Trials of the technique at eight major U.S. hospitals began in 1992, and found that the procedure significantly improved patients' angina and also reduced the number of times patients had to be admitted to hospitals for treatment.

The treatment remains in the experimental stage, but advocates believe it offers promise to people who cannot be helped with coronary bypass graft surgery or **angioplasty.**

Additional reading: Gibbs, "Helping Heartache"; Squires, "Treatment Brings New Blood to Ailing Hearts."

trauma center

Trauma centers are specialized **hospital** divisions that provide care for people with traumatic injuries.

The idea that trauma was treatable became widely accepted after the National Academy of Science's National Research Council released its 1966 report, "Accidental Death and Disability: The Neglected Disease of Modern Society."

Two years later, the first accident hospital in the United States, the Maryland Institute for Emergency Medical Service Systems, was established in Baltimore.

City hospitals began establishing trauma centers in the 1970s, and pilot programs in the early part of the decade proved that using helicopters to transport injured people via **air ambulance** to trauma centers was feasible. In 1973, trauma centers got a boost from the federal Emergency Medical Services Systems Act, which included funding for emergency medical service programs. Training centers for paramedics sprang up around the country soon afterwards. In 1976, the American College of Surgeons published a list of requirements for trauma centers. In 1978, the Lincoln Medical Education's Physicians Committee on Trauma, along with Southeastern Nebraska Emergency Medical Service, piloted the first Advanced Trauma Life Support Course.

R. Cowley (1917–) of the University of Maryland Medical School introduced the concept of the "golden hour," the first hours after an accident when emergency care could do the most good, in 1979. Specialized pediatric trauma centers began opening in the 1980s.

Additional reading: Doelp, *In the Blink of an Eye.*

trepanation

Trepanation, one of the earliest known surgical procedures, is the drilling of a hole in the skull to relieve distress. Evidence for the operation, in the form of trepanned fossil human skulls, dates back to 10,000 B.C.

The main methods for performing the operation were scraping away the bone, digging grooves in the skull, drilling several holes, or making overlapping incisions.

The trepanned fossil skulls usually are fractured, suggesting that the operation was performed to relieve pressure on the brain caused by the injury. These skulls often show evidence of healing, so patients frequently survived the procedure.

Trepanning remains in use for **head-injury treatment** to relieve pressure within the skull, although techniques for gauging when the operation is necessary have been greatly refined.

Additional reading: Finger, *Origins of Neuroscience,* pp. 4–6; Porter, ed., *Medicine,* pp. 118.

tretinoin

Tretinoin is a derivative of **vitamin A** that is used to treat acne and sun-damaged skin.

Tretinoin was synthesized in 1946. Researchers soon began investigating the chemical's dermatological applications because it was known that vitamin A deficiency could cause skin problems. In 1969, researchers found that an oral preparation of tretinoin helped treat acne. The **Food and Drug Administration (FDA)** approved a form of this preparation called Retin-A for marketing two years later.

In 1974, researchers found that tretinoin could shrink some skin **cancers**. This substance continues to be studied as an agent for preventing and treating cancer. Studies on using Retin-A to treat skin damaged by ultraviolet rays began in 1985. Retin-A is now also used to treat wrinkles and lighten the color of scars.

Additional reading: "Study Shows Danger to Skin and Gives Hope of a Savior," *The New York Times.*

triage

Triage is a strategy for rationing care in emergency rooms, **intensive care units (ICUs)**, and battlefields. Jean-Dominique Larrey (1766–1842) is credited with the first use of the term. During the Napoleonic wars, Larrey would treat wounded soldiers who could return to battle first, while the more severely injured would have to wait.

In ICUs and emergency rooms, the method is somewhat different: people who need care most urgently are treated first. Systems for allocating care for trauma patients were developed in the late 1960s and early 1970s.

The **National Institutes of Health (NIH)** made a consensus statement in 1983 which said the first priority for ICUs should be people with acute, reversible disease who aren't likely to survive without ICU intervention; next are people with a lower probability of survival even with ICU intervention; and last are people who are not critically ill but at risk of becoming critically ill.

Additional reading: Rutkow, *American Surgery,* pp. 340–41.

TSEs. See transmissible spongiform encephalopathies

tubal sterilization

Tubal sterilization is a surgical method for sterilizing women by blocking or severing the fallopian tubes leading from the ovaries to the uterus so that eggs cannot travel along the tubes and be fertilized.

Surgical sterilization is the most popular method of birth control in the United States, but it only became popular in the 1970s, thanks to the improvement of instrument and surgical techniques and changes in public attitudes.

James Blundell (1790–1898), a London physician, first proposed the idea of tubal sterilization in the 1820s. Some historians also credit him with performing the first such procedure around this time, although there is no direct evidence for this.

At the beginning of the twentieth century, sterilization became associated with eugenics as a method for preventing "undesirable" elements of society from bearing children. The Nazis were the most notorious practitioners of eugenic sterilization, but they weren't the only ones; another eugenics advocate was birth-control pioneer Margaret Sanger (1883–1966). Some experts argue that this problematic connotation has much to do with why it took decades for women to accept sterilization as a birth-control option.

With the development of **laparoscopy**, tubal sterilization could be performed in a short, uncomplicated operation, even in some cases on an outpatient basis, which also

eventually helped to make it more popular. The procedure did not become truly popular until the development of fiberoptics and better techniques for insufflating the abdomen (filling it with air to ease visualization and maneuvering). Tying off the tubes is called tubal ligation.

Patrick Steptoe (1913–1988), of test-tube baby fame, wrote the first textbook on laparoscopy in English, published in 1967. His book included reports on laparoscopic sterilizations performed by closing off the tubes with electrocoagulation. Problems with electrocoagulation—which could burn other organs—led to the development of clips and rings for closing off tubes in the 1970s.

Additional reading: Moss, *Contraceptive Sterilization.*

tuberculosis (TB)

Tuberculosis is a disease caused by infection with an airborne bacterium, usually *Mycobacterium tuberculosis.* Only 1 in 10 to 1 in 20 people infected with TB actually get sick, but it is an extremely difficult illness to treat once a person does become ill. TB infects the lungs, but it can spread to other parts of the body, including the spine, abdominal cavity, and joints.

The bacillus has been found in Egyptian mummies, so TB has most likely plagued humans since prehistoric times.

In ancient India, sadness, fasting, pregnancy, and exhaustion were all thought to be potential causes of tuberculosis. The ancient Chinese used moxibustion, in which herbs are burned at the surface of the skin, to treat tuberculosis. Hippocrates (c.460–c.377 B.C.), who may have coined the word "phthisis" (pulmonary tuberculosis) to describe TB, thought that tuberculosis was caused by growths in the lungs.

Rene Laennec's (1781–1826) **autopsy** studies of tuberculosis confirmed that the bacterium could infect various areas in the body. In 1865, Jean-Antoine Villemin (1827–1892) established that the disease was infectious; he injected rabbits with material from human tuberculosis lesions and the animals subsequently got sick. Robert Koch (1843–1910) isolated the TB bacillus in 1882.

Before drugs became available to treat tuberculosis, people with the disease often went to sanitariums in the mountains where the high altitude and fresh air, along with rest and plenty of food, were thought to be an effective treatment. The first TB spa in the United States was founded in 1884 on Saranac Lake in New York's Adirondack Mountains by Edward Livingston Trudeau (1848–1915), who himself had TB. The sanitariums were helpful for people with less advanced disease, often arresting the progress of the infection, but were of no help for people with more advanced TB.

Another treatment of the time was pneumothorax, in which a patient's lung was collapsed in order to let it rest.

Perhaps because the disease was so common and tragic, often striking young people, the symptoms of TB or "consumption," such as pallor, flushed cheeks, and emaciation, were considered romantic and attractive during the nineteenth century.

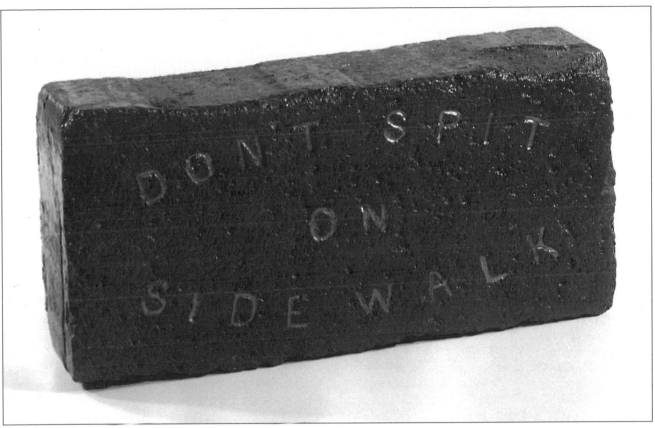

"Don't spit on the sidewalk" brick, part of anti-tuberculosis campaign in Kansas in 1908. (Courtesy of American Society for Microbiology Archives Collection.)

Reporting systems for TB infections were among the earliest forms of **public health** regulation. Spain required doctors to notify the government of any cases of infectious TB beginning in 1751, and Italy followed in 1780. England did not enact such regulations until 1903. Tuberculosis also was a major focus of U.S. public health efforts. The first voluntary health group in the United States was a tuberculosis association formed in 1892 in Philadelphia.

The **U.S. Public Health Service** began giving grants for TB control programs in 1947, and established a national case-reporting system for TB in 1953.

In 1890, Koch developed a substance he called tuberculin, which consisted of the material left after heat-killed TB bacteria were strained out of its culture and concentrated, and thought that it would provide an effective treatment for the disease. It did not, but in 1907 Clemens von Pirquet (1874–1929) found that tuberculin could be used in a skin test to determine if people had been exposed to the bacillus. By the 1920s, **X-rays** of the lungs were the standard method for screening people for active TB.

Researchers established in the mid-twentieth century that TB was spread by breathing air contaminated with the bacteria.

The first drug effective against TB was **streptomycin**, first given to a patient in 1944. Isoniazid, first tested at Sea View Hospital in Long Island in 1951, was found to work even better. Patients' fevers dropped within 24 hours, and chest X-rays of two-thirds of the patients given isoniazid cleared up within two or three months.

When isoniazid became generally available in 1953, TB hospitals began to clear out and close down. That year, there were 839 tuberculosis hospitals in the United States; by 1972, there were only four.

The rifamycin organism was isolated at the Lepetit Research Laboratories in Milan, Italy, in 1959. The first **antibiotic** drug for TB derived from it, rifampicin, was introduced in 1970.

Tuberculosis is much less of a threat today, but it is still a serious disease in many parts of the world. In 1990, 7.5 million people developed TB and 2.5 million died. One-third of the world's population is infected with TB. The disease is rampant in sub-Saharan Africa and southeast Asia. Other serious problems today include the development of drug-resistant strains of tuberculosis, as well as the risk of TB in people with weakened immune systems, such as **AIDS** patients. Surgeons are returning to old methods for tuberculosis treatment, such as the removal of part or all of the lung, to treat cases of the disease that do not respond to drugs.

Additional reading: Daniel, *Captain Death.*

tumor necrosis factor (TNF)

Tumor necrosis factor is a chemical produced by cells of the immune system to kill abnormal **tissue**. It causes blood vessels within tumors to adhere together, then cues a massive attack from the immune system that shuts down blood flow to the tumor and eventually causes a hemorrhage.

Elizabeth Carswell and Lloyd Olds, working at the Memorial Sloan Kettering Cancer Center in New York, discovered a substance that they named "tumor necrosis factor" in 1971 and published their discovery in 1975. This substance, when taken from the blood of mice and given to animals with tumors, wiped out the tumors.

Also in New York, researchers at Rockefeller University had discovered a substance they called "cachectin" that they believed caused wasting in patients with **cancer**, which was eventually found to be the same as TNF.

There was a great media stir about the possibilities of TNF for treating disease after David Goeddel (1951–) and his colleagues at Genentech cloned the TNF gene in 1984. But when **clinical trials** began the following year, TNF was discovered to be highly toxic, bringing down patients' **blood pressure** dramatically and dangerously. Many researchers dropped TNF completely.

Belgian researchers first tried a technique useful in **melanomas** that were limited to certain areas of the body—a small percentage—in 1988. The surgeons would "tie off" the person's cancerous limb or organ and flood it with TNF. The tumors would liquefy in hours, but, for many people, would ultimately appear elsewhere in the body. The technique has been dramatically successful in limited cancers, especially when combining TNF with a **chemotherapy** drug called melphalan and **interferon.**

Drugs that block TNF were developed in the 1990s and have been found to be an effective treatment for inflammatory conditions, such as **rheumatoid arthritis** and Crohn's disease. The first anti-TNF drug to go on the market, etanercept, was approved by the **Food and Drug Administration (FDA)** for treating rheumatoid arthritis in 1998.

Additional reading: Hall, *A Commotion in the Blood,* pp. 10–17, 409–20.

tumor-suppressor gene

A tumor-suppressor **gene** is a coding sequence in the **DNA** that, when functioning normally, serves to control cellular growth. A series of mutations in a tumor-suppressor gene can promote **cancer** by disabling this brake on cellular growth.

The first tumor-suppressor gene to be discovered was the retinoblastoma gene. This disease, an extremely rare cancer of the retina that strikes children younger than four, was invariably fatal until the **ophthalmoscope** was discovered in the 1800s. This made it possible to detect the disease and remove the tumor before it spread to the brain. Once people with retinoblastoma began surviving into adulthood, they began having children with the disease.

In 1971, Alfred Knudson (1922–) of the M.D. Anderson Hospital in Houston, Texas, suggested 1971 that retinoblastoma was caused by a recessive gene. According to Knudsen's two-hit model, a person would be born with one

mutated, recessive gene and a normal, dominant gene that prevented the disease; but if this dominant healthy gene was mutated during embryonic development or early childhood, the person would develop the disease. This would explain why the disease was extremely rare in nonfamilial cases, striking 1 out of 20,000 people; two mutations would have to occur in order for the disease to develop.

Jorge Yunis (1933–) of the University of Minnesota Medical School observed that pieces of a particular site on chromosome 13 were missing in retinoblastoma cells, and that people with the familial form of the disease had this deletion on chromosomes in all body cells. Researchers at the University of Utah showed in 1983 that a particular gene was missing in people with retinoblastoma. The actual gene responsible for retinoblastoma was discovered in 1986 by medical geneticist Thaddeus Dryja (1951–) of the Massachusetts Eye and Ear Infirmary, pediatrician Stephen Friend (1953–), and Robert A. Weinberg (1943–) of the Whitehead Institute in Cambridge, Massachusetts.

Mark Skolnick (1934–) of the University of Utah found a link between polyps and bowel cancer and a common gene. In 1988, Bert Vogelstein of Johns Hopkins University spelled out the series of four to six mutations through which this gene had to go in order for cancer to develop.

Vogelstein and his colleagues also discovered the most important tumor-suppressor gene known, the p53 gene. The team linked the gene to colon cancer in 1989, and found in a series of 1990 experiments that inserting a healthy version of the p53 gene into laboratory colonies of cancer cells will halt their growth.

The p53 gene has since been linked to many different forms of cancer. Researchers are investigating techniques for "switching on" this and other tumor-suppressor genes, or treating cancer patients by giving them a healthy version of the p53 gene. So far laboratory and animal experiments have shown promise, but actually delivering **gene therapy** to a human being and making it work has proven to be an extremely complex problem.

Additional reading: Lyon and Gorner, *Altered Fates,* pp. 330–37.

twilight sleep

Twilight sleep is a form of partial **anesthesia** with the drugs scopolamine and **morphine** that was given to women in labor during the first half of the twentieth century.

Physicians began giving women scopolamine and morphine during labor in 1915. Word spread, and a group of American women formed the National Twilight Sleep Association to encourage doctors to provide the method to all women; the association wrote articles in popular magazines and performed demonstrations in department stores.

Twilight sleep became very popular, but it was abandoned during the 1950s when it was found to be associated with prolonged labor, newborn asphyxia, hemorrhage after birth, and other side effects.

Additional reading: Caton, *What a Blessing She Had Chloroform,* pp. 130–51.

typhoid fever

Typhoid fever is caused by infection with *Salmonella typhi* and is fatal in 10 percent of cases if left untreated. People can carry and spread the infection without being sick themselves. "Typhoid" means "like **typhus**," and the two were thought until the nineteenth century to be the same disease.

Typhoid was first described by the Brussels anatomist Van den Spigelius (1578–1625) in 1624, and in 1669 Thomas Willis (1621–1675) made the first attempt to distinguish typhus from typhoid, noting many differences in the contagiousness and manifestations of the two diseases.

Nathan Smith (1762–1829) was the first person to describe typhoid fever in the United States. He observed in an 1824 essay that the disease was contagious and transmissible by water. Pierre-Charles-Alexandre Louis (1787–1872) introduced the term "typhoid fever" in 1829, while William Gerhardt (1809–1872) made the first clinical distinction between typhus and typhoid fever in 1837.

Edwin Klebs (1833–1913) and Karl Joseph Eberth (1835–1926) isolated the typhoid bacterium in 1880. The first typhoid vaccinations were developed in the 1890s, independently, by Sir Almroth Wright (1861–1947) in Great Britain and Richard Pfeiffer (1858–1945) in Germany.

The rate of typhoid fever declined in the late 1800s thanks to improved water treatment and sewage systems, so that the role of carriers became more important. Probably the most famous typhoid carrier was Mary Mallon (1870–1938), better known as "Typhoid Mary."

Mallon held a series of cooking jobs on Long Island and in New York City. She was arrested in New York in 1907 after **public health** officials traced several outbreaks of typhoid fever to her cooking. Mallon was the first confirmed carrier of the bacteria found in North America. She had infected 22 people, one of whom died. She refused to cooperate with public health officials, arguing that she hadn't spread the disease because she wasn't sick. Mallon was **quarantined** on an island in the East River.

Authorities agreed to release her three years later if she promised not to cook again; but she did, and authorities caught up with her again in 1915 at a maternity hospital in New York, alerted by 25 new cases of typhoid fever. Mallon was sent back to the island. She spent the rest of her life there, dying in 1938.

Up until the mid-twentieth century, treatment for typhoid fever consisted of bed rest and **hydrotherapy**. In 1948, chloramphenicol, the world's first completely synthetic **antibiotic,** was introduced and found to be an effective treatment for typhoid. There is still no completely effective typhoid fever **vaccine**.

Typhoid fever is now rare in the developed world but is endemic to certain parts of the developing world, especially South and Southeast Asia.

Additional reading: Kiple, *The Cambridge World History of Human Disease*, pp. 1071–77.

typhus

Typhus is a disease spread by lice and caused by a bacteria, most often a type called *Rickettsia prowazekii*. The name typhus comes from a Greek word meaning "cloudy" or "hazy," which is how people with a typhus infection often feel. If the infection is left untreated, mortality from typhus can be as high as 40 percent.

The disease was known in Europe as jail fever, ship fever, and famine fever. Typhus was rampant in Ireland and to a lesser degree in England from the Middle Ages on, but it was basically unknown in continental Europe. Charles Nicolle (1866–1936) identified louse feces as the source of typhus infection in 1909.

William Gerhardt (1809–1872) of Philadelphia first clearly distinguished between typhoid and typhus in 1837.

Typhus is now rare in the United States. Treatment consists of complete bed rest and broad-spectrum **antibiotics** such as chloramphenicol and the tetracyclines.

Additional reading: Kiple, *The Cambridge World History of Human Disease*, pp. 1080–88.

U

Ulcer. *See* H. pylori

ultrasound

Ultrasound is a technique for examining a fetus while it is still in the womb and also for detecting certain abnormalities within the body, such as ovarian cysts and prostate tumors. Ultrasound also is the basis of **echocardiography**, a commonly used method for examining the structure of the heart for defects.

Ultrasound technology comes from sonar, which was developed during World War I to locate submarines at sea. Waves of sound are pulsed into the area to be imaged. The returning waves are interpreted by a computer and recorded as an image on the monitor.

Two brothers from Austria, Karl (1908–) and Friedreich Dussik, were the first to attempt to use ultrasound to "look inside" the body in 1937. They made a transmission image of a patient's head.

William Fry led a Navy-funded team investigating ultrasound for therapeutic purposes after founding the Bioacoustics Laboratory at the University of Illinois in 1946. Fry had worked for the Navy on sonar during World War II. Douglas Howry at the University of Colorado built an ultrasound imaging machine from bomber parts and Navy surplus sonar equipment in 1949, and used it to image his own thigh. John Wild, a British surgeon who emigrated to work at the University of Minnesota, developed an ultrasound machine that used short pulses of sound to produce images, which was safer for patients than continuous high-intensity ultrasound.

In 1953, Swedish neurosurgeon Lars Lekskell (1907–1986) found that ultrasound waves could penetrate children's thin skulls. He used ultrasound to diagnose a hematoma in a comatose child. Subsequently, he developed a system for imaging the adult brain by sending the ultrasound waves into a relatively thin section of the skull near the ear. These waves bounced off the midline of the brain, and distortions in the reflected soundwaves could belie abnormalities in the brain.

Scientists at the University of Lund developed echocardiography in 1953. Researchers at Japan's Osaka University developed Doppler ultrasound in the mid-1950s. This technique is used to measure the velocity of blood flow.

Since their invention, **X-rays** had been used to provide images of the fetus in the womb, but a 1956 report linked in-utero X-ray exposure to later development of **leukemia** and other types of **cancer**. In the early 1950s, researchers began using ultrasound technology to image the fetus instead.

Ultrasound technology became commercially available to doctors in 1970. By the mid-1970s, advances in computer technology made it possible to create real-time ultrasound images. During this decade, ultrasound was used for high-risk pregnancies only, but by the 1980s ultrasound had become a regular part of **prenatal care** and was covered by most types of insurance.

Ultrasound can be used to gauge the age of a fetus, and may also be used with other diagnostic procedures such as **amniocentesis** in order to guide the instruments. Sonographers can identify anatomical features in an ultrasound image at 18 to 20 weeks, and may also be able to detect certain birth defects such as **Down syndrome** and **cystic fibrosis.**

Additional reading: Kevles, *Naked to the Bone,* pp. 228–50.

UNICEF (United Nations Children Fund)

UNICEF is the United Nation's Children Fund, an organization headquartered in New York City that is dedicated to protecting the rights and health of the world's children. UNICEF was established in 1946, and has 8 regional offices, 125 national offices, and 37 participating nongovernmental organizations.

UNICEF joined the **World Health Organization (WHO)** in sponsoring 1978's **Alma Ata International Conference on Primary Health Care**. A declaration resulting from this meeting called for nations to dedicate resources to **public health**, and for all of the world's people to have an acceptable level of public health by 2000. Although the health of the global population has indeed improved at the turn of the millenium, much work still needs to be done.

Much of UNICEF's mission, which includes attempting to provide children everywhere with preventive health care, good nutrition, access to education, and protection from violence, is based on the Declaration of the Rights of the Child. Drafting of the document began in 1979, and it was adopted by the United Nations' General Assembly in 1989. Currently only two U.N. member nations have not signed the declaration: Somalia and the United States.

UNICEF is also calling for the world's richer nations to ease their requirements on the poorest countries for paying back loans, which the organization says is crippling these countries and affecting children's health and education.

At the outset of the twenty-first century, UNICEF released a report featuring economic and social statistics on the well-being of children around the world. The report, "The State of the World's Children 2000," noted that major progress has been made in eliminating blindness from **vitamin A** deficiency, retardation from iodine deficiency, death from **measles** and neonatal **tetanus,** and paralysis and death from **polio.** But the report also points to serious problems that continue to face the world's children, such as **AIDS,** discrimination against female children, poverty, and the threat of violence from local and regional conflicts.

Additional reading: Black, *Children First.*

universal precautions

Universal precautions are a strategy for controlling infection in which medical professionals use gloves and other protective equipment while in contact with every patient. The precautions are called "universal" because the health care provider assumes that all patients are infected, and protects him or herself accordingly. The main purpose of universal precautions is to protect against infection with HIV, the **virus** that causes **AIDS,** and other blood-borne diseases such as **hepatitis.**

A version of universal precautions was first recommended around the turn of the nineteenth century, because medical professionals faced a serious risk of contracting **syphilis,** a common disease of the time. William Osler (1849–1919) warned doctors to be aware of the possibility of becoming infected while treating patients. The development of **rubber gloves** in 1890 helped doctors and nurses protect themselves and the evolution of goggles followed. Nurses were pioneers in this area. By World War I, nurses and doctors were using universal precautions when conducting examinations in which they might become infected (or they might infect a patient), such as pelvic exams. Although dentists also were warned against the potential for contracting syphilis in their work, dental professionals didn't begin adopting universal precautions until the AIDS epidemic began in the late 1980s.

The **Centers for Disease Control and Prevention (CDC)** first recommended methods by which medical and dental professionals could protect themselves while caring for patients with HIV infection in 1983. These methods stressed the isolation of AIDS patients. In 1987, the CDC first used the phrase "universal precautions," recommending that health care workers treat all patients as if they were infected with HIV, and guard themselves against exposure to blood and body fluids of all patients.

Additional reading: Donowitz, *Infection Control for the Health Care Worker.*

U.S. Children's Bureau

The U.S. Children's Bureau was established as part of the Department of Commerce and Labor by Congress in 1912 in order to study and promote the health of children.

Public health nursing pioneer Lillian Wald (1867–1940), along with Florence Kelley (1859–1932), Julia Lathrop (1858–1932), and Grace Abbott (1878–1939), formed the National Child Labor Committee in 1904. The group observed that the U.S. government had more information on the nation's agricultural products than on its young people; no agency kept track of births and deaths among children. The committee helped introduce a bill in 1906 to create a Children's Bureau to keep these and other statistics. President Theodore Roosevelt (1858–1919), at the behest of Wald and Kelley, called the first White House Conference on Dependent Children in 1908. The legislation to establish the bureau was finally passed in 1912, and Lathrop became director.

The bureau's first order of business was to create a birth registry, with the help of women's clubs throughout the nation. Within three years, 32 states had passed laws requiring birth registration. By 1929 all but two had, and death registration legislation was nearly complete.

The bureau also began conducting studies of infant mortality, which were published in its annual report. The bureau found that in 1915 infant mortality was 100 per 1,000 live births. The following year, they found that between 95,000 and 100,000 of the 230,000 infant deaths annually were directly related to the health of the mother and the care she received while pregnant. The bureau ranked the United States 14th among the world's 16th leading nations in infant mortality rates.

The bureau also began studying infant mortality in industrial towns, finding that the father's income correlated closely with infant mortality: the lower the income, the higher the mortality. Women in poorer families also tended to work outside the home and to return to work soon after giving birth. The bureau decided that infant mortality could be reduced by teaching women to care for themselves properly during pregnancy. By this point it was clear that by having regular checkups during pregnancy women could prevent most complications of pregnancy and labor. But from 1900 to 1913, childbirth was the leading cause of death of adult women, aside from **tuberculosis.**

The bureau published free pamphlets for doctors and families, including "**Prenatal Care**" and "Infant Care."

Nurses and doctors working for the bureau set up health conferences in rural areas. The bureau also sponsored "Baby Week" in 1916 and 1917 to highlight the health needs of infants and mothers.

In 1919, Congressmen Morris Sheppard (1875–1941) and Horace Mann Towner (1855–1932) introduced a bill to provide funding for maternal and child care, which was passed in 1921. The bill was based on a plan Lathrop and Abbot developed to prevent maternal and infant deaths and was intended to provide funding to educate women on prenatal care and support adequate community resources for this care.

The medical profession, including the American Medical Association (AMA), opposed the bill. The AMA's Pediatric Section supported Sheppard-Towner, however, and broke with the AMA to form the American Academy of Pediatrics as a result of this dispute.

Maternal deaths and infant morality fell in the years under Sheppard-Towner. However, the law was allowed to lapse by President Herbert Hoover (1874–1964). The Title V amendments to the **Social Security** Act, passed in 1935, restored funding for maternal and child care. However, the U.S. Children's Bureau was dismantled by Congress in 1946.

Today, the Administration for Children and Families of Health and Human Services oversees child and family health issues.

Additional reading: Lindenmeyer, *A Right to Childhood.*

U.S. Public Health Service (PHS)

The U.S. Public Health Service grew out of the Marine Hospital Fund (MHF), founded in 1798 to care for sick and disabled sailors. Sailors were taxed 20 cents a month to fund the program, making it the first **health insurance** program in this country.

In 1870, Congress reorganized the MHF under central control with a headquarters in Washington, D.C., renamed it the Marine Hospital Services (MHS), and created the position of "supervising surgeon" to head the services. The 1878 Quarantine Act gave the MHS responsibility for enacting **quarantine**, but these duties were shifted to the National Board of Health the following year.

Dr. Joseph Kinyoun (1860–1919) of the MHS opened a one-room Hygienic Laboratory at the Staten Island Marine Hospital in 1887. He intended to make the lab the "nucleus of one national in character," modeled on facilities he had visited in Germany.

In 1902, the MHS became the Public Health and Marine Hospital Service, and the "supervising surgeon" became the "surgeon general." The 1902 act also united federal and state **public health** efforts, put the surgeon general at their head, and gave regulatory control of **vaccine** and antitoxin production to the Hygienic Laboratory. The service's duties included screening immigrants at Ellis Island for disease, especially **mental illness**, mental retardation, and trachoma.

In 1912, the service's name was changed to the Public Health Service (PHS), and it was given the authority to "investigate the diseases of man and conditions influencing the propagation and spread thereof, including sanitation and sewage and the pollution, either directly or indirectly, of the navigable streams and lakes of the United States." In 1917, President Woodrow Wilson (1856–1924) made the PHS part of the United States's military forces. Its main actions during World War I were to control disease around troop encampments. The following year, a PHS Division of Venereal Diseases was established, with a $2 million budget.

In 1929, Congress established a Narcotics Division within the PHS and required that two facilities be built to study and treat addicts. The Ransdell Act established the **National Institutes of Health (NIH)** in place of the Hygiene Laboratory in 1930, with an initial appropriation of $750,000 for expansion.

Beginning in 1935, the PHS ran a National Health Survey. The results showed that chronic and disabling illnesses were much more common among families on relief. That year, the **Social Security** Act provided funds to PHS for maternal and child health and to establish a network of state and local health departments.

The Nurse Training Act of 1943 established the U.S. Cadet Nurse Corps, which sought to draw young women into nursing. The 1944 PHS act reorganized the service, and during the war the service doubled in size.

In 1946, the Hospital Survey and Construction Act provided funding for hospital construction through the PHS, and the National Mental Health Act was passed.

When President Dwight Eisenhower (1890–1969) took office in 1953 he organized the Department of Health, Education, and Welfare. The secretary of the department was made part of the president's cabinet. Health programs within the Bureau of Indian Affairs, a government organization dedicated to Native Americans, were made part of the PHS in 1955. Later in the decade, legislation provided funding for sanitation and hospital construction on reservations, which by 1960 had helped to cut the infant mortality rate among Native Americans living on reservations by 25 percent and halved the tuberculosis death rate.

In 1964, the PHS launched the first antismoking campaign, following the Advisory Committee on Smoking and Health conclusion after two years of study that smoking causes lung **cancer**. In 1968 the PHS was restructured, losing jurisdiction over water pollution and gaining responsibility for the **Food and Drug Administration (FDA)**.

The National Health Service Corps, proposed in 1969, began providing medical professionals with scholarship aid in exchange for their service in underserved areas in 1972. The program continues today.

In 1970, the National Institute of Occupational Safety and Health was created within the PHS, along with the Occupational Safety and Health Administration in the Department of Labor. These bureaus were intended to standardize worker protection and **industrial hygiene**. In 1973, further reorganization divided the PHS into six agencies: the **Centers for Disease Control**, the National Institutes of Health, the FDA, the Health Services Administration, the Health Resources Administration, and the Alcohol, Drug Abuse and Mental Health Administration. That year, a **HMO (health maintenance organization)** program also was set up and the PHS began giving out grants to stimulate the formation of HMOs in order to reduce health-care costs.

In 1981, the Omnibus Reconciliation Act shifted several PHS programs into block grants to states and cut its budget by 25 percent, trimming PHS staff and the size of the commissioned corps. In 1983, the PHS took on the responsibility of managing the health aspects of the Superfund Act. The Indian Health Service gained agency status in 1988, during the administration of Dr. Everett Rhoades (1931–), the PHS's first Native American director. Today, the PHS employs 40,000 people.

Additional reading: Mullan, *Plagues and Politics.*

U.S. Sanitary Commission

Civilian volunteers formed the U.S. Sanitary Commission during the Civil War to improve medical care for soldiers.

The Union Army's medical services were in great disarray. Military **hospitals** had to be improvised in churches, prisons, and other public buildings, as there were none in the United States and the largest hospital at any military post contained only 41 beds. The Army had no system for transporting the wounded or taking precautions to prevent the spread of infection. During the war's early battles, wounded soldiers often were left to die on the battlefield.

A group of doctors led by Henry Bellows (1814–1882) of New York, a Unitarian minister, asked the secretary of war to establish a civilian advisory board, which he created in 1861. The Secretary of War and President Abraham Lincoln (1809–1865) were initially unenthusiastic about the commission and called it the "fifth wheel on the coach."

The commission's first act was to call for a new surgeon general and a corps of medical inspectors. They began by inspecting Army camps near Washington and making suggestions for their improvement.

In 1862, William A. Hammond (1828–1900) replaced Clement A. Finley as surgeon general. Hammond required records to be kept on sick, wounded, and deceased soldiers; sped procurement of supplies; proposed an **ambulance** corps; recommended that a permanent hospital be established in Washington; and founded the Army Medical School. Jonathan Letterman (1824–1872) was named medical director for the Army of the Potomac, where he organized care for the wounded and established an ambulance system. Two years later, an ambulance corps was created by Congress for the rest of the Union army.

At the beginning of the war, there were roughly 100 Army doctors. This number swelled to 13,000, thanks to the efforts of the Sanitary Commission. The commission also helped to distribute supplies and donations and vaccinated 20,000 men against **smallpox**. During the war, the commission collected $7 million in contributions.

In 1862, the commission began keeping track of patients in hospitals in Washington, D.C., and Maryland. Relatives of soldiers could write to the commission for information on the soldier, and received a response by return mail. The commission also provided lodges where soldiers returning from the front could recuperate and helped the soldiers organize their affairs. By the end of the war, they had established 40 Soldiers' Homes, as they were called.

The commission also made recommendations for pensions for soldiers and support for widows and orphans.

Additional reading: Maxwell, *Lincoln's Fifth Wheel.*

V

vaccine

Vaccination is the introduction of a mild or "killed" form of a bacterium or **virus**, or pieces of the infectious agent, into a person's body to train his or her immune system to resist infection by the agent so that he or she can avoid developing the disease.

Edward Jenner (1749–1823) discovered the principle of vaccination in 1798. British dairy farmers had long known that people would become immune to the serious illness **smallpox** after a bout with cowpox, which is a mild disease in humans.

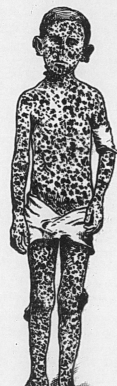

'VACCINATION A CURSE,"
And a Menace to Personal Liberty,"

BY J. M. PEEBLES, A. M., M. D., PH. D.

ECZEMA FROM VACCIN-ATION.

AN

INNOCENT

VICTIM

OF

THE

VACCINATOR'S

LANCE

Compulsory Vaccination
and the Result.

Does Vaccination Prevent Small-Pox.

I. Jenner's discovery of vaccination, from the horse, the cow, the heifer, and later the goat.

II. Facts, figures and proofs showing that vaccination utterly fails to protect against small-pox.

III. The Dangers, deformities and deaths from vaccination.

IV Court decisions against compulsory vaccination.

V Reasons why some doctors with an eye to their fees insist upon vaccination.

VI. Local contests and their victories against calf-lymph vaccination.

VII. The un-American and illegal conduct of health-boards in locking the public school doors against children because their parents conscientiously refused to have their childrens' blood poisoned with calf-lymph virus.

VIII. Eczema, cancer, tumors, carbuncles, boils, syphilis and skin diseases directly traceable to vaccination.

IX. The fight against vaccination in England resulting in the parliamentary enactment of the "optional conscience clause."

X. Decisive testimonies of distinguished American, English, French and Australian physicians and surgeons against this terrible scourge, vaccination.

The above subjects with others relating to cowpox and calf-lymph vaccination, are ably and medically discussed in this volume of 326 pages, cloth binding, gilt edges and handsomely illustrated, by Dr. J. M Peebles, M. D. For sale by Dr. Peebles & Co., Battle Creek, Mich., price $1.25.

"On the cover of this book is a picture in gold of a patient bound hand and foot—a doctor on the right side injecting the virus, and a policeman on the left with a club compelling the poor defenseless man to submit to the wickedness of poisoning his blood."—R. P. Journal, San Francisco.

Advertisement for J.M. Peebles' 1800 anti-vaccination tract. (Courtesy of American Society for Microbiology Archives Collection.)

To test this claim, Jenner collected pus from a cow-pox-infected woman and injected it into a boy, who he later injected with smallpox. The boy didn't get sick.

Jenner called the technique "vaccination," after the Latin word for cow, *vacca*. This was an advance from variolation, a folk smallpox treatment in which people were intentionally exposed to material from smallpox-infected individuals, such as pus or powdered scabs from sores. The greatest risk of vaccination was that a person might catch cowpox, but people treated with variolation risked developing smallpox.

After a serious epidemic of smallpox, Britain passed a law in 1841 making vaccinations free for all. In 1853, another law made infant vaccination against smallpox compulsory.

Louis Pasteur (1822–1895) expanded on Jenner's knowledge while working to find cures for chicken **cholera**, swine erysipelas, and anthrax in livestock. Pasteur found that injecting chickens with cultures of cholera that had been grown for several generations protected them against getting the disease. In a dramatic experiment on 24 sheep in 1881, he proved the effectiveness of his **anthrax vaccine**. He also later developed a vaccine against **rabies**.

Today there are vaccines for many infectious diseases, including **poliomyelitis, mumps, measles, rubella,** and **influenza.** Children and adults in many countries now receive regularly scheduled **immunizations** to protect them against deadly diseases.

Scientists are now working on developing **cancer vaccines**. These won't prevent people from getting **cancer**, but will help people with cancer to fight off the disease by training their immune system to recognize and kill cancer cells. In trials, cancer vaccines for **melanoma** and lymphoma have been able to shrink tumors in patients with advanced disease. A 1998 trial of a **colorectal cancer** vaccine found that patients who received it were less likely to develop a recurrence of disease. Vaccines also are being investigated for preventing infection with HIV, the virus that causes **AIDS.**

Additional reading: Friedman and Friedland, *Medicine's 10 Greatest Discoveries,* pp. 65–93.

valve repair

There are several sets of valves that regulate blood flow within the chambers of the heart, and they may need to be repaired or replaced with artificial material if they malfunction seriously. Valvulotomy is an operation to "unstick" malfunctioning valves in the heart.

In the early twentieth century, Boston surgeon Elliot Cutler (1888–1947) performed a series of experimental valvulotomies in dogs with some success, but his colleagues' single attempt to operate on a human resulted in the patient's death.

Samuel Levine (1891–1966) and Cutler performed the first successful valvulotomy for mitral stenosis in a human in 1923, in a 12–year-old girl. This operation and several that followed were imperfect; they basically involved mak-

ing a tight valve leaky. Charles P. Bailey (1910–1993), after some failures, performed a more successful version of the operation that he named a "commissurotomy," in 1950.

Once the **heart-lung machine** made it possible to operate directly on the heart, not blindly, in 1954, procedures for repairing heart valves were much improved.

Surgeons working with artificial heart valves began to have some success during the late 1950s. Today, dozens of types of artificial heart valves are available, made from materials ranging from pig flesh to titanium.

Additional reading: Shorter, *The Health Century,* pp. 172–74; Comroe, *Exploring the Heart,* pp. 172–75.

vascular endothelial growth factor (VEGF)

Vascular endothelial growth factor is a natural substance that spurs the growth of new blood vessels.

Researchers are investigating the use of VEGF to promote blood vessel growth for treating heart disease.

In 1997, Jeffrey Isner (1947–) and his colleagues at St. Elizabeth Medical Center in Boston showed that injecting the gene for VEGF directly into the heart of patients with **angina pectoris** helped ease pain and allowed patients to exert themselves. Angina occurs because vessels aren't able to supply enough blood to the heart muscle, and VEGF eases chest pain by promoting the growth of new blood vessels to feed the muscle. Subsequent studies have found treatment with VEGF safe and effective. No feared side-effects, such as the growth of **cancers** or development of eye problems, have developed in patients treated with the **growth factor**.

Additional reading: Mitka, "High Tech Angina Relief Explored in Treatment Trials."

vascular surgery

Vascular surgery is the repair and sometimes reconstruction of the blood vessels. The unquestioned pioneer of vascular surgery was Alexis Carrel (1873–1944), who only once operated on a human being. Working on dogs at the Rockefeller Institute in New York, Carrel devised nearly every vascular surgical technique now in use.

Carrel reconnected arteries and veins, grafted blood vessels to one another, and developed artificial materials to serve as blood vessels. He invented his own equipment. He also paved the way for transplants by developing techniques for reconnecting severed blood vessels and devised a method for "banking" donor vessels by freezing them. During his internship, he had studied with an embroiderer.

Carrel won the 1912 Nobel Prize for his work. His techniques were not widely used in humans until the 1940s, when the development of the **heart-lung machine** made it possible to perform operations on the heart itself and also made operating on other parts of the vascular system easier.

Additional reading: Wangensteen, *The Rise of Surgery,* pp. 255–74.

vasectomy

Vasectomy is an operation in which the vas deferens, the tube carrying sperm from the testes to the penis, is cut or blocked to produce sterility.

The first vasectomy on a human patient was performed in 1893. Most early vasectomies were performed under the mistaken belief that sterilization would be rejuvenating, or could keep men—especially reform-school inmates—from masturbating.

There were laws on the books allowing vasectomy for a variety of causes in 23 states in 1933. This was also the first year in which National Socialist sterilization laws went into effect in Germany, and 28,000 vasectomies were performed in that country.

Voluntary vasectomy for family planning became popular in the 1950s and 1960s. Today, there are roughly 500,000 vasectomies performed in the United States each year.

Additional reading: Moss, *Contraceptive Sterilization.*

VEGF. *See vascular endothelial growth factor.*

Viagra. *See impotence treatment.*

vinca alkaloids

Vinca alkaloids are anticancer drugs derived from the leaves of the Jamaican periwinkle plant. They stop cell division by binding to the mitotic spindle.

Scientists originally began examining the plant as a treatment for **diabetes**, because a tea made from periwinkle leaves was used as a folk remedy for the disease. Researchers in James Collip's (1892–1965) lab at the University of Western Ontario in Toronto began examining the plant in the early 1950s. They found that periwinkle plant extract decreased white blood cell counts in mice, while increasing the number of **red blood cells** and platelets.

This led the researchers to theorize that the substance might be useful for treating **leukemia** and lymphoma, diseases in which the white blood cell counts are much higher than normal. After investigation of various components within the plants, vinblastine was isolated and identified in 1957.

The following year, Canadian researchers began working with the American drug company Eli Lilly, where the related substance vincristine was isolated and identified. **Cancer** trials of vinblastine began in the late 1950s.

The two substances are nearly identical in their molecular structure, but have very different properties. Vinblastine can effectively treat lymphomas, and damages bone marrow, while vincristine treats leukemia in children and damages the peripheral nervous system. (*See also* chemotherapy)

Additional reading: Sneader, *Drug Discovery,* pp. 356–59.

virus

Viruses are infectious agents, too small to be seen with a conventional **microscope**, that are only capable of repro-

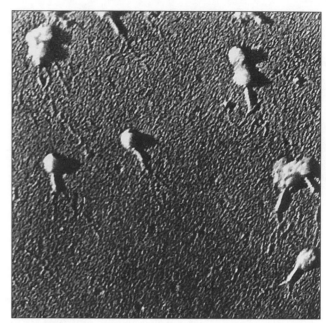

E. coli phage shadowed with gold. This virus infects bacteria. (American Society for Microbiology Archives Collection.)

ducing themselves by infecting another organism. Viruses have a single strand of genetic material, either **DNA** or RNA.

Martinus Beijerinck (1851–1931), a Dutch botanist, was the first person to discover that organisms smaller than bacteria existed that could cause disease. In 1898 he proved this by grinding up an infected tobacco plant, filtering the resulting material through holes so tiny they did not allow bacteria to pass, and infecting a healthy plant with the fluid. He named the substance a "contagious living fluid," and later said the fluid contained a "filterable virus." Virus is the Latin word for "poisonous slime."

Once the **electron microscope** became available in the 1930s, it was possible to see viruses.

Viruses infect animals and plants, and may be spread by insects. Viruses often cause disease, including some **cancers**, while others can exist peacefully inside their host without sickening them. There are few effective **antiviral** drugs; generally, the most effective treatment for virus is preventive, with vaccination. (*See also* vaccine)

Additional reading: Henig, *A Dancing Matrix,* pp. 58–71

vision test

Vision tests are used to gauge the strength of vision and the health of the eyes.

Dr. Hermann Snellen (1834–1909), a Dutch ophthalmologist, developed the famous eye chart with a series of letters of descending size, as well as one for illiterate individuals with the letter "E" facing in various directions. He invented the charts, which he called Optotypes, in 1862. The test remains in use worldwide.

The first school-based vision-testing program in the United States was initiated in Connecticut in 1899.

Additional reading: "Watching Out for Eyes," *Los Angeles Times.*

visiting nurse association (VNA)

Visiting nurse associations are nursing organizations that provide care to patients at home.

William Rathbone (1819–1902), a wealthy Englishman, developed a prototype of the VNA. A skilled nurse had cared for his wife before her death in 1859, and he thought such relief would be very helpful to the poor. He began by sending the nurse who had cared for his wife to the homes of poor people in Liverpool, and subsequently established a visiting nurse system in the city to serve the poor. In 1887, Queen Victoria (1819–1901) donated 70,000 pounds to help establish the Queen Victoria Jubilee Institute for Nurses, which funded visiting nurse services.

In the United States, early visiting nurse groups were associated with religious denominations. The country's first nondenominational VNA was the Women's Branch of the New York City Mission, established in 1877. Groups followed in Boston and Philadelphia (1886) and in 1889 in Chicago. These groups were also known as instructive district nursing associations, because nurses who worked for them would teach hygiene and sanitation practices to their patients.

Lillian Wald (1867–1940) moved to New York's Lower East Side in 1893 to care for poor families living in the tenement district there. Her Henry Street Nursing Service provided care to all, regardless of their ability to pay. Wald was a pioneer in **public health** nursing. She and her colleagues not only cared for the sick; they also fought for legal rights for tenement residents and exposed child labor and poor working conditions.

Other nursing settlements were founded in Richmond, Virginia, and San Francisco in 1900 and Orange, New Jersey, in 1903.

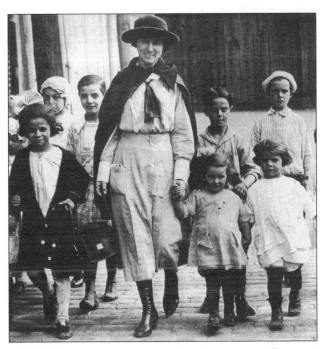

Visiting nurse of the 1920s with some of her young patients. (Courtesy of Visiting Nurse Association of Washington, DC.)

In 1909, the Metropolitan Life Insurance Company collaborated with the Henry Street Settlement to provide visiting nurse services to its industrial policy holders. The program was a success, and by 1912 there were nearly 600 visiting nurse departments in the United States.

By 1920, the two arms of visiting nursing—public health nursing and visiting nurses—had diverged. Public health nurses were employed by city health departments, while visiting nurses served the private sector.

The first **hospital**-based home-care agency, which employed visiting nurses to care for patients at home, was established at Montefiore Hospital in the Bronx. The number of VNAs remained steady for several years until two shifts in health care led to a boom in home-care services: the birth of **Medicare/Medicaid** in 1965, which provided funding for health care for the elderly, poor, and disabled; and 1990s efforts to cut health care costs by providing care at home rather than in the hospital.

There were approximately 1,700 home care agencies in the United States in 1967. By 1974, there were more than 2,200, and today there are more than 18,000 agencies in the United States serving 7 million patients. Much of the growth during the 1990s was due to thousands of private companies joining nonprofit VNAs in the home-care business. (*See also* U.S. Children's Bureau)

Additional reading: Hardy, *William Rathbone and the Early History of District Nursing.*

vitamin

Vitamins are organic substances present in minute amounts in natural foodstuffs and that are necessary for animal nutrition. Unlike fats, proteins, or carbohydrates, which act as fuel and are converted into energy, vitamins must be consumed to trigger or facilitate several different vital biochemical reactions. For a substance to be classified as a vitamin for human nutrition, people must not be able to synthesize it on their own. Vitamins are divided into two groups: fat-soluble (A, D, E, K) and water-soluble (B, C).

The effect of deficiencies of certain types of foods—even though the responsible components were not known—was long understood as disease. Famine, warfare, and poverty tended to produce these deficiency diseases. Folk wisdom also held that eating certain foods could cure certain diseases; for example, liver was known from Hippocrates' (c.460–377 B.C.) time to be an effective treatment for night blindness. We now understand that this is because liver is rich in **vitamin A.**

J.B.A. Dumas (1800–1884) published a paper in 1871 describing the health of infants living on extremely restricted diets in Paris while the city was under siege by the Germans. Attempts were made to feed babies on artificial milk made from carbohydrates, fats, and protein, but the infants died. Dumas concluded that real milk contained some unknown substances that were necessary for life.

In 1896, Christian Eijkman (1858–1930) proposed after a series of experiments that the well-known neurological disease **beriberi** was caused by eating rice from which the outer coat had been removed. He had observed that fowl that ate the milled rice would develop paralysis, but would recover after eating rice with an intact husk. He equated this paralysis in birds with beriberi in humans. However, Eijkman believed that there was something toxic within the rice that was neutralized by material in the husk.

Frederick Gowland Hopkins (1861–1947) conducted a series of experiments during the first decade of the twentieth century in which he investigated the results of feeding animals on purified artificial diets with some additions of natural substances. His experiments proved that natural foods contained tiny amounts of some unknown substances that were necessary for health. He published his findings in 1912.

The German chemist Casimir Funk (1884–1967) concluded in a widely read 1912 paper that beriberi, **pellagra**, and **scurvy** were actually caused by a deficiency in "special substances which are of the nature of organic bases, which we will call vitamines." Funk's word continues to be used today, without the "e" at the end.

During the 1930s and 1940s, it became possible to synthesize and extract vitamins commercially, and these vitamin products went on the market as soon as they became available. In 1931, about $12 million worth of vitamins were sold in the United States; by 1942, annual vitamin sales had reached $130 million. Manufacturers also began to enrich certain foods with vitamins, including grain products and milk.

Today, many people take multivitamin preparations to supplement their nutritional needs. The medical establishment is divided on whether this is necessary; many nutrition experts argue that getting the right nutrients from fresh foods is healthier and more nutritious.

Additional reading: Combs, *The Vitamins*, pp. 3–116.

vitamin A

Vitamin A, which is formed in the body from plant pigments called carotenes, is essential for normal growth and development of epithelial **tissue**, teeth, and bones, as well as the health of the eyes. It is fat-soluble and is stored in the liver.

Elmer V. McCollum (1879–1967) and his colleague Marguerite Davis (1887–1967) at the University of Wisconsin discovered what would become known as **vitamin A** during a series of experiments in rats. They reported in 1913 that rats allowed a certain amount of butter fat or egg yolk would grow and thrive, while those on a purified artificial diet would not. Up to this point, fat had been thought to be nutritionally useful only as a fuel. They eventually separated the nutrient factor from butter fat and named it fat-soluble A. They also learned that this vitamin was present in certain plants and in kidney and other glandular organs. Thomas Osborne (1859–1929) and Lafayette B. Mendel (1872–1935) found shortly afterwards that cod-liver oil also contained A.

Research in animals and humans soon revealed that eye disease was a consequence of vitamin A deficiency, and that one of the first signs of this deficiency is degradation of the epithelial tissue.

Researchers working in the 1930s found that vitamin A is important in vision because it is a component of visual purple, or **rhodopsin**, a pigment that the retina uses to adapt to low-light conditions. A person who lacks sufficient vitamin A will not be able to restore depleted rhodopsin, and will thus have difficulty seeing in the dark.

Efforts began in the 1920s to isolate vitamin A from fish livers. These preparations were powerful but tended to also have a strong fishy smell. Paul Karrer (1889–1971) of Zurich University isolated a nearly pure preparation of vitamin A in 1931 and reported the vitamin's chemical structure two years later.

Harry N. Holmes (1879–1958) of Oberlin College isolated pure vitamin A in 1937. Ten years later, scientists at the pharmaceutical company Hoffmann-La Roche invented a process for synthesizing the vitamin in large quantities.

Additional reading: McCollum, *A History of Nutrition*, pp. 229–41.

vitamin B

Vitamin B is actually a set of vitamins collectively called the B complex. All are water soluble. They are necessary for a number of metabolic processes, as well as for growth and development. The B complex includes thiamin (B1), riboflavin (B2), folic acid, niacin, pantothenic acid, biotin, pyroxidine (B6), and cyanocobalamin (B12).

A disease called **beriberi** was known to be associated with a diet of milled rice. Christian Eijkman (1858–1930) and colleagues reported in 1906 that feeding pigeons a substance found in rice hulls would cure them of the disease. They described the substance, which came to be called thiamin or vitamin B1, and noted that it was water soluble. The vitamin was synthesized and its chemical structure characterized in 1937.

The second B **vitamin** to be found, riboflavin, was discovered by Elmer McCollum (1879–1967) at the University of Wisconsin in 1913, in the course of experiments in which he fed rats artificial diets. The substance was isolated by German researchers in 1933, and synthesized by Paul Karrer (1889–1971) in Zurich and Richard Kuhn (1900–1967) at Heidelberg. Karrer won the Nobel Prize for Chemistry in 1937, and Kuhn was awarded the Nobel Prize the following year, but the Nazi government did not allow him to accept it.

Niacin, or nicotinic acid, was isolated in the late 1800s and was discovered in 1937 to be the substance responsible for preventing **pellagra.**

The next B vitamin to be discovered was B6, which was isolated in 1938. Biotin and pantothenic acid, deficiencies of which were found to be responsible for dermatitis and hair problems in rats, were discovered in the 1930s. Vitamin B12 was identified as the "essential factor," the absence of which caused **pernicious anemia**, in the 1940s.

Scientists at Glaxo Laboratories and Karl Folkers (1906–1997) at the drug company Merck isolated B12 in

1948, and Merck began making it for sale in 1949. B12 contains cobalt, so it was given the name cyanocobalamin. A team of researchers at Cambridge and Oxford universities and Glaxo characterized the molecule in 1955. Alexander Todd (1907–1997) of Cambridge and Dorothy Hodgkin (1910–1994) of Oxford won the Nobel Prize for Chemistry for this accomplishment, Todd in 1957 and Hodgkin in 1964. B12 is most effective when given by intramuscular injection.

Researchers in the 1930s noticed that deficiency in some as-yet-unidentified vitamin produced **anemia** and stunted growth, apparently due to abnormally developed **red blood cells**. Scientists at the Detroit drug company Parke-Davis isolated the responsible substance in 1942. Meanwhile, Esmond Snell (1914–) and Herschel Mitchell (1913–), in the course of searching for an extract of yeast to promote bacterial growth in culture, isolated a similar substance from spinach that they called folic acid, from the Latin *folium* for leaf. Conrad Elvehejm (1901–1962) at the University of Wisconsin confirmed that folic acid prevented anemia in chickens. The vitamin was synthesized in 1945 by Lederle Laboratories scientists.

It is now known that pregnant women who consume enough folic acid virtually eliminate the chance that their fetus will develop spina bifida and other **birth defects** in which the spinal column is not properly formed. For this reason, the United States passed laws that went into effect in 1998 requiring all grain products to be fortified with folic acid.

Additional reading: Kirschmann, *Nutrition Almanac*, pp. 17–43.

vitamin C

The body requires vitamin C, or ascorbic acid, for many processes, including immune-system and endocrine function and wound healing.

The effect of vitamin C deficiency—**scurvy**—was known long before the substance itself was identified. Sailors began developing the disease in the 1400s, when marine technology made it possible for them to go to sea for long journeys, where they depended on preserved food.

James Lind (1716–1794) proved with the first-ever **clinical trial** that citrus fruit could cure scurvy. But it was not until the era of **vitamin** research began at the outset of the twentieth century that inroads were made into defining what would became known as vitamin C and confirming the cause of scurvy.

In a series of experiments with guinea pigs between 1907 and 1912, Norwegian researcher Axel Holst (1861–1931) and his colleagues found that fresh fruit, fresh vegetables, and vegetable and fruit juices would prevent scurvy in animals on grain-only diets. They found that although many fruits lost their antiscorbutic properties upon being heated or losing their freshness, lemon juice retained this power, while dried beans became antiscorbutic if they were soaked and allowed to sprout. The Norwegians also proved that the antiscorbutic substance could be dissolved in water.

Workers at the Lister Institute of Preventive Medicine began making extracts of the antiscorbutic substance in 1918, coming up with a concentrated, powerful preparation in 1923. Charles King (1896–1988) at the University of Pittsburgh further refined the extract and was able to isolate the vitamin from lemon juice in crystal form in 1931. Albert Szent-Gyorgi (1893–1986), working in the Cambridge University laboratory of Frederick Gowland Hopkins (1861–1947), had isolated a similar substance from **adrenal glands,** cabbage, and oranges. The Hungarian researcher proved that the substance prevented scurvy in guinea pigs. Szent-Gyorgyi, with Walter Haworth (1883–1950), proposed that the vitamin be called ascorbic acid. Szent-Gyorgi won the 1937 Nobel Prize in Medicine and Physiology for his discovery.

The vitamin was synthesized in 1933, and Hoffmann-La Roche began commercial manufacture of vitamin C the following year.

Linus Pauling (1901–1994), who won the Nobel Prize for his work on discovering the cause of **sickle-cell anemia,** became an advocate for consuming large amounts of vitamin C to prevent and treat **cancer.** Pauling's claims for vitamin C as a cancer-fighting agent remain controversial and unconfirmed, but many people do take the vitamin to stave off or treat the common cold. The effectiveness of the vitamin for this purpose has not been scientifically proven or disproven.

Additional reading: Kirschmann, *Nutrition Almanac*, pp. 44–49.

vitamin D

Vitamin D is necessary for normal bone formation and other vital functions. This **vitamin** helps deposit minerals in bone by regulating levels of **calcium** and phosphorus in the blood. It may be consumed in food, and also can be produced in the skin by sunlight. The active form of vitamin D is produced with a two-step process: hydroxylation in the liver and then the kidneys.

The disease that led to the discovery of vitamin D's necessity—and ultimately the actual vitamin—was **rickets**. The bones of children with rickets fail to form properly, so their legs are bowed and crooked. In the late 1900s, as the Industrial Revolution forced more people into crowded, dark city dwellings, rickets began to appear at epidemic levels in Northern European, North American, and Northern Asian children.

Frederick Gowland Hopkins (1861–1947) suggested in 1912 that rickets was caused by deficiency in an accessory food factor, or vitamin. The concept of vitamins had just been developed.

In 1919, Sir Edward Mellanby (1884–1955) showed that rickets could be healed with cod-liver oil, but he thought that the responsible nutrient was **vitamin A**.

In 1922, Elmer McCollum (1879–1967) proved that the therapeutic properties of cod-liver oil came from a new vitamin that he discovered and named vitamin D. Vitamin D was isolated in 1931.

Researchers working in the 1960s and early 1970s determined that vitamin D does not act directly on the bones, as had been thought, but cues the kidneys and intestine to allow more calcium and phosphorous to enter the bloodstream when levels of these minerals drop. The function of this vitamin—which acts more like a **hormone**—is still being studied.

Additional reading: Kirschmann, *Nutrition Almanac*, pp. 49–52.

vitamin E

Vitamin E is an antioxidant vitamin that is essential for normal reproductive function and may also protect against heart disease.

In 1922, Herbert McLean Evans (1882–1971) reported that rats raised on an experimental diet were less fertile than normal, while the rats born of this generation were totally sterile. He found that feeding the animals lettuce, wheat germ, or dried alfalfa would restore fertility, and they named the unknown nutrient contained in these foods "substance X." Evans and his colleagues subsequently found that E-deficient animals ovulated and became pregnant normally, but that the fetus would develop blood vessel and liver abnormalities and would eventually die of asphyxiation. Giving vitamin E to the rat even a few days into pregnancy would save the fetus. Further research found that deficiency in the **vitamin** could impair nerve development.

Evans, H.P. Emerson and Gladys Anderson Emerson (1903–1984) isolated a substance from wheat germ that they named alpha-tocopherol. This turned out to be the elusive vitamin E. Paul Karrer (1889–1971) and colleagues synthesized the vitamin in 1938.

Today, vitamin E is believed to play an important role in the proper metabolism of fats. Large studies in humans strongly suggest that the vitamin can protect against **atherosclerosis,** and may even reverse the arterial plaque buildup that characterizes this condition.

Additional reading: Kirschmann, *Nutrition Almanac*, pp. 52–58.

vitamin K

Vitamin K is a nutritional substance required for normal blood clotting. It is found in fats, fish, some grains, and alfalfa, and may also be formed by bacteria in the intestines. It assists in blood clotting by helping the body to form a substance called prothrombin.

In 1913, while conducting experiments on fat-soluble **vitamins**, Robert G. McFarlane (1907–) and colleagues found that chickens fed on a diet of **ether**-extracted fish meal often died of hemorrhage, and that their blood didn't clot even when kept overnight in the laboratory.

In work that began in 1929, Henrik Dam (1895–1976), discovered a new deficiency disease that appeared in chickens fed an artificial diet and was distinct from **scurvy** or other known vitamin deficiencies. He described the disease in 1934, and noted that the hemorrhage-preventing substance was fat soluble. He suggested naming it vitamin K, for the German word "koagulation." Dam showed that hog liver fat, cereals, fruits, vegetables, and fats contained the **vitamin**. By 1935, Dam had further specified the role of vitamin K. He found that animals deficient in the vitamin had lower-than-normal levels of prothrombin, which could be remedied by feeding them preparations containing vitamin K.

Herman James Almquist (1903–) and E.L. Robert Stokstad (1913–) reported that same year that bacterial growth seemed to increase vitamin K content in certain preparations.

Dam and several other groups of researchers were able to purify and isolate vitamin K in the late 1930s. Soon after that, vitamin K was found to be useful in treating certain types of hemorrhagic disease, especially in newborns born without the vitamin. Now infants are given an injection of Vitamin K at birth.

Additional reading: McCollum, *A History of Nutrition*, pp. 376–83.

VNA. *See* visiting nurse association

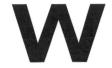

warfarin

Warfarin is an **anticoagulant** drug derived from a substance found in spoiled sweet clover hay.

Beginning in the 1920s, several epidemics of hemorrhagic disease struck herds of cows throughout the United States. In 1922, Alberta veterinarian F.W. Schofield showed that the disease was caused by the spoiled hay. Veterinary pathologist Lee M. Rodcrick observed in 1931 that cows with the disease had very low levels of prothrombin, a protein found in the blood that is required for normal clotting.

In Wisconsin, Karl Paul Link (1901–1978) began searching for the substance that caused the disorder after a farmer brought him a bucket of unclotted blood. The farmer's cattle were bleeding to death after having their horns shorn or being castrated. He identified the coagulant, reporting his discovery in 1941.

The drug companies Abbott and Eli Lilly began marketing the drug, which they called dicoumarol, the following year.

Link synthesized a similar compound, naming it warfarin, for the initials of the Wisconsin Alumni Research Foundation, which licensed it as a rat poison. The drug was found to actually be a more effective anticoagulant than dicoumarol after a U.S. soldier tried to kill himself by taking rat poison. Today, warfarin is given to people with an abnormal heart rhythm called atrial fibrillation in order to prevent stroke.

Additional reading: Callahan, et al., *Classics of Cardiology, Volume III,* pp. 415–30.

weight-loss drugs

Weight-loss drugs are medications used to fight obesity by reducing the appetite. They work by increasing levels of certain neurotransmitters associated with appetite and satiety, mainly serotonin and norepinephrine.

The first drugs used as appetite suppressants were amphetamines, which were effective but were also addictive and had harmful side effects. Aminorex fumarate, an amphetamine-like drug, was withdrawn from the Swiss market in the late 1960s after it was found to increase a person's risk of developing primary pulmonary hypertension 20-fold. This condition is potentially fatal.

Fenfluramine (sold as Pondimin), a drug that worked by increasing serotonin levels, was introduced in 1964 and approved by the Food and Drug Administration (FDA) for sale in the United States in 1973 as a controlled substance, and then as a regular prescription drug in 1995.

Dexfenfluramine (sold as Redux), a similar drug, was launched in 1987 and approved by the FDA in 1996. After its release, U.S. doctors wrote 85,000 dexfenfluramine prescriptions weekly. A combination of dexfenfluramine and the drug phentermine, known as Fen/Phen, became extremely popular.

However, reports that these drugs were associated with heart-valve disorders and primary pulmonary hypertension led to their being withdrawn from the U.S. market in September 1997.

Sibutramine (Meridia), a drug sold by Knoll Pharmaceutical Company, was approved by the FDA in November 1997. The drug was first synthesized in 1980, and had been developed initially as an antidepressant. It is a serotonin-norepinephrine reuptake inhibitor, and some studies suggest it may also work by speeding up the metabolism.

Additional reading: Schwartz, John, "FDA approves new diet drug for obese with warning about monitoring," *Washington Post.*

WHO. *See* World Health Organization.

WIC

The Special Supplemental Nutrition Program for Women, Infants and Children (WIC) is a federal program that was launched in 1974 to ensure adequate nutrition for pregnant women, nursing mothers, and children. WIC provides funding to low-income women and children up to five years old who are at risk of poor nutrition.

In 1975, there were roughly 344,000 people enrolled in WIC and funding for the program was $85 million. In

1994, there were approximately 7.4 million women and children participating in the program, at a cost of about $3.7 billion.

WIC enrollees receive purchasing vouchers for foods rich in nutrients usually lacking in low-income individuals' diets, including **vitamins A** and **C**, **calcium**, protein, and iron, as well as nutrition and health counseling. The total value of WIC vouchers for each person is about $45 a month.

Numerous studies have found that women who participate in WIC while pregnant are less likely to have low birthweight babies, and children in the WIC program are less likely to be anemic and more likely to grow normally than poor children who do not participate. Some critics argue that women who participate may be healthier for other reasons—such as that they may be less likely to smoke and better able to care for themselves than those who do not.

WIC legislation was enacted in 1972 in response to several studies in the 1960s that found low-income children were smaller and weighed less than their higher-income counterparts. The program was an amendment of the 1966 Child Nutrition Act. After a two-year pilot program, the program was established nationwide, with local clinics required to apply for grants through state health departments. The U.S. Department of Agriculture determines a person's eligibility, and also decides which foods can be bought with WIC vouchers. A law passed in 1978 required that women and children be at risk of poor nutrition as well as meeting income requirements.

Ten years later, WIC benefits were mandated for homeless women and children in the Hunger Prevention Act. Income requirements for WIC vary state-by-state, but generally are set at below 185 percent of the U.S. poverty level.

Additional reading: Walker, "Feeding Babies vs. Fueling Competition."

workers compensation

Workers compensation is a legal system for reimbursing workers—and some cases their families—who suffer injury or death on the job.

In 1825, Alabama passed the first law making an employer liable for a worker injured through another worker's carelessness. Montana passed a workers compensation law in 1909 and New York followed in 1910, but these laws were declared unconstitutional.

The first lasting workers compensation law was passed in Illinois in 1911. It required that companies compensate workers who developed diseases caused by exposure to poisonous fumes, gases, and dust in the workplace, and required that workers using dangerous materials such as zinc, lead, arsenic, brass, and mercury have monthly medical exams. Nine other states passed similar laws that year.

These laws forced companies to insure themselves against workers' claims, and insurance companies then pressured the companies to improve working conditions to reduce the chances that such claims would be made.

By 1940, 47 of the nation's 48 states had workers compensation laws. Today, all 50 states have workers compensation laws requiring companies to insure themselves against a worker being injured on the job, but these laws are not uniform. Some require only companies with a certain number of employees to buy workers compensation insurance. In some states, only workers in fields that are considered hazardous are covered. Household workers, agricultural workers, and employees of interstate railroads are often excluded from state plans. Workers compensation insurance within a state may be organized under a state fund or administered by private insurance companies.

Additional reading: Bellamy, *A History of Workmen's Compensation, 1898–1915.*

World Health Organization (WHO)

The World Health Organization, founded in 1948, is an agency of the United Nations (UN) devoted to public health. WHO is responsible for establishing international sanitary regulations, controlling epidemics of disease, and strengthening the **public health** programs of its member nations. It is headquartered in Geneva, Switzerland.

The World Health Assembly meets annually to make policy for WHO. An executive board runs the organization. The board is made up of specialists in health who serve for three-year terms. There are also WHO field offices worldwide, staffed by regional officers and administered by the Secretariat.

Member organizations fund WHO, which also has recieved funding from the UN's expanded technical assistance program since 1951.

Dr. Geraldo de Paula Souza (1889–1951) of Brazil was responsible for including "health" in the UN charter, and requested the international conference on health held in July 1946 that led to the forming of WHO. The WHO constitution was signed by representatives of 61 governments.

WHO took on some of the duties that had been carried out by its predecessor, the Health Organization of the League of Nations, which was founded in 1923, and Paris's International Office of Public Health, founded in 1909.

In 1948, the first World Health Assembly gave top priority to **malaria**, **tuberculosis**, venereal disease, and maternal and child health, as well as sanitary engineering and nutrition. The assembly also approved a $5 million budget for 1949.

In 1978, WHO and **UNICEF** sponsored the **Alma Ata International Conference on Primary Health Care.** Participants at the meeting resolved to work toward establishing the goal of an acceptable level of health for all of the world's people by 2000, which has not been achieved.

One of WHO's major achievements was the complete eradication of **smallpox** in 1980. The organization's current goals include eradicating dracunculiasis and **poliomyelitis** and eliminating **leprosy**, neonatal **tetanus**, **Chagas' disease**, and iodine deficiency. Eradication means completely wiping out the disease, while eliminating it means to bring the prevalence of the disease down to extremely low levels. WHO is seeking to accomplish these goals by improving immunization and sanitation and in some cases destroying populations of insects that spread a particular disease.

WHO also is currently seeing to establish global standards for the production of food, biological products, and drugs.

Additional reading: Beigbeder, *The World Health Organization.*

X–Y

X-rays

X-rays are high-energy electromagnetic waves capable of penetrating most solid objects and of acting on film. They are used to create images of the inside of the body and to treat **cancer**.

In 1895, Wilhelm Konrad Roentgen (1845–1923) first described X-rays, which are also called Roentgen rays. X-rays are produced by directing high-velocity electrons at a target in a vacuum tube, which Roentgen had done by chance while working with a cathode ray tube. He made the first radiograph of a human, of his wife's hand, soon afterwards. Roentgen won the first Nobel Prize for Physics in 1901 for his discovery.

In 1896, Henri Becquerel (1852–1908) discovered natural radiation when he observed that pitchblende (an ore that contains uranium) produced an image on photographic film, even on a cloudy day. In Canada that year, the X-ray was used for the first time to locate a bullet in a young man's leg; the exposure took 45 minutes, and the image was used in court.

At the beginning of the twentieth century, X-rays took a long time to make—at least 20 minutes—and exposed the subject to large amounts of radiation. Early X-ray researchers suffered gruesome effects from their frequent exposure to radiation, including severe deterioration of their exposed body parts and virulent cancers.

Refinements of the technique over this century have brought down the radiation dose a person receives with an X-ray to near-insignificance. Specialized X-ray machines are used to perform **mammography** screening for **breast cancer**. X-rays have also given rise to more sophisticated, detailed imaging techniques such as **CAT scanning**, **PET scanning**, **angiography**, and more, and they are still used commonly today in **dentistry** and to detect bone fractures and abnormalities.

Additional reading: Friedman and Friedland, *Medicine's 10 Greatest Discoveries*, pp. 115–32; Kevles, *Naked to the Bone*, pp. 9–141.

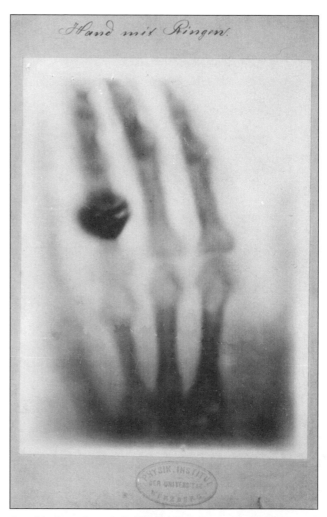

One of the first radiographs by Wilhelm Konrad Roentgen, the discoverer of X-rays, Dec. 22, 1895. The hand is probably his wife's. (Courtesy of The Wellcome Trust Medical Photographic Library, London.)

xenograft

A xenograft is a transplant of **tissue** or an organ from one species to another. Xenografting is now a hotly debated topic because of the short supply of human organs available for transplantation, recent successes in inter-species transplants, and the fear that an epidemic of a previously unknown human disease could be launched if a person becomes infected by a **virus** from another animal. Many people also have ethical concerns about the implications of breeding animals for the purpose of harvesting their organs.

The first recorded xenograft was performed in 1682, when a Russian nobleman received a piece of skull from a dog to repair his own skull. The surgery was reported to have worked, but because the Russian Church threatened to excommunicate the man, he had the graft removed. In the seventeenth and eighteenth centuries, a number of animal-to-human **blood transfusions** were performed, with varying but generally bad results.

Peter Medawar's (1915–1987) research in the 1940s on immunologic rejection proved why this occurred. People reject transplants from humans who are not genetically identical to them, and implants from another species are even less tolerable. **Antibody** molecules hitch on to the alien tissue, which cause complement proteins in the blood to be activated and the foreign organ to be destroyed. Medawar won the Nobel Prize for his work in studying immune-system function.

In the 1960s, before dialysis became widely available to replace kidney function, Keith Reemtsma (1911–), then at Tulane University, transplanted chimpanzee kidneys into 13 human patients. One patient survived six months. Thomas Starzl (1926–) transplanted humans with kidneys and livers from baboons in 1964 and 1993, respectively. All of the kidney patients died of infections, probably due to the massive immunosuppressive treatment necessary to prevent them from rejecting the organs.

In 1984, an infant girl known as "Baby Fae" received a baboon heart to replace her deformed heart in an operation performed by Leonard Bailey (1942–) at Loma Linda Medical Center in California, and lived for 20 days. In 1992, some humans received baboon livers, and three years later an **AIDS** patient, Jeff Getty (1957–), was given immune cells from baboons. He is currently alive and healthy, although it is unclear if the baboon-cell transplant helped.

In 1997, patients with **Parkinson's disease** received transplants of dopamine-producing fetal nerve cells from pigs, with some success. The cells lived in one person's brain for seven months.

Scientists have also been genetically engineering animals in attempts to make their organs more tolerable to humans. Another strategy would be to somehow splice out the substance to which the human would react, or removing all antibodies to the organ from the human's blood. (*See also* immunosuppression)

Additional reading: Caplan and Coelho, eds., *The Ethics of Organ Transplantation,* pp. 121–32.

yellow fever

Yellow fever is a viral disease transmitted by mosquitoes, with symptoms that include jaundice, vomiting, and fever. It commonly appears in the tropics.

The first recorded epidemic of yellow fever struck the West Indies and Central America in the late 1640s. The disease is believed to have originated among nonhuman primates.

Yellow fever has been known by approximately 150 names, including yellow jack for the yellow **quarantine** flag flown by ships, black vomit, and Barbados distemper.

Carlos Finlay (1833–1913) suggested in 1878 that yellow fever was spread by the *Aedes aegypti* mosquito. Max Theiler (1899–1972), a South African-born microbiologist, developed an attenuated strain of the yellow fever virus while working at Harvard Medical School. He moved on to the Rockefeller Institute for Medical Research in New York, where he and his colleagues developed and improved a yellow fever **vaccine** from 1930 to 1964. Theiler won the 1951 Nobel Prize for this achievement, and his vaccine is still used today.

Mosquito eradication programs run by U.S. Army surgeon William Gorgas (1854–1920) in Cuba and Panama rid these nations of the disease. The last cases of yellow fever in North America appeared in New Orleans in 1905 and Barbados three years later.

Today a small number of cases occur every year in people who live near Central and South American forests, while epidemics strike African cities every few years.

Additional reading: Kiple, *The Cambridge World History of Human Disease,* pp. 1100–07.

Timeline

Boldfaced words can be found as entries in this book.

c.10,000 B.C. First evidence of **trepanation**.

c.3500 B.C. First description of **migraine**.

c.3100 B.C. First reported use of Chinese herb Ma Huang, also known as **ephedrine**.

c.2500 B.C. Earliest known **skin graft**.

2737 B.C. First mention of **marijauna** as medication.

1400 B.C. Light-sensitizing plant material psoralen is used in **phototherapy**.

1350 B.C. Earliest recorded epidemic of **smallpox**.

600 B.C. **Reserpine's** medicinal use is described.

Rabies is described.

Reconstructive **rhinoplasty** is mentioned in medical literature.

420–370 B.C. Seventy works constituting the **Hippocratic Corpus** are written.

c.400 B.C. First connection drawn between swamps and **malaria**.

400–300 B.C. **Pineal gland** is described.

c.300 B.C. Human body is dissected.

c.200 B.C. **Lithotomy** is performed.

c.100 A.D. Location of lens within the eye is described.

c.200 A.D. **Asthma** attack is described.

Diabetes mellitus is described.

335 Emperor Constantine decrees that infirmaries (early hospitals) must be built in Rome.

341 First reported use of Chinese herb qinghaosu to treat **malaria**.

390 First surgical repair of **cleft lip**.

700s–800s First asylums (early version of **mental hospital**) are built.

900s First clinical description of **leprosy**

927 First reported surgery to remove a **brain tumor**.

c.1000 Arab physicians recommend plaster casts for broken bones.

First mention of **opium** abuse.

1200s **Eyeglasses** are invented.

1353 Worst epidemic of **bubonic plague**, known as the Black Death, begins.

1371 First **quarantine** is enacted, against **bubonic plague**.

1400s Pope Sixtus IV permits **autopsies** at Bologna and Padua medical schools.

First regulation of **midwifery**.

1500s First descriptions of **atherosclerosis**.

1507 *The Hidden Causes of Disease*, Antonio Benevini's book describing 111 cases (including 15 **autopsies**) is published.

1521 Appendix is described.

1529 French surgeon ties off blood vessel to stop bleeding after leg **amputation**.

1530 **Contagion theory** of disease is articulated.

1543 First work of modern **anatomy** is published.

1563 First book on dental anatomy is published.

1564 First description of the **adrenal glands**.

Leg **prosthesis** with knee joint is described.

1578 First recorded epidemic of **pertussis**.

1582	First description of use of **ergot** to accelerate labor.
c.1590	Compound **microscope** is invented.
early 1600s	Cinchona, early **malaria** treatment, is introduced to Europe.
1600s	**Forceps** are introduced.
	First description of **reflex** action.
1610	**Cesarean section** performed on a living woman.
1623	Book on **eyeglasses** and **vision testing** is published.
	Lymph system is discovered.
1624	**Typhoid fever** is described.
1628	**Circulation** is described.
1642	First European account of **beriberi**.
Late 1640s	**Yellow fever** epidemic is recorded.
1658	First suggestion of a link between brain blood vessels and apoplexy (**stroke**).
1660	Definitive description of **rickets**.
1660s	First observation and description of **red blood cells**.
1665	Scientific journals begin publication.
1667	First recorded **blood transfusions** in humans, using animals as donors.
	London doctor suggests that epileptic seizures originate in the cerebellum.
1682	First recorded **xenograft**.
1699	First regulation of **dentistry** is introduced.
1700	**Thermometer** is invented.
Early 1700s	Variolation, technique for preventing **smallpox**, is introduced to Europe from the Ottoman Empire.
1700s	First **orthodontia** appliances are introduced.
	Bristle **toothbrushes** are introduced.
1725	Dental key, a tool for pulling teeth, is introduced.
1728	Cordon sanitaire, for preventing spread of **bubonic plague**, is established. Lasts until 1872.
1730	**Pellagra** is described.
1735	First surgical removal of an inflamed appendix (**appendectomy**).

1747	First **clinical trial**, of citrus fruit for treating **scurvy**, is conducted.
1747–1748	First extraction of **cataract**.
1750	Word "antiseptic" is first used.
1751	Giovanni Morgagni's *On the Seats and Causes of Disease as Investigated by Anatomy*, containing life and post-mortem observations on 700 patients, is published.
1758	**Measles** is proven to be contagious.
1770s	**Hypnotherapy**, then known as "animal magnetism," is developed.
1772	**Nitrous oxide** is discovered.
1775	First description of occupational **carcinogen**, coal dust exposure among chimney sweeps.
1784	Tenotomy, cutting of Achilles tendon to treat **club foot**, is performed.
1785	First clinical description of **chicken pox**.
	First description of **digitalis's** effects on the heart.
	First reported case of **artificial insemination** in human.
	Placebo is described.
1788	Damage to pancreas is proposed as cause of **diabetes mellitus**.
1790	Dental chair is invented.
1798	Marine Hospital Fund is established (precursor of **U.S. Public Health Service**).
1794	**Cesarean** section is performed in United States.
1796	First intentional cowpox infection of human to prevent **smallpox**. Technique named vaccination.
1800	First description of **tissues**, then called "membranes."
1803	**Morphine** isolated from **opium**.
1806	**Melanoma** is identified and described.
1809	First **ovariotomy** is performed.
	Schizophrenia is described.
1810	Scientific (**medical**) **journal** devoted entirely to medicine is published.
1816	First surgical repair of **cleft palate**.
	Stethoscope is invented.
1817	Active substance in ipecacuanha (**ipecac**) root, emetine, isolated.
	Parkinson's disease is described.

1819	Iodine is found to cure **goiter**.
c.1820	Achromatic **microscopes** are available.
1820s	First description of **diphtheria**. **Tubal sterilization** is proposed.
1820	**Quinine** and cinchonine are isolated from cinchona bark.
1821	Connecticut passes first U.S. law banning **abortion**.
1826	First description of **osmosis**.
1827	**Bright's disease** (glomerulonephritis) is described.
1830s	Incubators first used for **premature infant care**.
1831	Cell nucleus is discovered.
1832	**Hodgkin's disease** is described.
1833	Term "**atherosclerosis**" is introduced. **Mental hospital**, dedicated to treatment rather than confinement, is established in United States.
1835	First U.S. college of **homeopathy**. **Glaucoma** is linked to increased pressure within eyeball. **Graves' disease** is described.
1836	Iodine is used as antiseptic. **Neurons** are described.
1837	First distinction between **typhoid** disease and **typhus**.
1839	Idea that cells are the essential unit of all living things is introduced as "**cell theory**." Vulcanization is discovered, making rubber **condoms** possible.
1840	First dental college is founded, in Baltimore.
1841	First description of **leukemia**.
1842	Surgery is performed using **ether anesthesia**.
1844	**Nitrous oxide** used as an anesthetic in dental surgery.
1845	Scottish physician uses a **biopsy** to determine nonmalignancy of a woman's breast ulcer.
1846	**Down syndrome** is described. Germany and Vienna issue laws regulating exposure to phosphorous fumes.

1847	**Nitroglycerin** is synthesized.
1848	**Chloroform** is used as an anesthetic. Viennese physician Ignaz Semmelweis orders surgeons in his hospital to use antiseptic techniques.
1851	Cause of **schistosomiasis**, infection of the blood by parasitic flukes, is discovered. Mechanism of **curare's** paralyzing action, at the site where motor nerves connect with muscle, is described.
1852	**Ophthalmoscope** is invented.
1853	**Syringe** for injecting medication into the skin is invented.
1854	Cause of **gout** (kidney abnormality) is described.
1855	British physician Thomas Addison describes a disease resulting from **adrenal gland** insufficiency that is later named "Addison's disease." The condition is characterized by weakness, darkening of the skin, and abnormally high levels of white blood cells. Cell division is first described. John Snow's *On the Mode of Communication of **Cholera*** is published.
1856	First anatomical description of **thyroid gland**.
1857	Bromides, first drugs for treating epileptic seizures, introduced.
1859	Louis Pasteur suggests that fermentation is caused by living organisms, and that human disease is caused by a similar process.
1860s	Louis Pasteur proposes heating food and drink to destroy bacteria, process now known as **pasteurization**. Commercial baby foods are invented.
1860	Causes of **asthma** attacks are described. **Otoscope** is invented.
1861	Location of the center for speech within the brain is described. **U.S. Sanitary Commission** is established.
1862	**Apoptosis**, or planned cell death, is observed during toad metamorphosis. **Cocaine** isolated from coca leaves. Optotype **vision test** is invented.
1863	First clinical use of **physostigmine**.

| 1863 | International Committee of the **Red Cross** is founded. |

1864 Barbituric acid, compound on which **barbiturate** drugs are based, is synthesized.

1865 Mendel publishes his work on inheritance.

1866 First **public health** organization is established in New York.

United States' first urban **ambulance** system is established at New York City's Bellevue Hospital.

1867 **Amyl nitrate** is discovered to be effective treatment for angina.

Joseph Lister reports on treating 11 patients with carbolic acid to prevent "hospitalism," now known to be infection.

Short clinical **thermometer** is introduced.

1868 Electric dentist's drill is introduced.

First employee- and employer-sponsored **health insurance** program is established.

1869 **Chloral hydrate's** properties as a sedative and sleeping draught are discovered.

1870 French physiologist Paul Bert publishes *Barometric Pressure,* a summary of his pioneering studies of the effects of high and low pressure on human physiology.

1871 **Anxiety disorder** is first described, as "irritable heart."

1872 Weight criteria is established for premature birth.

1873 Bacterium that causes **leprosy** isolated.

Comstock Law is passed, making distribution of **contraception** information by mail illegal in the United States.

First full, accurate description of nerve cells (**neurons**).

Iodoform is shown to kill anthrax bacteria.

1875 Union of sperm and egg nuclei during fertilization is observed.

1876 Cortical map, along with neurological symptoms, is used to locate tumor within brain.

Visual pigment **rhodopsin** is discovered.

1877 First nondenominational **visiting nurse association** in United States is established.

1878 Description of the synthesis of **acetaminophen**, the drug that would become Tylenol, is published.

Endotracheal intubation is used during surgery.

First treatment of angina with **nitroglycerin**.

1879 Bacteria that causes **gonorrhea** is discovered.

1880 Crede prophylaxis, preventing gonorrheal infection in newborn babies' eyes with silver nitrate solution drops, is invented.

Parathyroid gland is described.

Plasmodium, parasite that causes **malaria**, is discovered.

1881 First successful **gastrectomy**.

Louis Pasteur demonstrates **anthrax vaccine**.

Robert Koch discovers how to grow bacteria in culture, an advance for testing potential **antibiotics**.

Rubella is recognized as disease.

Shunt proposed as treatment for **hydrocephalus**.

Tay-Sachs disease is described.

1882 Bacillus that causes **tuberculosis** is isolated.

United States signs Geneva Convention.

1883 **Multiple sclerosis** is described and identified.

1884 **Cocaine** is used as a local anesthetic in eye surgery.

Endotracheal intubation is used to save a child with **diphtheria**.

Phagocytosis is observed and described.

"Suggestion therapy," using **hypnotherapy**, is introduced.

1885 First **rabies vaccine**.

1886 First modern surgery to treat **epilepsy**.

1887 **Ephedrine** is isolated from desert shrub.

First **contact lens** is made.

Recording of heart's electrical activity as measured on surface of the body (**ECG**) is published.

1889 Baltimore surgeon suggests that his nurse wear **rubber gloves** during surgery.

Rubber gloves are introduced for surgeons and other medical personnel.

"Seed and soil" theory, in which particular types of **cancer** are proposed to spread to specific types of **tissue**, is put forth by James Paget.

1890s Surgeons develop techniques for performing **biopsies** during surgery.

1890 **Antibodies,** then called antitoxins, are discovered.

Cause of dental caries is discovered.

First radical mastectomy is performed.

1891 **Diphtheria** antitoxin is given to patient; first use of **serum therapy**.

Spinal tap technique is perfected.

1893 Johns Hopkins School of Medicine, first U.S. medical school to require students to have a bachelor's degree and to study for four years, opens in Baltimore.

Ralph Stockman shows that **anemia** can be treated with iron supplements.

1894 American School of **Osteopathy** is founded.

Extracts of **adrenal glands** are reported to raise **blood pressure**.

1895 **X-rays** are discovered.

1896 First use of **radiation therapy** to treat **cancer**.

Radium is discovered.

Sphygmomanometer is invented for measuring **blood pressure**.

1897 **Epinephrine** isolated.

1898 **Acetylcholine,** the first neurotransmitter to be discovered, is isolated from **ergot**, a fungus that grows on spoiled wheat.

Battery-powered **hearing aid** becomes available in United States.

Experiments demonstrate existence of infectious organism smaller than bacteria, later identified as a **virus**.

First **cancer center** founded in the United States in Buffalo, New York.

First school of **chiropractic** medicine is established.

First **vasectomy**.

Heroin is released as a cough suppressant.

Kidney extracts are shown to raise **blood pressure**.

1899 **Aspirin** is introduced.

1900 **Blood types** are discovered.

First school of **orthodontia** is founded.

International Association for Labor Legislation is established to improve **industrial hygiene**.

1901 First recording of heart's electric activity with an **electrocardiograph**.

Freud's *The Interpretation of Dreams* is published.

Patent filed for first electric **hearing aid**.

1902 **Anaphylaxis** is observed and described.

Inflatable rubber suit is introduced to treat **shock**.

Radiation is used to treat **Hodgkin's disease**.

1903 Number of **chromosomes** observed to be halved in sperm and egg cells.

Several nations sign International Sanitary Agreement to prevent the spread of **yellow fever**, **cholera**, and **bubonic plague**.

1904 Edinburgh doctor reports that alcohol, lead, and **morphine** given to a pregnant woman can harm developing fetus.

First insertion of radium in tumor to treat **cancer**.

First removal of prostate gland to treat **prostate cancer**.

1905 First **corneal transplant** is performed.

Tonometer is introduced.

Word "**hormone**," from the Greek "to urge on" or "set in motion," is coined.

1906 **Alzheimer's disease** is described.

Bacterium that causes **pertussis** is isolated.

Mass production of synthetic **epinephrine** begins.

Pure Food and Drug Act, first federal legislation on food and drug safety, is passed.

Word "**allergy**" is coined.

1907 First **tissue** culture.

1908 Harvey Cushing publishes comprehensive book on neurosurgery.

Idea of **inborn errors of metabolism** is described.

Russian scientists show that feeding animals cholesterol-rich food causes them to develop **atherosclerosis**.

1909 **Chagas' disease** is discovered.

1909	Role of **capillaries** in gas exchange is discovered.
	Word "**gene**" is coined to describe units of inheritance
1910	First **gene** mapped to a **chromosome**.
	First National Conference on Industrial Diseases in United States.
	First sex-linked genetic mutation is observed, in fruit flies.
	Flexner report is published.
	Salvarsan, first drug effective against syphilis, is introduced.
	United States bans importation of smoked **opium**.
1911	**Bone grafts** used to treat spinal deterioration caused by **tuberculosis**.
	Chemical composition of **cerebrospinal fluid** is described.
	First clinic for **prenatal care** opens in the United States.
	First lasting **workers compensation** act is passed, in Illinois.
	Histamine is isolated.
	Measles proven to be caused by a **virus**.
1912	Phenobarbital is used to control epileptic seizures.
	U.S. Children's Bureau is founded.
	Word "**vitamines**" is coined to describe nutrients, deficiencies of which cause disease.
1913	Congress passes Harrison Act to regulate **cocaine** distribution.
	First description of **mammography**.
	First genetic linkage map is published, of fruit fly **chromosome**.
	James B. Watson's manifesto on **behaviorism** published.
	Vitamin A is discovered.
	Vitamin B2, riboflavin, is discovered.
1914	Congress passes Harrison Act, which taxes production of **cocaine** and **opium**.
	First detailed description of **cerebrospinal fluid** circulation.
	First use of spinal fusion to treat **scoliosis**.
	Researchers discover adding citrate to blood keeps it liquid so it can be stored.
	U.S. Public Health Service forms Division of Occupational Health.

1915	First known air medical transport takes place as the Serbian army retreats from Albania.
	"**Twilight sleep**," anesthetic for women in labor, is introduced.
1916	**Heparin** is discovered.
1917	Mathematical process for converting multiple two-dimensional **X-ray** images into a single three-dimensional image is invented.
1918	**Ergotamine** is isolated.
	First **arthroscopic** investigations are performed.
	U.S. Public Health Service creates Venereal Disease Division
1919	**Rickets** attributed to dietary deficiency, shown to be preventable and curable with cod liver oil.
1920s	Dick test is developed to check for **scarlet fever** immunity.
	First **intrauterine devices (IUD)** are invented.
	Magnesium sulfate first used to treat **eclampsia**.
	Rabies vaccine for pets is invented.
1921	First professional organization for plastic surgeons is founded.
	Human receives **BCG vaccine** for the first time.
	Prausnitz-Kustner reaction is described.
1922	Cures of **cancer** with radiotherapy are reported.
	Insulin is isolated.
	Vitamin D is discovered.
	World's first organized blood donation system established in London.
	X-ray cannons make it possible to use this energy in **radiation therapy** for **cancer**.
1923	First successful repair of heart valves.
1924	First **dialysis** of human patient.
	Iodized salt is introduced to prevent **goiter**.
	Last outbreak of **bubonic plague** in United States begins. Last reported U.S. case of human-to-human plague transmission occurs.

Recording of electrical activity in the human brain with an **electroencephalograph**.

Varicella zoster virus isolated.

1925   **Colposcope** is invented.

Sympathectomy is performed to treat **hypertension**.

1926   Electrocoagulation is introduced to stop bleeding in brain surgery.

Ephedrine is approved for clinical use in United States.

First successful treatment for **pernicious anemia** is described.

1927   Patent is issued for shoe store **fluoroscope**.

Pregnancy test is invented.

1928   **Penicillin** is discovered.

Pituitary gland hormones oxytocin and vasopressin are isolated.

Sunscreen is introduced commercially.

1929   **Estrogen** is isolated.

First **cardiac catheterization** is performed.

First **HMO** is established.

1930s   Pain mechanism involved in **migraine** headache is described.

1930   First breast **prosthesis** is produced.

Public Health Service's Hygiene Laboratory is renamed the **National Institutes of Health**.

1931   **Androgen hormone** is isolated.

Electron microscope is built.

First **angiogram** is made.

First planned surgery to repair **aneurysm**.

First report of use of **epidural anesthesia**.

Sedative, **blood pressure**-lowering effects of rauwolfia are described.

1932   Cushing publishes system for classifying **brain tumors**.

First **amphetamine** drug, Benzedrine, is introduced to U.S. market.

First semi-flexible **gastroscope** is produced.

1933   First flu virus (**influenza**) is isolated.

First removal of entire lung to treat **lung cancer**.

Heparin is purified.

Streptokinase, first **thrombolytic** drug, is discovered.

Thyroid-stimulating **hormone** is isolated.

1934   **Anticholinesterase** drugs are introduced.

Commercial manufacture of **vitamin C** begins.

Convulsive therapy is used to treat **mental illness**.

Cortisone is isolated from the **adrenal gland** cortex.

Mumps are shown to be caused by **virus**.

Phenylketonuria, most common **inborn error of metabolism**, is discovered.

Progesterone is isolated.

Vitamin K is described.

1935   **Alcoholics Anonymous** is founded.

Congress passes **Social Security** Act.

First **lobotomy** is performed.

Prontosil, first effective drug for **puerperal fever**, is introduced.

Prostaglandin is isolated.

1936   **Cystic fibrosis** is described.

Dilantin, a drug for controlling epileptic seizures, is discovered.

1937   **Drinker respirator**, or iron lung, is built.

First reversal of malignant **hypertension**.

First U.S. **blood bank** is established in Chicago.

First use of **ultrasound** to image the interior of the body.

Marihuana Tax Act is passed banning nonmedical use of drug.

National **Cancer** Act, establishing National Cancer Institute, is founded.

Pellagra preventive factor, niacin, is isolated.

Vitamin A is isolated.

1938   Aminophylline is introduced for treating acute **asthma** attacks.

Biotin (**vitamin B6**) is discovered.

Electroconvulsive therapy, or "shock treatment," is used on a human patient.

First **hip replacement**.

Timeline

1938   Food, Drug and Cosmetic Act is passed.
LSD is synthesized.

1939   Gamma globulin is discovered.

Early 1940s   Dapsone, first effective treatment for **leprosy**, is introduced.

Late 1940s   **Stereotactic surgery** is introduced.

1940   **Actinomycin**, an **anti-tumor antibiotic**, is discovered.

Contrast agent Pantopaque is used for **myelography**.

One of four viruses that cause **dengue** fever is discovered.

1941   Classification of "open-angle" and "angle-closure" introduced to describe different types of **glaucoma**.

Osteoporosis is described.

Rubella infection in pregnant women is shown to cause **birth defects**.

1942   **Antihistamines** are introduced.

Curare is first used as a muscle relaxant during surgery.

Marketing of anti-clotting drug **warfarin** begins.

1943   First use of **LSD**.

Streptomycin is discovered.

1944   **Blalock-Taussig procedure** to treat heart defect in children is performed for the first time.

Human growth hormone is isolated.

Penicillin is introduced as **syphilis** treatment.

1945   American Cancer Society endorses **Pap smear** for **cervical cancer** prevention.

B vitamin folic acid is synthesized.

Cephalosporin is isolated.

Commercial sales of **penicillin** begin.

First water **fluoridation** program is launched in Michigan.

Helicopter is used as an **air ambulance** to evacuate an injured pilot from the Burmese jungle.

Immune tolerance is observed.

Simple test of urine's sugar content is introduced to help people with **diabetes** control blood sugar levels.

Scientists synthesize **cortisone** and develop a technique for manufacturing commercial quantities of the artificial **hormone**.

1946   **Clinical trials** of **streptomycin** for **tuberculosis** begin.

Communicable Disease Center, which developed into the **Centers for Disease Control and Prevention**, is founded.

Norepinephrine is isolated.

Tretinoin is synthesized.

United Nations' Children's Fund (UNICEF) is established.

1947   **Antabuse** is discovered.

First successful open-chest **defibrillation**.

First U.S. center established for **burn treatment**.

Isolette incubator is introduced.

Nuremburg Code is promulgated.

1948   Aminopterin, an **antimetabolite cancer drug**, is found to produce remission in children with **leukemia**.

Chloramphenicol, first effective drug for **typhoid fever**, is introduced.

Diphtheria-pertussis-tetanus (DPT) **vaccine** is introduced.

Serotonin is isolated and identified.

Vitamin B12 (cyanocobalamin) is isolated.

World Health Organization is founded.

1949   Abnormal hemoglobin molecule is discovered as cause of **sickle cell anemia**.

Barr body is discovered.

Cortisone is used to treat patients.

Effectiveness of **lithium** in treating manic-depression is discovered.

Framingham Heart Study is launched.

Plastic lens is introduced to replace lens removed for **cataract surgery**.

U.S. automobile maker Nash introduces **seat belts**.

1950s   First **intensive care units** are established.

First **telemedicine** programs are established.

1950   Beta-2 agonists (for treating **asthma**) are introduced.

Chinese government announces it wants to reconcile traditional **Chinese medicine** and Western medicine into a single system.

First use of **ultrasound** to image the heart.

Hyperbaric oxygenation is shown to have therapeutic effects.

Studies conclude there is strong evidence that smoking cigarettes causes **lung cancer**.

1951 First **growth factor**, nerve growth factor, is discovered.

Phenylbutazone and probenecid, drugs for **gout**, are introduced.

X-ray machine used specifically for **mammography** is introduced.

1952 First edition of the **Diagnostic and Statistical Manual of Mental Disorders (DSM)** is published.

First state, Oregon, passes air pollution control regulation.

Marketing of chlorpromazine, first **antipsychotic drug**, begins.

1953 **Apgar score** is published.

First all-transistor **hearing aid** becomes available.

First human impregnation using frozen sperm.

First poison information center is opened.

Halothane, today's most widely used **anesthetic**, is synthesized.

Heart-lung machine is used successfully during surgery.

Linear accelerators are introduced for **radiation therapy**.

Operating **microscopes** become available commercially.

Public Health Service establishes national case-reporting for **tuberculosis**.

Rapid eye movement (REM) during sleep is described.

Reserpine is introduced.

Shoe store **fluoroscopes** are banned because of radiation exposure.

Structure of **DNA** is discovered.

1954 Clinical use of **anti-tumor antibiotic Actinomycin** D begins.

Fiberoptic **endoscope** is built.

Field trials of **polio vaccine** begin.

First **carotid endarterectomy** is performed.

First **kidney transplant**.

1955 **Acetaminophen** (Tylenol) becomes available without prescription in the United States.

Cancer Chemotherapy National Service Center is established.

Chlorothiazide, first nonmercurial **diuretic** drug, is synthesized.

Congress passes first federal law addressing air pollution, the Air Pollution Control Act.

First **bone marrow transplants** are performed in humans.

1956 Experimental **autoimmune disease** is induced in an animal.

First **cancer** cure with **chemotherapy**, of gestational choriocarcinoma.

First report of closed-chest, or external, **defibrillation**.

1957 American Medical Association recognizes **alcoholism** as a disease.

Existence of "slow **virus**" (later identified as **prion**) is proposed as cause of kuru.

Fiberoptic **gastroscope** is produced.

First **antidepressant** drug, iproniazid, is discovered.

First **cochlear implant** is performed.

Interferon is discovered.

Vinblastine, a **vinca alkaloid cancer** drug, is isolated and identified.

1958 **Antipsychotic drug** haloperidol is synthesized.

CPR is discovered.

Development of cine-**angiography** begins.

First clinical use of **human growth hormone**.

First internal pacemaker is implanted.

Melatonin is isolated and identified.

1959 **Brain death** is described.

Trisomy 21, genetic defect that causes **Down syndrome**, is discovered.

1960s First **beta-blocker**, propanolol, is developed.

Surgical telescopes are invented.

T cells are discovered.

1960 **FDA** approves a drug containing artificial **progesterone** and **estrogen**, popularly known as "the Pill," as a **contraceptive**.

Method for preventing erythroblastosis fetalis, fatal disease caused by **Rh-factor** incompatibility, is introduced.

1960   **Opiate antagonist** naloxone is synthesized.

      Philadelphia **chromosome** is discovered.

1961   Denis Burkitt reports discovery of lymphoma caused by Epstein-Barr **virus** infection, later called **Burkitt's lymphoma**.

      Sets of three **DNA** bases, or "codons," shown to be basic unit of **genetic code**.

1962   Clomid found to stimulate ovulation.

      First **cingulotomy** is performed to treat chronic pain.

      First edition of *Mendelian Inheritance in Man* is published.

      First **kidney transplant** from nonrelated donor is performed.

      First partial meniscectomy (removal of cartilage within knee) is performed using **arthroscopy**.

      Rabies virus is observed.

      Rubella virus is isolated.

      Severed arm is "replanted" surgically.

1963   **Anti-tumor antibiotic** daunomycin's first clinical use in United States, to treat **leukemia**.

      Community Mental Health Centers act is passed.

      First **Clean Air Act** is passed.

      First **liver transplant**.

      Flexible sigmoidoscope is introduced.

      Indomethacin and allopurinol, drugs for treating **gout**, are is introduced.

      Measles vaccine is licensed for general use in United States.

      THC, active ingredient in **marijuana**, is identified.

      Valium is introduced to U.S. market.

1964   First **calcium channel blocker** is discovered.

      First **methadone** maintenance program for **heroin** addicts is established.

      U.S. Public Health Service launches its first antismoking campaign.

1965   Australia **antigen**, used to test blood for **hepatitis** B, is discovered.

      Congress passes Drug Abuse Control Act.

      Congress passes legislation creating **Medicaid** and **Medicare**.

      Cryoprecipitate, concentrated clotting factor used to treat **hemophilia**, is invented.

      First successful open **fetal surgery**.

      Positron emission tomography (PET scan) is used in humans.

1966   Congress passes National Traffic and Motor Vehicles Safety Act, establishing federal regulation of automobile design and manufacture.

      FDA requires drug manufacturers to test products for teratogenic effects.

      First member of **anti-tumor antibiotic** family the bleomycins is discovered.

1967   First reported **bypass surgery** is performed.

      First successful **liver transplant.**

      Genetic code (61 codons for 20 amino acids) is cracked.

      Mumps vaccine is licensed.

1968   Alabama senator makes first U.S. **911** call.

      Criteria for judging **brain death** is established.

      First **cardiac ablation** is performed to treat heart arrhythmia.

      First successful **heart transplant**.

      Gamma knife is used in patients.

Early 1970s   First reported cases of **Lyme disease**.

      Widespread **rubella** vaccination of children begins.

1970s   **DNA fingerprinting** is developed.

      Oral rehydration therapy is introduced worldwide.

      Self-tests for blood **glucose** are introduced.

1970   **Chromosome banding** is invented.

      Environmental Protection Agency founded.

      FDA approves **lithium** for treating manic depressive illness.

      First surgical laser is built.

      Laser surgery for **glaucoma** is introduced.

      Name of Communicable Disease Center changed to **Center for Disease Control (CDC)**. ("Centers" was pluralized in 1980.)

      Ultrasound technology becomes commercially available.

1971   Australia passes first law requiring **seat belt** use.

Clinical trials of etoposide, **cancer** drug derived from **podophyllotoxin**, begin.

First **CAT scan** of a human patient, used to locate a tumor within the brain.

Herb used in ancient **Chinese medicine** to treat **malaria**, quinghaosu, is proven to be effective.

Measles-mumps-rubella (MMR) **vaccine** is licensed.

Nonsteroidal anti-inflammatory drugs (NSAIDs) are shown to work by inhibiting **prostaglandin** synthesis.

Test for identifying **Tay-Sachs disease** carriers are introduced.

Tumor necrosis factor is discovered.

1972   American Hospital Association releases *A Patient's Bill of Rights,* document addressing **informed consent**.

First hospital-based **air ambulance** program is founded in Denver, Colorado.

Clean Water Act is passed.

1973   Congress passes **Health Maintenance Organization** act.

Endorphin binding sites in the brain are discovered.

Fetal alcohol syndrome is described.

First **DNA** recombination.

First freestanding **hospice** in United States is founded.

Supreme Court passes *Roe vs. Wade*, a law legalizing first-term **abortion** and leaving the regulation of second- and third-term abortions in state hands.

Tamoxifen is introduced as **breast cancer** treatment.

U.S. Congress passes Emergency Medical Services Systems Act, which funds **ambulance** services in most of nation's cities.

1974   Congress passes Safe Drinking Water Act.

Federal government launches Special Supplemental Nutrition Program for Women, Infants and Children (**WIC**)

Heimlich maneuver is used to save choking person.

Ibuprofen is introduced in United States.

Relaxation response is described.

World Health Organization (WHO) establishes Expanded Programme on Immunization.

1975   First case of **E. coli 0157:H7** is reported.

First hybridoma, cell that produces **monoclonal antibodies**, is created.

Scientists at the U.S. drug company Bristol-Myers Squibb synthesize the first effective angiotensin converting-enzyme **(ACE) inhibitor**, captopril.

1976   Existence of **oncogenes** is reported.

First mass flu vaccine **(influenza)** program is launched.

Operating **arthroscope** is introduced.

1977   Anti-ulcer drug Tagamet (**cimetidine**) goes on market.

First **angioplasty** is performed.

First peripheral **stem cell** transplantation.

1978   First **rapid opiate detoxification** is performed.

First "test-tube baby," conceived by **in vitro fertilization**, is born.

Hepatitis A is grown in culture.

Refractive surgery is performed in United States.

World Health Organization (WHO) sponsors the **Alma Ata International Conference on Primary Health Care.**

1979   **Bulimia nervosa** is described.

First computer-assisted **stereotactic surgery**.

Gamete intrafallopian transfer (GIFT) is performed for the first time.

National Alliance for the Mentally Ill is founded.

Retrovirus infecting humans is discovered.

1980s   "Riflip" technology for quickly sequencing **genes** is introduced.

1980   American Medical Association changes its code to allow members to refer their patients to **chiropractors**.

Automatic implantable cardiac **defibrillator** is implanted in a human.

Congress passes Superfund act, formally known as the Comprehensive Environmental Response, Compensation, and Liability Act.

Cyclosporine is introduced.

1980	Image of brain is produced with **magnetic resonance imaging (MRI).**
	Last case of **smallpox** is reported.
1980–81	First human **oncogene** is isolated.
1981	**Botulism toxin** is used to treat strabismus.
	First custom-designed **anti-idiotype antibodies** are used to treat a patient with lymphoma.
	First description of **AIDS** is published in *Mortality and Morbidity Weekly Report.*
	First **heart-lung transplant.**
	First laparoscopic **appendectomy** performed.
1982	First **artificial heart** is implanted in human patient.
	RU-486, an artificial progestin antagonist that induces **abortion**, is synthesized.
1983	Burn patients receive grafts of **artificial skin**, grown from cultured cells.
	Medicare begins paying for **hospice** care.
	Retinoblastoma gene, a mutated form of a **tumor-suppressor gene**, is identified.
1984	First **needle exchange program** is introduced in Amsterdam.
	First successful pregnancies using donated eggs.
	Role of **H. pylori** in causing ulcers is confirmed.
1985	**Azidothymidine (AZT)** first used in **AIDS** patients.
	First nonsedating **antihistamine**, Seldane (terfenadine), is introduced.
	Production of recombinant **erythropoietin** begins.
	Researchers genetically sequence human immunodeficiency **virus**, the organism that causes **AIDS.**
1986	American Medical Association recognizes drug **addiction** as a disease.
	First **stent** is implanted.
	First use of **transmyocardial revascularization.**
1987	**Centers for Disease Control** and Prevention recommend universal precautions for preventing the spread of infection.
	Electricity first used in **cardiac ablation.**

	FDA approves lovastatin, a **cholesterol-lowering drug**, for sale in the United States.
	Ivermectin, an **antiparasitic** drug for treating river blindness, is introduced.
	Prozac is introduced.
1988	Congress bans use of federal funds for **needle exchange programs.**
	Congress passes Hunger Prevention Act, guaranteeing **WIC** benefits for homeless women and children.
	Human Genome Project is launched.
	Polymerase chain reaction (PCR) is introduced.
1989	**CDC** becomes Centers for Disease Control and Prevention.
	Cystic fibrosis gene is identified.
	FDA approves gancyclovir, **antiviral drug** for treating cytomegalovirus.
	First successful **liver transplant** using portion of living donor's organ.
	Hepatitis C **antibody** test is developed.
	Spiral **CAT scanning** is introduced.
1990s	Drugs introduced for treating **osteoporosis.**
Early 1990s	First **public health** recommendations urging women to have regular mammograms.
	Functional **MRI** is developed.
	Test for detecting telomerase, the enzyme that maintains **telomere** length, is developed.
	Whole-body **PET scanning** is introduced.
1990	**BRCA1**, the **breast cancer** gene, is located on **chromosome** 17.
	Clozapine, an **antipsychotic drug**, is introduced in the United States.
	Congress passes Nutrition Labeling and Education Act, requiring all food products to carry detailed labels describing nutritional content.
	FDA approves Norplant.
	First use of **gene therapy.**
	Methotrexate is introduced for **immunosuppression.**
	Pre-implantation genetic diagnosis first performed.

Food and Drug Administration approves methylprednisolone for **spinal cord injury treatment.**

1991 FDA approves foscarnet, an **antiviral** drug for treating cytomegalovirus infection.

"Healthy People" 2000 is released.

World Health Organization (WHO) publishes *Guidelines for the Assessment of Herbal Medicines.*

1992 FDA approves Depo-Provera.

First report on sentinel node **biopsy** for **breast cancer**.

National Institutes of Health (NIH) forms Office of **Alternative Medicine.**

1993 The **Food and Drug Administration (FDA)** approves nonsedating **antihistamine** Claritin for sale in the United States.

1994 **BRCA2**, second **breast cancer** gene, located and identified.

Congress passes Dietary Supplement Health and Education Act, barring the **FDA** from regulating **herbal medicines**.

First permanent international **telemedicine** link is established.

Standardized methods for **prostate-specific antigen** testing are issued.

1995 **Hepatitis** A **vaccine** is introduced.

Protease inhibitors are introduced.

World Health Organization (WHO) confirms the link between human papillomavirus and **cervical cancer**.

1996 Enzyme cyclooxygenase-2 (**COX-2**) is discovered.

FDA approves latanoprost, drug for **glaucoma**.

1997 **Air bags** become mandatory for all cars made in the United States.

First report on angina patients treated with **vascular endothelial growth factor** gene.

1998 FDA approves celecoxib, the first **COX-2 inhibitor** sold in the United States.

FDA approves **Herceptin**, first monoclonal **antibody** for treating **breast cancer**.

FDA approves Viagra.

Fetal surgery performed at 23 weeks gestation to repair spina bifida.

"Healthy People 2010" is released.

Human embryonic **stem cells** are cultured.

Lyme Disease vaccine is approved by **FDA**.

NIH's Office of **Alternative Medicine** becomes the National Center for Complementary and Alternative Medicine.

Tamoxifen is shown to prevent **breast cancer**.

1999 Washington University in St. Louis researchers show that treating rats' injured spinal cords with immature nerve cells grown from **stem cells** helps restore some function. The research suggests this technique could one day be used in human **spinal cord injury treatment.**

Fetal cell implants found to help some patients with **Parkinson's disease.**

National Cancer Institute announces that a **cancer vaccine** for lymphoma will enter large-scale clinical trials.

2000 National Cancer Institute reports that testing for human papilloma virus can help screen patients for **cervical cancer.**

Clinical trials launched by the **National Institutes of Health** to determine whether **COX-2 inhibitors** can help slow mental deterioration in **Alzheimer's disease.**

First clinical trial of use of **robotic surgery** to perform heart bypass operation finds the technique is safe and feasible for some patients.

U.S. **Environmental Protection Agency** signs agreement with 26 other nations to bring down emissions of several chemicals in order to reduce smog, acid rain, and other types of environmental damage. The agreement created the first multinational, comprehensive structure dedicated to controlling air pollution.

Bibliography

"Abdominal Aortic Aneurysms Run in the Family." *Harvard Heart Letter* (August 1999).

Abel, Ernest L. *Marihuana: The First Twelve Thousand Years.* New York: Plenum Press, 1980.

Abt, Arthur F. *Abt-Garrison History of Pediatrics.* Philadelphia: W.B. Saunders Company, 1965.

Acierno, Louis J. *The History of Cardiology.* London: The Parthenon Publishing Group, 1994.

Ackerknecht, Erwin H. *A Short History of Psychiatry.* New York: Hafner Publishing, 1959.

Aggarwal, Bharat B. and Raj K. Puri. *Human Cytokines: Their Role in Disease and Therapy.* Cambridge, MA: Blackwell Science, 1995.

Aird, Robert B. *Foundations of Modern Neurology: A Century of Progress.* New York: Raven Press, 1994.

Albee, Fred Houdlett. *Bone Graft Surgery in Disease, Injury and Deformity.* New York; London: D. Appleton-Century Co., Inc., 1949.

Albert, Daniel and Diane Edwards, eds. *The History of Ophthalmology.* Cambridge, MA: Blackwell Science, 1996.

Alberts, Nuna. "When Sex Gets Sidelined." *Good Housekeeping* (June 1998): 72

Aldridge, Susan. *The Thread of Life: The Story of Genes and Genetic Engineering.* Cambridge: Cambridge University Press, 1996.

Alexander, Eben, Jay S. Loeffler, and Dade L. Lunsford, eds. *Stereotactic Radiosurgery.* New York: McGraw-Hill, Health Professions Division, 1993.

Alexander, Howard. "Hearing Aids: Smaller and Smaller." *The New York Times* (November 26, 1998): G6.

Alpert, Philip R. "The Thyroid Gland." *Healthline* (July 1995).

Altman, Lawrence K. *Who Goes First?: The Story of Self Experimentation in Medicine.* New York: Random House, 1987.

————. "With AIDS Advance, More Disappointment." *The New York Times* (January 19, 1997):1.

Anders, George. *Health and Wealth: HMOs and the Breakdown of Medical Trust.* Boston: Houghton Mifflin, 1996.

Anderson, Linda. *What You Can Do about Adrenal Insufficiency.* Bethesda, MD: National Institutes of Health, 1988.

Andreason, Nancy C. *The Broken Brain: The Biological Revolution in Psychiatry.* New York: Harper & Row, 1984.

————., ed. *Schizophrenia: From Mind to Molecule.* Washington, DC: American Psychiatric Association, 1994.

Andrews, Anthony T. *Electrophoresis: Theory, Techniques, and Biochemical and Clinical Applications.* Oxford [Oxfordshire]: Clarendon Press; New York: Oxford University Press, 1986.

Andrews, Richard N.L. *Managing the Environment, Managing Ourselves: A History of American Environmental Policy.* New Haven, CT: Yale University Press, 1999.

Angier, Natalie. *Woman: An Intimate Geography.* Boston: Houghton Mifflin Company, 1999.

Annas, George J. and Michael A. Groden. *The Nazi Doctors and the Nuremberg Code: Human Rights in Human Experimentation.* New York: Oxford University Press, 1992.

Apple, Rima D. *Vitamania: Vitamins in American Culture.* New Brunswick, NJ: Rutgers University Press, 1996.

Appleton, William S. *Prozac and the New Antidepressants: What You Need to Know about Prozac, Zoloft, Paxil, Wellbutrin, Effexor, Serzone, Luvox and More.* New York: Plume/Penguin, 1997.

Arno, Peter S. and Karyn L. Feiden. *Against the Odds: The Story of AIDS Drug Development, Politics and Profits.* New York: HarperCollins Publishers, 1992.

Austin, Gregory A. *Perspectives on the History of Psychoactive Substance Use.* Rockville, MD: National Institute on Drug Abuse, 1979.

Barazansky, Barbara and Norman Gevitz, eds. *Beyond Flexner: Medical Education in the Twentieth Century.* Westport, CT: Greenwood Press, 1992.

Baurac, Deborah. "Joint Exchange: Recent Implants Just Keep Going and Going." *Modern Maturity* (September/October 1997): 68.

Bazell, Robert T. *HER-2: The Making of Herceptin, A Revolutionary Treatment for Breast Cancer.* New York: Random House, 1998.

Begley, Sharon. "Blood, Hair and Heredity." *Newsweek* (July 11, 1994): 24.

Beigbeder, Yves. *The World Health Organization.* The Hague, The Netherlands: M. Nijhoff, 1998.

Bellamy, David and Andrea Pfister. *World Medicine: Plants, Patients and People.* Oxford: Blackwell Publishers, 1992.

Bellamy, Paul B. *A History of Workmen's Compensation, 1898–1915: From Courtroom to Boardroom.* New York: Garland Publishing, 1997.

Benson, Herbert. *The Relaxation Response.* New York: Morrow, 1975.

Berkowitz, Edward D. *Mr. Social Security: The Life of Wilbur J. Cohen.* Lawrence: The University Press of Kansas, 1995.

Bindra, Jasit S. and Daniel Lednicer, eds. *Chronicles of Drug Discovery,* vol. 1. New York: John Wiley & Sons, 1982.

———. *Chronicles of Drug Discovery,* vol. 2. New York: John Wiley & Sons, 1983.

Bing, Elisabeth D. *The Adventure of Birth: Experiences in the Lamaze Method of Prepared Childbirth.* New York: Simon & Schuster, 1970.

Birk, Lee. *Biofeedback: Behavioral Medicine.* New York: Gruen & Stratton, 1973.

Black, Maggie. *Children First: The Story of UNICEF, Past and Present.* New York: Oxford University Press, 1996.

Bliss, Michael. *The Discovery of Insulin.* Chicago: University of Chicago Press, 1984.

Bodmer, Walter and Robin McKie. *The Book of Man: The Human Genome Project and the Quest to Discover Our Genetic Heritage.* New York: Scribner, 1995.

Bonner, Thomas Neville. *Becoming a Physician: Medical Education in Britain, France, Germany, and the United States, 1750–1945.* New York: Oxford University Press, 1995.

Booth, Martin. *Opium: A History.* New York: Simon & Schuster, 1996.

Boraker, D.K. "The Syringe." *Medical Heritage* vol. 2 (September-October 1986): 341–48.

Bottcher, Hellmuth Maximilian. *Miracle Drugs: A History of Antibiotics.* London: Heinemann, 1963.

Brandt, J.D. and M. Packer. "Ophthalmology's Botanical Heritage." *Survey of Ophthalmology* vol. 36 (March-April 1992): 357–65.

Breimer, Douwe D. *Pharmakokinetics of Hypnotic Drugs: Studies on the Pharmakokinetics and Biopharmaceutics of Barbituates and Chloral Hydrate In Man.* Nijmegen, The Netherlands: Drukkerij-Uitgeverij Brakkenstein, 1974.

Brody, Jane E. "Calcium Takes Its Place as a Superstar of Nutrients." *The New York Times* (October 13, 1998): D1.

———. "Device Transforms Brain Surgery." *The New York Times* (July 5, 1995): C9.

———. "A Study Guide to Scientific Studies." *The New York Times* (August 11, 1998): F7.

Bromberg, Walter. *Man above Humanity: A History of Psychotherapy.* Philadelphia: Lippincott, 1954.

Brown, Malcolm W. "Chemical Found to Absorb Radar." *The New York Times* (August 18, 1987): C1.

Brumberg, Joan Jacobs. *Fasting Girls: The History of Anorexia Nervosa.* New York: Plume, 1989.

Bryner, Gary C. *Blue Skies, Green Politics: The Clean Air Act of 1990.* Washington, DC: CQ Press, 1995.

Brzezinski, Amnon. "Melatonin in Humans." *New England Journal of Medicine* vol. 336 (January 16, 1997): 186.

Burkett, Elinor. *The Gravest Show on Earth: America in the Age of AIDS.* Boston; New York: Houghton Mifflin Company, 1995.

Burros, Marian. "U.S. Food Regulation: Takes from a Twilight Zone." *The New York Times,* (June 10, 1987): C1.

Bynum, William F. *Science and the Practice of Medicine in the Nineteenth Century.* New York: Cambridge University Press, 1994.

Bynum, William F., ed. *Medical Journals and Medical Knowledge: Historical Essays.* New York: Routledge, 1992.

Bynum, William F., Christopher Lawrence, and Vivian Nutton. *The Emergence of Modern Cardiology.* London: Wellcome Institute for the History of Medicine, 1985.

Callahan, John A., Thomas Edward Keys, Jack D. Key, and Frederick A. Willus. *Classics of Cardiology, Volume III.* Malabar, FL: Krieger, 1983.

Campion, Margaret Reid. *Hydrotherapy: Principles and Practice.* Boston: Butterworth-Heinemann, 1997.

"Can the Private Sector Help to Put Health Care Right?" *The Economist* (U.S.) (October 24, 1998).

Caplan, Arthur L. and Daniel H. Coelho, eds. *The Ethics of Organ Transplants.* Amherst, NY: Prometheus Books, 1998.

Carpenter, Mary. "Learning to Hear Takes More Than Hardware." *The Washington Post* (September 2, 1997): WH9.

Casper, Monica J. *The Making of the Unborn Patient: A Social Anatomy of Fetal Surgery.* New Brunswick, NJ: Rutgers University Press, 1998.

Cassileth, Barrie R. *The Alternative Medicine Handbook: The Complete Reference Guide to Alternative and Complementary Therapies.* New York: W.W. Norton & Company, 1999.

Caton, Donald. *What a Blessing She Had Chloroform: The Medical and Social Response to the Pain of Childbirth.* New Haven, CT: Yale University Press, 1997.

Cautela, Joseph R. and Waris Ishaq. *Contemporary Issues in Behavior Therapy: Improving the Human Condition.* New York: Plenum Press, 1996.

"Cholesterol Drugs." *Consumer Reports* vol. 63, no. 10 (October 1998): 54.

Christopherson, W.M. "Cytologic Detection and Diagnosis of Cancer: Its Contributions and Limitations." *Cancer* vol. 51 (April 1983): 1201–08.

Cimons, Marlene. "Should She Take Tamoxifen?" *Los Angeles Times* (February 6, 1999): A1.

Clark, William R. *At War Within: The Double-Edged Sword of Immunity.* New York: Oxford University Press, 1995.

———. *A Means to an End: The Biological Basis of Life and Death.* New York: Oxford University Press, 1999.

Clarke, Joe T.R. *A Clinical Guide to Inherited Metabolic Disease.* Cambridge; New York: Cambridge University Press, 1996.

Colburn, Don. "Propping Arteries Open Lets Blood flow; Implanted 'Stents' Have Become a Surgical Commonplace, But One Doctor Calls Them Overused." *The Washington Post* (December 15, 1998): WH7.

Combs, Gerald F. *The Vitamins: Fundamental Aspects in Nutrition and Health.* San Diego, CA: Academic Press, 1992.

Comroe, Julius H. Jr. *Exploring the Heart: Discoveries in Heart Disease and High Blood Pressure.* New York: W.W. Norton & Company, 1983.

Cone, Thomas E. *History of the Care and Feeding of the Premature Infant.* Boston: Little, Brown and Company, 1985.

Cook, Allan R., ed. *Allergies Sourcebook.* Detroit, MI: Omnigraphics, 1997.

Corsini, Raymond J., ed. *Encyclopedia of Psychology,* 2d ed. New York: John Wiley & Sons, 1994.

Cotton, Peter B. and Christopher B. Williams. *Practical Gastrointestinal Endoscopy.* Oxford; Cambridge, MA: Blackwell Science, 1996.

Courtwright, David T. *Dark Paradise: Opiate Addiction in America Before 1940.* Cambridge, MA: Harvard University Press, 1992.

Cowley, Geoffrey. "A Little Help from Serotonin." *Newsweek* (December 29, 1997/January 5, 1998): 78.

Crooke, Stanley T. and Archie W. Prestayko, eds. *Cancer and Chemotherapy Volume III: Antineoplastic Agents.* New York: Academic Press, 1981.

Bibliography

Curzon, G. "How Reserpine and Chlorpromazine Act: The Impact of Key Discoveries on the History of Psychopharmacology." *Trends in Pharmacological Science* vol. 11 (February 1990): 61–63.

Dahlburg, John-Thor. "Simple Oral Therapy Helps Third World in Fight Against Diarrhea." *Los Angeles Times* (December 4, 1995): A11.

Daniel, Thomas M. *Captain Death: The Story of Tuberculosis.* Rochester, NY: University of Rochester Press, 1997.

Daniels, Ken and Erica Haimes. *Donor Insemination: International Social Science Perspectives.* New York: Cambridge University Press, 1998.

Dao, James. "Paramedics Can Practice Life-Saving Process on Cats." *The New York Times* (August 9, 1995): B5.

Davenport, Horace W. *A History of Gastric Secretion and Digestion: Experimental Studies to 1975.* New York: Oxford University Press, 1992.

David, Shari I. *With Dignity: The Search for Medicare and Medicaid.* Westport, CT: Greenwood Press, 1985.

Davis, Joel. *Endorphins: New Waves in Brain Chemistry.* Garden City, NY: Dial Press, 1984.

Day, Michael. "Poor Vaccine Ruled Out in TB Puzzle." *New Scientist* (July 13, 1996).

Dekking, H.M. and H.D. Coster. "Dynamic Tonometry." *Ophthalmologica* vol. 154 (1967): 59–74.

de Moulin, Daniel. *A Short History of Breast Cancer.* Boston: Kluwer, 1983.

DePrince, Elaine. *Cry Bloody Murder: A Tale of Tainted Blood.* New York: Random House, 1997.

Despain, J.J. "A Stitch in Time: Sutures Help Wounds Heal." *Current Health 2* (March 1999).

Division of Cancer Research Resources and Centers, National Cancer Institute. *The Cancer Centers Program.* Washington, DC: U.S. Department of Health, Education, and Welfare, Public Health Service, National Institutes of Health, 1974.

Doelp, Alan. *In the Blink of an Eye: Inside a Children's Trauma Center.* New York: Prentice Hall, 1989.

Donahue, M. Patricia. *Nursing, The Finest Art: An Illustrated History.* St. Louis, MO: The C.V. Mosby Company, 1985.

Donowitz, Leigh G. *Infection Control for the Health Care Worker.* Baltimore, MD: Williams & Wilkins, 1994.

Duffy, John. *From Humors to Medical Science: A History of American Medicine,* 2d ed. Urbana: University of Illinois Press, 1993.

"East Meets West." *Consumer Reports* vol. 58, no. 2 (February 1993): 108.

Earle, A. Scott, ed. *Surgery in America: From the Colonial Era to the Twentieth Century,* 2d ed. New York: Praeger Special Studies, Praeger Scientific, 1983.

Edwards, Robert and Patrick Steptoe. *A Matter of Life: The Story of a Medical Breakthrough.* London: Hutchinson Publishing Group, 1980.

Eisenberg, Ronald L. *Radiology: An Illustrated History.* St. Louis, MO: Mosby Year Book, 1992.

Ellis, Harold. *Famous Operations.* Media, PA: Harwal Publishing Company, 1984.

Emili, J. Milic. *Basics of Respiratory Mechanics and Artificial Ventilation.* Milan, NY: Springer, 1999.

Enkin, Murray. *A Guide to Effective Care in Pregnancy and Childbirth.* New York: Oxford University Press, 1995.

Environmental Health Criteria Series no. 18. Geneva: World Health Organization, 1991.

Epstein, Randi Hutter. "Poison Control." *Ladies Home Journal* (July 1998).

Etheridge, Elizabeth. *The Butterfly Caste: A Social History of Pellagra in the South.* Westport, CT: Greenwood Press, 1972.

Fackelmann, Kathleen. "Arsenic: A Novel Cancer Remedy?" *Science News* (April 11, 1998): 239.

Fancher, Raymond E. *The Intelligence Men: Makers of the I.Q. Controversy.* New York: W.W. Norton & Company, 1985.

Fernandez, Humberto. *Heroin.* Hazelden Information Education, 1998.

Fields, William S. *A History of Stroke: Its Recognition and Treatment.* New York: Oxford University Press, 1989.

Finger, Stanley. *Origins of Neuroscience: A History of Explorations into Brain Function.* New York: Oxford University Press, 1994.

Fischer, Bernd, Kewal K. Jain, Erwin Braun, and Siegfried Lehrl. *Handbook of Hyperbaric Oxygen Therapy.* Berlin: Springer-Verlag, 1988.

Fisher, Lawrence M. "Biology Meets High Technology; Biochips Signal a Critical Shift for Research and Medicine." *The New York Times* (December 21, 1999): C1.

Fisher, William Albert. *Ophthalmoscopy, Retinoscopy and Refraction with a New Chapter on Orthoptics.* Chicago: H.G. Adair Printing Company, 1937.

Flieger, Ken. "Mad Dogs and Friendly Skunks." *FDA Consumer* vol. 24, no. 5 (June 1990): 22.

Floyer, Sir John. *The Physician's Pulse-Watch.* London: S. Smith & B. Walford, 1707–10.

Ford, Brian J. *Single Lens: The Story of the Simple Microscope.* New York: Harper & Row, 1985.

Foster, William Derek. *A Short History of Clinical Pathology.* Edinburgh: Livingstone, Ltd., 1961.

Fox, Nicols. *Spoiled: Why Our Food Is Making Us Sick and What to Do about It.* New York: Penguin, 1997.

Foye, William O., ed. *Cancer Chemotherapeutic Agents.* Washington, DC: American Chemical Society, 1995.

Franklin, Jon and John Sutherland. *Guinea Pig Doctors.* New York: Morrow, 1984.

Free, Alfred H. and Helen M. Free. "Self-Testing: An Emerging Component of Clinical Chemistry." *Clinical Chemistry* (June 30, 1984): 829–38.

Friedman, Howard S. *Encyclopedia of Mental Health.* San Diego, CA: Academic Press. 1998.

Friedman, Meyer and Gerald W. Friedland. *Medicine's 10 Greatest Discoveries.* New Haven, CT: Yale University Press, 1998.

Fujimura, Joan H. *Crafting Science: A Sociohistory of the Quest for the Genetics of Cancer.* Cambridge, MA: Harvard University Press, 1996

Fuller, Terry. *Surgical Lasers: A Clinical Guide.* New York: Macmillan Publishing Company, 1987.

Fye, W. Bruce. "T. Lauder Brunton and Amyl Nitrate: A Victorian Vasodilator." *Circulation* vol. 74 (1996): 222–29.

Gaby, Alan R. *Preventing and Reversing Osteoporosis.* Rocklin, CA: Prima Health, 1993.

Gadsby, Patricia. "Fear of Flu." *Discover* vol. 20, no. 1 (January 1999): 82.

Galasso, George J. et al., eds. *Antiviral Agents and Human Viral Diseases.* Philadelphia: Lippincott-Raven Publishers, 1997.

Galton, Lawrence. *Med Tech: The Layperson's Guide to Today's Medical Miracles.* New York: Harper & Row, 1985.

Ganz, Jeremy C. *Gamma Knife Surgery.* Vienna: Springer, 1997.

Garrett, Laurie. *The Coming Plague: Newly Emerging Diseases in a World out of Balance.* New York: Penguin, 1995.

———. "The Future of Medicine." *Minneapolis Star Tribune* (March 3, 1999): 14A.

Geison, Gerald L. *The Private Science of Louis Pasteur.* Princeton, NJ: Princeton University Press, 1995.

Gevitz, Norman. *The D.O.s: Osteopathic Medicine in America.* Baltimore, MD: Johns Hopkins University Press, 1991.

Gibbs, W. Wayt. "Helping Heartache; Surgeons Blast Holes Through the Heart to Relieve Chest Pain." *Scientific American* (July 1997).

Gilman, Sander L. *Making the Body Beautiful: A Cultural History of Aesthetic Surgery.* Princeton, NJ: Princeton University Press. 1999.

Glasser, Ronald. *The Light in the Skull: An Odyssey of Medical Discovery.* Boston: Faber & Faber, 1997.

Glaz, Edith and Paul Vecsei. *Aldosterone.* Oxford; New York: Pergamon Press, 1971.

Glionna, John M. "Heimlich Helper." *Los Angeles Times* (October 8, 1997): B1.

Gonzalez-Crussi, F. *Suspended Animation. Six Essays on the Preservation of Bodily Parts.* San Diego, CA: Harcourt Brace & Company, 1995.

Gordon, Richard. *The Alarming History of Medicine.* New York: St. Martin's Press, 1993.

Gorman, Jack M. *The Essential Guide to Psychiatric Drugs.* New York: St. Martin's Press, 1997.

Gosden, Roger. *Designing Babies: The Brave New World of Reproductive Technology.* New York: W.H. Freeman and Company, 1999.

Gould, Steven J. *The Mismeasure of Man.* Revised and Expanded Edition. New York: W.W. Norton & Company, 1996.

Grace, Eric S. *Biotechnology Unzipped: Promises and Realities.* Washington, DC: Joseph Henry Press, 1997.

Grady, Denise. "Live Donors Revolutionize Liver Care." *The New York Times* (August 2, 1999): A1.

Grmek, Mirko D. *History of AIDS: Emergence and Origin of a Modern Pandemic.* Princeton, NJ: Princeton University Press, 1990.

Gutkind, Lee. *Many Sleepless Nights.* New York: Norton, 1988.

Gwei-Djen, Lu and Louis Needham. *Celestial Lancets: A History and Rationale of Acupuncture and Moxa.* Cambridge: Cambridge University Press, 1980.

H. Pylori and Peptic Ulcer. Bethesda, MD: National Digestive Diseases Information Clearinghouse, October 1997.

Haiken, Elizabeth. *Venus Envy: A History of Cosmetic Surgery.* Baltimore, MD: The Johns Hopkins University Press, 1997.

Hall, Stephen S. *A Commotion in the Blood: Life, Death and the Immune System.* New York: Henry Holt and Company, 1997.

Haller, John S. *Farmcarts to Fords: A History of the Military Ambulance, 1790–1925.* Carbondale, IL: Southern Illinois University Press, 1992.

Hallowell, Edward M. and John J. Ratey. *Driven to Distraction.* Simon & Schuster, 1995.

Hammonds, Evelynn Maxine. *Childhood's Deadly Scourge: The Campaign to Control Diphtheria in New York City, 1880–1930.* Baltimore, MD: Johns Hopkins University Press, 1999.

Handbook of Nonprescription Drugs, 11th ed. Washington, DC: American Pharmaceutical Association, 1996.

Harden, Victoria A. *Inventing the NIH: Federal Biomedical Research Policy, 1887–1937.* Baltimore, MD: Johns Hopkins University Press, 1986.

Hardy, Gwen. *William Rathbone and the Early History of District Nursing.* Ormskirk, Lancashire, UK: G W & A Hesketh, 1981.

Harper, Barbara. *Gentle Birth Choices.* Rochester, VT: Inner Traditions International, Ltd., 1994.

Harrington, Anne, ed. *The Placebo Effect: An Interdisciplinary Exploration.* Cambridge, MA: Harvard University Press, 1997.

Harris, Henry. *The Birth of the Cell.* New Haven, CT: Yale University Press, 1999.

Hart, Matthew. "The Flying Rescuers." *McClean's* (December 9, 1985): T1.

Heath, John K. *Growth Factors.* Oxford; New York: IRL Press, 1993.

Heidel, William Arthur. *Hippocratic Medicine: Its Spirit and Method.* New York: Columbia University Press, 1941.

Hellman, Samuel and Everett E. Vokes. "Advancing Current Treatments for Cancer." *Scientific American* (September 1996).

Henig, Robin Marantz. *A Dancing Matrix: How Science Confronts Emerging Viruses.* New York: Vintage Books, 1994.

———. *The People's Health. A Memoir of Public Health and Its Evolution at Harvard.* Washington, DC: Joseph Henry Press, 1997.

Hentoff, Nat. *A Doctor among the Addicts.* New York: Rand McNally, 1968.

Herbert, Wray. "Psychosurgery Redux." *U.S. News and World Report* (Nov. 3, 1997).

Hoizey, Dominique and Marie-Joseph. *A History of Chinese Medicine.* Vancouver: University of British Columbia Press, 1993.

Hopkins, Karen. *Understanding Cystic Fibrosis.* Jackson: University Press of Mississippi, 1998.

Horvitz, Leslie Alan. "Dialing for Diagnoses." *Insight on the News* (May 5, 1997).

"How Humans Learnt to See in Red, Green and Blue." *The Economist* (May 3, 1986).

"How To Find Help." *Consumer Reports* vol. 58, no. 2 (February 1993): 391.

Hutchinson, John F. *Champions of Charity: War and the Rise of the Red Cross.* Boulder, CO: Westview Press, 1996.

James, Dinah M. *Human Antiparasitic Drugs: Pharmacology and Usage.* New York: John Wiley & Sons, 1985.

Jankovic, Joseph, and Eduardo Tolosa. *Parkinson's Disease and Movement Disorders.* Baltimore: Williams & Wilkins, 1993.

Jeffries, D.J. and Erik DeClercq, eds. *Antiviral Chemotherapy.* New York: John Wiley & Sons, 1995.

Jones, James H. *Bad Blood: The Tuskegee Syphilis Experiment.* New York: Free Press, 1992.

Jordaens, Luc. *The Implantable Defibrillator: From Concept to Clinical Reality.* Basel; New York: Karger, 1996.

Jouvet, Michel. *The Paradox of Sleep: The Story of Dreaming.* Cambridge, MA: MIT Press, 1999.

Kalisch, Beatrice J. and Philip A. Kalisch. *The Advance of American Nursing,* 3d ed. Philadelphia: J.B. Lipincott Company, 1995.

Kaplan, Henry S. *Hodgkin's Disease.* Cambridge, MA: Harvard University Press, 1980.

Karch, Steven B. *A Brief History of Cocaine.* Boca Raton, FL: CRC Press, 1997.

Karczmar, Alexander George. "Anticholinesterase Agents." In *ternational Encyclopedia of Pharmacology and Therapeutics,* no. 13. New York: Pergamon Press, 1970.

Karlen, Arno. *Man and Microbes: Disease and Plagues in History and Modern Times.* New York: Putnam, 1995.

Keefe, Richard S.E. and Philip D. Harvey. *Understanding Schizophrenia.* New York: Free Press, 1994.

Keller, Evelyn Fox. *A Feeling for the Organism: The Life and Work of Barbara McClintock.* San Francisco: W. H. Freeman, 1983.

Kent, Christina. "Report: Seatbelts, Helmets Save Lives and Health Costs." *American Medical News* (March 4, 1996).

Kevles, Bettyann Holtzmann. *Naked to the Bone: Medical Imaging in the 20th Century.* Reading, MA: Addison-Wesley, 1997.

Khan, M. Gabriel and Henry J.L. Marriott. *The Heart Trouble Encyclopedia.* Toronto: Stoddart Publishing Company, 1996.

Kilner, John F., Rebecca D. Pentz, and Frank E. Young, eds. *Genetic Ethics: Do the Ends Justify the Genes?* Grand Rapids, MI: William B. Eerdmans Publishing Company, 1997.

King, Lester S. and Marjorie C. Meehan. "A History of the Autopsy: A Review." *American Journal of Pathology* vol. 73, no. 2 (1973): 514–41.

Kiple, Kenneth F., ed. *The Cambridge World History of Human Disease.* Cambridge: Cambridge University Press, 1993.

Kirschmann, John D. and Lavon J. Dunne. *Nutrition Almanac.* New York: McGraw-Hill, 1990.

Klasen, Henk J. *History of Free Skin Grafting: Knowledge or Empiricism?* Berlin; New York: Springer-Verlag, 1981.

Klein, Donald F. *Understanding Depression: A Complete Guide to Its Diagnosis and Treatment.* New York: Oxford University Press, 1993.

Kolata, Gina. "Drug Makers Say New Painkillers Work Without Side Effects." *The New York Times* (November 11, 1998): A18.

Kolata, Gina. "Next Up: Surgery by Remote Control." *The New York Times* (April 4, 2000): 1.

Kolker, Aliza and B. Meredith Burke. *Prenatal Testing: A Sociological Perspective.* Westport, CT: Bergin & Garvey, 1994.

Koller, William C., ed. *Handbook of Parkinson's Disease,* 2d ed. New York: Marcel Dekker, 1992.

Koprowski, Hilary and Michael B.A. Oldstone, eds. *Microbe Hunters Then and Now.* Bloomington, IL: Medi-Ed Press, 1996.

Kosslyn, Stephen M. and Olivier Koenig. *Wet Mind: The New Cognitive Neuroscience.* New York: Basic Books, 1992.

Kramer, Peter. *Listening to Prozac.* New York: Penguin Books, 1993.

Krantz, John C. Jr. *Historical Medical Classics Involving New Drugs.* Baltimore, MD: The Williams & Wilkins Company, 1974.

Kuczynski, Alex. "Anti-Aging Potion or Poison?" *The New York Times* (April 12, 1998): 1.

Kurian, George T., ed. *A Historical Guide to the U.S. Government.* Oxford: Oxford University Press, 1998.

Landy, Mark K., et al. *The Environmental Protection Agency: Asking the Wrong Questions: From Nixon to Clinton.* New York: Oxford University Press, 1994.

"Laxatives–and Alternatives." *Consumer Reports on Health* (April 1998): 8.

Le Vay, David. *The History of Orthopaedics.* Lancashire, UK: The Parthenon Publishing Group, 1990.

Leahey, Thomas Hardy. *A History of Psychology: Main Currents in Psychological Thought.* Upper Saddle River, NJ: Prentice Hall, 1997.

Leaman, Thomas L. *Healing the Anxiety Disorders.* New York: Plenum Press, 1992.

Leary, Warren E. "A Federal Panel Suggests Restriction on an Herbal Stimulant." *The New York Times* (August 29, 1996): D18.

Lednicer, Daniel, ed. *Chronicles of Drug Discovery,* vol. 3. Washington, DC: American Chemical Society, 1993.

Lender, Mark Edward and James K. Martin. *Drinking in America: A History.* New York: Free Press, 1987.

Levi-Montalcini, Rita. *The Saga of the Nerve Growth Factor: Preliminary Studies, Discovery, Further Development.* Singapore; River Edge, NJ: World Scientific, 1997.

Lickey, Marvin E. and Barbara Gordon. *Drugs for Mental Illness: A Revolution in Psychiatry.* New York: W.H. Freeman, 1983.

Lindenmeyer, Kriste. *A Right to Childhood: The U.S. Children's Bureau and Child Welfare, 1912–1946.* Urbana: University of Illinois Press, 1997.

Litovitz, Tony. "In Defense of Retaining Ipecac Syrup as an Over-the-Counter Drug." *Pediatrics* vol. 82 (September 1998): 514–16.

Loeb, Penny. "Very Troubled Waters: Despite Clean Water Act, Quality of Rivers Worsens." *U.S. News and World Report* (September 28, 1998).

Long, Esmond R. *A History of Pathology.* Baltimore, MD: The Williams & Wilkins Company, 1928.

Longman, Jere. "Lifesaving Drug Can Be Deadly When Misused." *The New York Times* (July 26, 1998): S11.

Loo, Marcus H. and Marian Betancourt. *The Prostate Cancer Sourcebook: How to Make Informed Choices.* New York: John Wiley & Sons, 1998.

Lowenstein, Werner R. *The Touchstone of Life.* New York: Oxford University Press, 1999.

Lyon, Jeff and Peter Gorner. *Altered Fates: Gene Therapy and the Retooling of Human Life.* New York: W.W. Norton & Company, 1995.

Mainwaring, W.I.P. *The Mechanism of Action of Androgens.* New York: Springer-Verlag, 1977.

Majno, Guido. *The Healing Hand: Man and Wound in the Ancient World.* Cambridge, MA: Harvard University Press, 1975.

Major, Ralph H., ed. *Classic Descriptions of Disease,* Springfield, IL: Charles C. Thomas Publishers, 1932.

Mannon, James M. *Caring for the Burned: Life and Death in a Hospital Burn Center.* Springfield, IL: Thomas, 1985.

Marks, John. *A Guide to The Vitamins: Their Role in Health and Disease.* Baltimore, MD: University Park Press, 1975.

Marsh, Margaret and Wanda Ronner. *The Empty Cradle: Infertility in America from Colonial Times to the Present.* Baltimore, MD: Johns Hopkins University Press, 1996.

Martin, Frederick. *Introduction to Audiology.* Englewood Cliffs, NJ: Prentice Hall, 1991.

Marwick, Charles. "New Focus on Children's Environmental Health." *Journal of the American Medical Association* (March 19, 1997).

Massie, Robert and Suzanne Massie. *Journey.* New York: Knopf, 1975.

Matthews, Jay. "A Solution of Substance for Substance Abuse?" *The Washington Post* (December 3, 1996): C1.

Maxwell, William Quentin. *Lincoln's Fifth Wheel: The Political History of the United States Sanitary Commission.* New York: Longmans, Green & Company, 1956.

McAuley, J.E. "The Hypodermic Syringe." *Dental History* vol. 32 (May 1997): 40–41.

McBeath, Andrew A. "Total Joint Replacement." *Healthline* (January 1998).

McCann, Samuel McDonald, ed. *Endocrinology: People and Ideas.* Bethesda, MD: American Physiological Society, 1988.

McCollum, Elmer Verner. *A History of Nutrition: The Sequence of Ideas in Nutrition Investigations.* Boston: Houghton Mifflin, 1957.

McCormick, Joseph B. *Level 4: Virus Hunters of the CDC.* Atlanta, GA: Turner Publishing, 1996.

McGraw-Hill Encyclopedia of Science and Technology, vol. 13, 8th ed. New York: McGraw-Hill, 1997.

McGrew, Roderick E. *Encyclopedia of Medical History.* New York: McGraw-Hill, 1985.

McHenry, Lawrence C. Jr. and Fielding H. Garrison. *Garrison's History of Neurology.* Springfield, IL: Charles C. Thomas Publishers, 1969.

Medvei, Victor Cornelius. *The History of Endocrinology.* Lancaster, UK: MTP Press Limited, 1982.

Mestel, Rosie. "Sexual Chemistry." *Discover* (January 1999): 32.

Miller, J.M. "William Stewart Halsted and the Use of Rubber Gloves." *Surgery* vol. 92 (September 1982): 541–43.

Mitka, Mike. "High Tech Angina Relief Explored in Treatment Trials." *Journal of the American Medical Association* vol. 281 (April 14, 1999): 1258.

Mofenson, Howard C. and Thomas R. Caraccio. "Benefits/Risks of Syrup of Ipecac." *Pediatrics* vol. 77 (April 1986): 551–52.

Monroe, Judy. "Defenders Against the World's Smallest Attackers." *Current Health 2* (March 1995): 18.

Moore, Keith L., ed. *Before We Are Born: Essentials of Embryology and Birth Defects,* 5th ed. Philadelphia: W.B. Saunders Company, 1998.

Morrison, Gale. "Advances in the Skin Trade." *Mechanical Engineering* (February 1999).

Morrow, David J. "Struggling to Spell Relief: Though Promising, Sales of Migraine Drugs Face Hurdles." *The New York Times* (December 29, 1998): C1.

Moser, Rod. *Ears: An Owner's Manual. Coping With Ear Infections: How to Use an Otoscope.* Fair Oaks, CA: Selfcare Educational Systems, 1994

Moss, William M. *Contraceptive Sterilization.* Amityville, NY: Essential Medical Information Systems, 1988.

Mullan, Fitzhugh. *Plagues and Politics: The Story of the U.S. Public Health Service.* New York: Basic Books, 1989.

Murphy, James S. *The Condom Industry in the United States.* Jefferson, NC: McFarlane and Company, 1990.

"A New Clot Buster." *Harvard Heart Letter* (August 1997).

"New Life for Old Hips." *Consumer Reports on Health* (December 1995).

Nichols, Buford L. Jr., Angel Ballabriga, and Norman Kretchmer, eds. *History of Pediatrics: 1850–1950.* New York: Raven Press, 1991.

Normand, Jacques, et al., eds. *Preventing HIV Transmission: The Role of Sterile Needles and Bleach.* Washington, DC: National Academy Press, 1995.

"Now Hear This." *University of California Berkeley Wellness Letter* (September 1998).

O'Dell, Lynne. "Watching Out for Eyes: School Vision Tests Catch Many, But Not All, Problems That Can Affect Learning." *Los Angeles Times,* Orange County Edition (October 27, 1997): 2.

O'Dowd, Michael J. and Elliott E. Philipp. *The History of Obstetrics and Gynaecology.* New York: Parthenon Publishing Group, 1994.

Okie, Susan. "Can Hormones Stop Aging?" *The Washington Post* (February 24, 1998): WH12.

———. "Herbal Relief: St. John's Wort May Ease Mild to Moderate Depression." *The Washington Post* (October 14, 1997): WH12.

O'Leary, James L. and Sidney Goldring. *Science and Epilepsy: Neuroscience Gains in Epilepsy Research.* New York: Raven Press, 1976.

Oppenheim, Joost J. and Stanley Cohen, eds. *Interleukines, Lymphokines, and Cytokines: Proceedings of the Third International Lymphokine Workshop.* New York: Academic Press, 1983.

"Oral Antidiabetes Drugs: One Size Does Not Fit All." *Patient Care* (February 15, 1998).

"Overactive Thyroid: Is Your Thyroid 'Hyper'?" *Mayo Clinic Health Letter* (January 1999).

Owen, Alan Robert George. *Hysteria, Hypnosis and Healing: The Work of J.-M. Charcot.* New York: Garrett Publications, 1971.

Pain, I.D. "Progress in Ophthalmological Instruments." *International Ophthalmology Clinics* vol. 8 (Spring 1968): 117–31.

Papaspyros, N.S. *The History of Diabetes Mellitus.* Stuttgart, Germany: G. Thieme, 1964.

Park, Gilbert and Keiron Saunders. *Fighting for Life: An Introduction to the Intensive Care Unit.* Oxford; New York: Oxford University Press, 1996.

Paul, John R. *A History of Poliomyelitis.* New Haven, CT: Yale University Press, 1971.

Perl, Peter. "Poisoned Package." *Washington Post Magazine* (January 16, 2000): W8.

Persaud, T.V.N. *Early History of Human Anatomy: From Antiquity to the Beginning of the Modern Era.* Springfield, IL: Charles C. Thomas, 1984.

———. *A History of Anatomy: The Post-Vesalian Era.* Springfield, IL: Charles C. Thomas, 1997.

Pickstone, J.V. "Discovering the Movement of Life: Osmosis and Microstructure in 1926." *International Journal of Microcirculation and Clinical Experimentation* vol. 14 (January-April 1994): 77–82.

Pittinger, Charles B. *Hyperbaric Oxygenation.* Springfield, IL: Charles C. Thomas Publishers, 1966.

Plaud, Joseph J. and George H. Eifert. *From Behavior Theory to Behavior Therapy.* Boston: Allyn and Bacon, 1998.

Podolsky, M. Lawrence. *Cures out of Chaos.* Amsterdam: Harwood Academic Publishers, 1997.

Poole, Catherine M. *Melanoma: Prevention, Detection and Treatment.* New Haven, CT: Yale University Press, 1998.

Porter, Roy, ed. *The Cambridge Illustrated History of Medicine.* New York: Cambridge University Press, 1996.

———. *Medicine: A History of Healing.* New York: Marlowe and Company, 1997.

——— and Mikulas Teich, eds. *Drugs and Narcotics in History.* London: Cambridge University Press, 1995.

"The Pre-Halstedian and Post-Halstedian History of the Surgical Rubber Glove." *Surgery, Gynecology and Obstetrics* vol. 167 (October 1988): 350–56.

Prescott, Laurie F. *Paracetamol (Acetaminophen): A Critical Bibliographic Review.* London: Taylor & Francis, 1996.

Primary Health Care: Report of the International Conference on Primary Health Care, Alma-Ata. "Health or All" series, no. 1. Geneva: World Health Organization, 1978.

Rabinow, Paul. *Making PCR: A Story of Biotechnology.* Chicago: University of Chicago Press, 1997.

Bibliography

Radetsky, Peter. *The Invisible Invaders.* Boston: Little, Brown and Company, 1994.

Rasmussen, Nicolas. *Picture Control: The Electron Microscope and the Transformation of Biology in America, 1940–1960.* Stanford, CA: Stanford University Press, 1997.

Ravitch, Mark M. et al. *Current Practice of Surgical Stapling.* Philadelphia: Lea & Febiger, 1991.

Restak, Richard. *Brainscapes: An Introduction to What Neuroscience Has Learned about the Structure, Function and Abilities of the Brain.* New York: Hyperion, 1995.

Rey, Roselyne. *The History of Pain.* Cambridge, MA: Harvard University Press, 1998.

Rhodes, Richard. *Deadly Feasts.* New York: Touchstone, 1998.

Richards, Raymond. *Closing the Door to Destitution: The Shaping of the Social Security Acts of the United States and New Zealand.* University Park, PA: Pennsylvania State University Press, 1994.

Riddle, John M. *Contraception and Abortion from the Ancient World to the Renaissance.* London: Harvard University Press, 1992.

Riese, Walther. *A History of Neurology.* New York: M.D. Publications, 1959.

———. *Eve's Herbs: A History of Abortion and Contraception in the West.* Cambridge, MA: Harvard University Press, 1997.

Ring, Malvin E. *Dentistry: An Illustrated History.* New York: Harry N. Abrams, Inc., Publishers, 1985.

Risse, Guenter B. *Mending Bodies, Saving Souls: A History of Hospitals.* London: Oxford University Press, 1999.

Robertson, Nan. *Getting Better: Inside Alcoholics Anonymous.* New York: William Morrow & Company, 1988.

Rogers, Adam and Jerry Adler. "The New War Against Migraines." *Newsweek* (January 11, 1999): 46

Roloff, Tricia Ann. *Moving Through a Strange Land: A Book for Brain Tumor Patients and Their Families.* Sheffield, MA: Option Indigo Press, 1995.

Root-Bernstein, Robert and Michele Root-Bernstein. *Honey, Mud, Maggots and Other Medical Miracles.* Boston: Houghton Mifflin, 1997.

Rose, F. Clifford and William F. Bynum, eds. *Historical Aspects of the Neurosciences: A Festschrift for Macdonald Critchley.* New York: Raven Press, 1982.

Rosen, George. *A History of Public Health.* Baltimore, MD: Johns Hopkins University Press, 1993.

Rosen, Marty. "Surgery Spurs Hope, Questions." *St. Petersburg Times* (August 24, 1997): 1B.

Rosenthal, M. Sara. *The Gynecological Sourcebook.* Los Angeles: Lowell House, 1999.

Roth, Jack A., James D. Cox, and Waun Ki Hong, eds. *Lung Cancer.* Malden, MA: Blackwell Science, 1998.

Rutkow, Ira M. *American Surgery: An Illustrated History.* Philadelphia: Lippincott-Raven Publishers, 1998.

Saltus, Richard. "Out of Sight." *The Boston Globe Magazine* (March 14, 1999): 8.

Saunders, Carol Silverman. "In Case of Shock." *Current Health 2* (November 1996).

Schindler, Rudolf. *Gastroscopy: The Endoscopic Study of Gastric Pathology.* New York: Hafner Publishing Co., 1966

Schmeck, Harold. "Sight Restored for Thousands Yearly." *The New York Times* (December 11, 1984): C4.

Schwartz, John. "FDA Approves New Diet Drug for Obese with Warning about Monitoring." *The Washington Post* (November 25, 1997): A3.

Scott, Donald F. *The History of Epileptic Therapy: An Account of How Medication Was Developed.* Lancashire, UK: The Parthenon Publishing Group, 1993.

Selleck, Henry B. and Alfred H. Whittaker. *Occupational Health in America.* Detroit, MI: Wayne State University Press, 1962.

Sellers, Christopher C. *Hazards of the Job: From Industrial Disease to Environmental Health Science.* Chapel Hill: University of North Carolina Press, 1997.

Shaffer, Marianne L. *Bone Marrow Transplants: A Guide for Cancer Patients and Their Families.* Dallas: Taylor Publications, 1994.

Shorter, Edward. *The Health Century.* New York: Doubleday, 1987.

———. *A History of Psychiatry: From the Era of the Asylum to the Age of Prozac.* New York: John Wiley & Sons, 1997.

———. *A History of Women's Bodies.* New York: Basic Books Inc., 1982.

Shute, Nancy. "No More Hard Labor: High Tech and High Touch Remedies for Easing the Pain of Childbirth." *U.S. News and World Report* (November 10, 1997).

Siebold, Cathy. *The Hospice Movement: Easing Death's Pain.* New York: Maxwell McMillan Int., 1992.

Silvers, Robert B., ed. *Hidden Histories of Science.* New York: New York Review Books, 1995.

Silverstein, Arthur M. *A History of Immunology.* San Diego, CA: Academic Press, 1989.

———. "Paul Ehrlich's Passion: The Origin of His Receptor Immunology." *Cellular Immunology* vol. 194 (June 15, 1999): 213–21.

Singer, Igor, ed. *Interventional Electrophysiology.* Baltimore, MD: Williams & Wilkins, 1997.

Skouge, John W. *Skin Grafting.* New York: Churchill Livingstone, 1991.

Smith, Mickey C. *Small Comfort: A History of the Minor Tranquilizers.* New York: Praeger Publishers, 1985.

Smith, Wesley D. *The Hippocratic Tradition.* Ithaca, NY: Cornell University Press, 1979.

Sneader, Walter. *Drug Discovery: The Evolution of Modern Medicines.* Chichester, NY: John Wiley & Sons, 1985.

Speaker, Susan L. and M. Susan Lindee. *A Guide to the Human Genome Project: Technologies, People and Institutions.* Philadelphia: Chemical Heritage Foundation, 1993.

Speert, Harold. *Obstetric & Gynecologic Milestones Illustrated.* New York: Parthenon Publishing Group, 1996.

———. *Obstetrics and Gynecology: A History and Iconography.* San Francisco: Normal Publishing, 1994.

Spillane, John D. *The Doctrine of the Nerves: Chapters in the History of Neurology.* Oxford: Oxford University Press, 1981.

Squires, Sally. "Report on Prevention Project is Mixed Bag." *The Washington Post* (April 18, 1995): Z6.

———. "Surgery to Prevent Strokes." *The Washington Post* (October 4, 1994): Z10.

———. "Treatment Brings New Blood to Ailing Hearts; When Bypass Operations Don't Succeed, Some Doctors Are Experimenting with Lasers." *The Washington Post* (April 8, 1997): WH7.

Starr, Douglas. *Blood: An Epic History of Medicine and Commerce.* New York: Knopf, 1998.

Stephenson, Patricia and Marsden G. Wagner, eds. *Tough Choices: In Vitro Fertilization and the Reproductive Technologies.* Philadelphia: Temple University Press, 1993.

Sternberg, Steve. "Impotence Treatment Keeps Urologists Busy; Erectile Problems are a Common Side Effect of Surgery for Prostate Cancer." *The Washington Post* (November 5, 1996): WH8.

Stevens, Jay. *Storming Heaven: LSD and the American Dream.* New York: Atlantic Monthly Press, 1987.

Stine, Susan and Thomas R. Kosten, eds. *New Treatments for Opiate Dependence.* New York: Guilford Press, 1997.

Stix, Gary. "Growing a New Field: Tissue Engineering Comes into Its Own." *Scientific American* (October 1997).

Stolberg, Sheryl Gay. "President Decides Against Financing Needle Programs; Bitter Internal Debate; Ban on Assistance for Addicts Continues Despite Success Against Spread of AIDS." *The New York Times* (April 21, 1998): A1.

Strauss, Evelyn. "Help for the Weary." *Health* (April 1999).

"Study Shows Danger to Skin and Gives Hope of a Savior." *The New York Times* (January 25, 1996): A19.

Tarimo, E. and E.G. Webster. *Primary Health Care: Concepts and Challenges in a Changing World, Alma-Ata Revisited.* Geneva: World Health Organization, 1997.

Taylor, J.A. *History of Dentistry.* Philadelphia: Lea & Febiger, 1922.

Temin, Peter. *Taking Your Medicine: Drug Regulation in the United States.* Cambridge, MA: Harvard University Press, 1980.

Temkin, Owsei. *The Falling Sickness: A History of Epilepsy from the Greeks to the Beginnings of Modern Neurology,* 2d ed. Baltimore, MD: Johns Hopkins University Press, 1971.

Therman, Eeva. *Human Chromosomes: Structure, Behavior, Effects.* New York: Springer-Verlag, 1992.

Thomson, Angus, ed. *The Cytokine Handbook,* 2d ed. New York: Academic Press, Harcourt, Brace & Company, 1994.

Timmis, G.M. *Chemotherapy of Cancer: The Antimetabolite Approach.* London: Butterworths, 1967.

Tomes, Nancy. *The Gospel of Germs: Men, Women and the Microbe in American Life.* Cambridge, MA: Harvard University Press, 1998.

Toporek, Chuck et al. *Hydrocephalus: A Guide for Patients, Families, and Friends.* Sebastopol, CA: O'Reilly & Associates, 1999.

"Trial and Error." *The Economist* (U.S.) (October 31, 1998).

Tyler, Varro E. "The Two Faces of Ma Huang." *Prevention* (May 1997): 78.

Ullman, Dana. *The Consumer's Guide to Homeopathy.* New York: G.P. Putnam's Sons, 1995.

Underwood, James Cresec Elphinstone. *Introduction to Biopsy Interpretation and Surgical Pathology.* Berlin: Springer-Verlag, 1987.

Valenstein, Elliot S. *Great and Desperate Cures: The Rise and Decline of Psychosurgery and Other Radical Treatments for Mental Illness.* New York: Basic Books, 1986.

Vos, Rein. *Drugs Looking for Diseases.* Dordrecht, The Netherlands; Boston, MA: Kluwer Academic Publishers. 1991.

Wade, Nicholas. "Discovery Bolsters a Hope for Regeneration; Biotechnology Firm Converts Basic Cells into Bones and Cartilage." *The New York Times* (April 2, 1999): A18.

Waldholz, Michael. *Curing Cancer: The Story of the Men and Women Unlocking the Secrets of Our Deadliest Illness.* New York: Simon & Schuster, 1997.

Waldman, Amy. "When You Want to Live, But You Can't Afford It: Hit and Miss AIDS Care on the Margins." *The Washington Post* (April 27, 1997): C1.

Walker, Sam. "Feeding Babies vs. Fueling Competition." *The Christian Science Monitor* (August 22, 1996): 4.

Wangensteen, Owen H. and Sarah D. Wangensteen. *The Rise of Surgery.* Minneapolis: University of Minnesota Press, 1978.

Wardwell, Walter I. *Chiropractic: History and Evolution of a New Profession.* St. Louis, MO: Mosby Year Book, 1992.

Watanabe, Masaki et. al. *Atlas of Arthroscopy,* 2d ed. Tokyo: Igaku Shoin, Ltd. 1969.

Watkins, Elizabeth Siegel. *On the Pill: A Social History of Oral Contraceptives.* Baltimore, MD: Johns Hopkins University Press, 1998.

Weatherall, Miles. *In Search of a Cure: A History of Pharmaceutical Discovery.* Oxford: Oxford University Press, 1991.

Weir, Neil. *Otolaryngology: An Illustrated History.* London: Butterworths, 1990.

Weinberg, Robert A. *One Renegade Cell: How Cancer Begins.* New York: Basic Books, 1998.

———. *Racing to the Beginning of the Road: The Search for the Origin of Cancer.* New York: Harmony Books, 1996.

Weinberger, Bernhard Wolf. *An Introduction to the History of Dentistry.* St. Louis, MO: The Mosby Company, 1948.

Weiss, Peter. "Curbing Air Bags' Dangerous Excesses." *Science News* (September 26, 1998): 206.

Weisse, Alan B. *Medical Odysseys: The Different and Sometimes Unexpected Pathways to Twentieth-Century Medical Discoveries.* New Brunswick, NJ: Rutgers University Press, 1991.

Wertz, Richard W. and Dorothy C. Wertz. *Lying In: A History of Childbirth in America.* New Haven, CT: Yale University Press, 1989.

Westphal, Sylvia Pagan. "The Promise of Stem Cells." *Los Angeles Times* (July 8, 1999): B2.

White, William L. *Slaying the Dragon: The History of Addiction Treatment and Recovery in America.* Bloomington, IL: Chestnut Health Systems, 1998.

Williams, Greer. *Virus Hunters.* New York: Knopf, 1959.

Wilson, A. Bennett Jr. *Limb Prosthetics,* 6th ed. New York: Demos Publications, 1989.

Wilson, Charles B. "Sensors 2010." *British Medical Journal* (Nov. 13, 1999): 1288.

Winslow, Ron. "Heroin Remedy to be Marketed for Alcoholism." *The Wall Street Journal* (January 17, 1995): B1.

Wintrobe, Maxwell M. *Hematology, The Blossoming of a Science.* Philadelphia: Lea & Febiger, 1985.

Wolman, Benjamin B. *Encyclopedia of Psychiatry, Psychology, and Psychoanalysis.* New York: Henry Holt, 1996.

Wright, J.R. Jr. "The Development of the Frozen Section Technique, the Evolution of Surgical Biopsy, and the Origins of Surgical Pathology." *Bulletin of the History of Medicine* vol. 59 no. 3 (1985): 295–326.

Wynbrandt, James. *The Excruciating History of Dentistry: Toothsome Tales and Oral Oddities from Babylon to Braces.* New York: St. Martin's Press, 1998.

Ziegler, Michael G. and Raymond Lake, eds. *Norepinephrine.* Baltimore, MD: Williams & Wilkins, 1984.

Zimmerman, Leo M. and Ilza Veith. *Great Ideas in the History of Surgery.* New York: Dover Publications, 1967.

Zuger, Abigail. "Surgery Leaves OR for the Office." *The New York Times* (May 18, 1999): C1.

Index

by Dottie M Jahoda

Page numbers in **bold** indicate main entries for those topics.

Anne Harding specializes in writing on health, medicine, and science. Her work has appeared in the *Boston Globe*, *Harvard Health Letter*, *Consumer Reports on Health*, Mount Sinai's *Focus on Healthy Aging*, and several other print and Web-based publications. She has a bachelor's degree from Amherst College and a master's degree from Columbia University's Graduate School of Journalism.